DECODING THE
HUMAN BODY-FIELD

"An innovative and fascinating book that describes the biomedical structure of the human body based upon the true energy wave structure of matter. This book lays the groundwork for a new branch of medicine!"

MILO WOLFF, PH.D.,
AUTHOR OF *EXPLORING THE PHYSICS OF THE UNKNOWN UNIVERSE*

"We are indeed on the verge of a Medical and Health Renaissance, one in which a comprehensive and energetic analysis is coupled with an equally comprehensive correction of the imbalances. Conventional medical treatments often carry risks and are less effective in chronic diseases than in acute ones. Fraser's theory is remarkably inclusive and integrative. NES is safe and efficacy studies will ultimately provide the proof of the pudding."

C. NORMAN SHEALY, M.D., PH.D.,
AUTHOR OF *LIFE BEYOND 100: SECRETS OF THE FOUNTAIN OF YOUTH*,
FOUNDING PRESIDENT OF THE AMERICAN HOLISTIC MEDICAL
ASSOCIATION, AND PRESIDENT OF THE INTERNATIONAL SOCIETY
FOR THE STUDY OF SUBTLE ENERGY AND ENERGY MEDICINE

DECODING THE HUMAN BODY-FIELD

The New Science of
Information as Medicine

PETER H. FRASER AND
HARRY MASSEY

WITH JOAN PARISI WILCOX

Healing Arts Press
Rochester, Vermont

Healing Arts Press
One Park Street
Rochester, Vermont 05767
www.HealingArtsPress.com

Healing Arts Press is a division of Inner Traditions International

Nutri-Energetics, Nutri-Energetics Systems, NES, NES–Professional, Infoceuticals, Energetic Driver, Energetic Integrator, and Energetic Terrain are registered trademarks.

Note to the reader: This book is intended as an informational guide. The remedies, approaches, and techniques described herein are meant to supplement, and not to be a substitute for, professional medical care or treatment. They should not be used to treat a serious ailment without prior consultation with a qualified health care professional.

Library of Congress Cataloging-in-Publication Data
Fraser, Peter H.
   Decoding the human body-field : the new science of information as medicine / Peter H. Fraser and Harry Massey with Joan Parisi Wilcox.
      p. cm.
   Includes bibliographical references and index.
   Summary: "A revolutionary system that reestablishes the proper flow of information to the body's energetic fields to promote health"—Provided by publisher.
   ISBN: 978-1-59477-225-2 (pbk.)
   1. Energy medicine. I. Massey, Harry. II. Wilcox, Joan Parisi. III. Title.
   RZ421.F73 2008
   615.5'3—dc22

                                                                                    2007047745
Printed and bound in Canada by Transcontinental Printing

10 9 8 7 6 5 4 3 2 1

Text design and layout by Virginia Scott Bowman
This book was typeset in Garamond Premier Pro with Copperplate and Avant Garde as
   display typefaces.
All chapter 8 illustrations created by and used with the permission of Steven Lehar. His
   illustration of the Chladni figures in 8.2c is based on the work of Mary D. Waller.
Figure 13.5 is a reproduction of an image created by physicist Florian Marquardt and posted
   in color on *Wikipedia, The Free Encyclopedia,* at www.wikipedia.org/wiki/Interference.
All other illustrations created by Melissa James/MrsToast for NES (© Nutri-Energetics
   Systems, LTD).

CONTENTS

PART THREE
The NES Model of the Human Body-Field

◆

NOTE TO READER

Because of the biographical nature of parts of this book and the long time span involved in the retelling of certain aspects of Peter's research efforts, the passage of time has been compressed.

Client cases have been submitted by NES practitioners with the consent of their clients, although all client names have been changed to maintain their privacy.

Nutri-Energetics Systems does not diagnose, cure, prevent, or treat disease. If you have a medical condition or concern, please consult the appropriate health care professional. Also, NES and its claims have not been evaluated by any government agency or regulatory organization.

ACKNOWLEDGMENTS

Thanks to my dog, Pedro, for accompanying me on long walks to work on the puzzle; to Chetan for playing the didgeridoo for me on the beach; to Harry for his rescue mission; and to Joan for her detailed and time-consuming work on this book.

PETER H. FRASER

I am grateful to the numerous people over the past ten years who have supported making both NES and this book a reality. I especially want to acknowledge the following people: my family, especially my mother, who put up with me when I was ill and for initially funding NES; my various business partners, who helped keep NES going through those first difficult years; and Peter, who cured me. My thanks, too, to our NES practitioners and their clients, who put their faith in our system, and to Joan and Bruce, who took on the difficult task of making NES understandable.

HARRY MASSEY

Special thanks to Joyce Cary for her tireless work in establishing and nurturing NES in the United States and to Bruce Robertson for all his work in sorting through NES research and making such good sense of it. To Peter and Harry, I extend my sincerest appreciation for their trust and friendship. To my soul partner, John, I offer my deepest gratitude for thirty years of love, support, and growth.

JOAN PARISI WILCOX

INTRODUCTION

WHEN YOU THINK OF YOUR BODY, you probably think of the heft and substance of it—flesh, muscles, bone. When you think of illness and disease, you ask, "What is the matter with me?"—speaking quite literally in physical terms about the real *matter* of your body. Your knee or elbow aches. Your throat is sore. Your stomach is upset. Your head is throbbing. It's counterintuitive to imagine your body at more discrete levels, such as at the levels of cells, molecules, or atoms. You are unlikely to hear a person with diabetes complain that "my beta cells are malfunctioning."

You get our point; it is almost impossible for us to view our bodies as vast networks of cells and molecules, much less as webs of interacting particles and waves. However, the beautiful mystery of nature is that at our most fundamental level, waves and particles are exactly what we are.

In grasping this reality, our problems are ones of perception and scale, for in the course of our everyday lives it appears that particles and waves have no relevance to us. However, as quantum physics reveals, everything is connected—the world is a vast web of interconnected relationships. We compartmentalize ourselves at our own risk. For example, where once we thought the body was machinelike, regulating itself independently of the mind, research now has proved that thoughts, beliefs, emotions, and attitudes profoundly influence the functions of our cells, organs, and immune system—processes that are vital to our health and overall sense of wellness. Science has birthed a new mind-body medicine, and we can no longer deny that such immaterial aspects of ourselves as thoughts, beliefs, hopes, and desires can change the chemistry of our bodies. We can no longer afford to ignore the web of relationships that determine just about everything we are on a physical level.

With this new frame of reference, we can begin to seek an even deeper understanding of our bodies and our health. We are motivated to find the mechanisms, processes, rules, and relationships that define and determine our state of being. Through the work of innovators such as Peter Fraser,* we can begin to peel back the different aspects of the body like layers of an onion, moving from the macro to the micro scales, and then even deeper to the subatomic scale. What we find is a radically different body at each level. The deeper we go, the less substance there is to the body. Tissues and organs give way to molecules and atoms, which, when you probe deeply into their nature, give way to fuzzy clouds of subatomic particles, some real and some virtual, with those virtual particles popping out of nothingness and returning there after only a whiff of existence.

As we probe into the subatomic realm, we find that the brain, blood, and bone of the body give way to invisible forces, fields, and particles whose interactions underlie not only the human body but all of matter. Molecules give way to atoms that dissolve into subatomic particles, so that our bodies are governed not only by the laws of everyday chemistry but also by the paradoxical principles of quantum electrodynamics.

---

*Coauthoring a book makes for some awkward narrative problems, such as using pronouns that will make it clear to readers which one of us is "speaking" at particular points in the text. This especially becomes a problem throughout part 2, in which we tell the stories of our individual journeys toward health and collaboration to create NES. Therefore, simply as a matter of narrative convenience, we have chosen to refer to ourselves in the text by first name.

When we probe to these levels of the body, our practical questions take on seemingly metaphysical overtones. How does a thinking, feeling, creative, intelligent human being arise from the fog of quantum particles? Where is the boundary at which the deterministic laws of chemistry give way to the quirky, probabilistic laws of quantum physics? At what level of being does illness first gain its foothold—at the quantum level of electrons and photons or only at the level of deoxyribonucleic acid (DNA) and cells? Is there such a thing as "quantum health," and if so, do we have any influence over it? Which mechanisms shift our bodies from health to illness and back toward health? These are among the myriad questions that are prompting researchers in biology and medicine to forge boldly forward, extending our understanding of how the body works and creating a new kind of health care in the process.

Nutri-Energetics Systems (NES*)—the system of health care that is the result of Peter Fraser's decades of research and his collaboration with Harry Massey—is pioneering this twenty-first-century health revolution. Their model of the human body-field integrates physics and biology to reveal a stunning new vision of how the body works. Peter's research over the past twenty-five years has expanded our understanding of how the body has two interdependent aspects: the biochemical (which is the basis of most modern Western medicine) and the bioenergetic (which has been the province of alternative and complementary medicine). The body and its physiology are stimulated by fields of energy, called Energetic Drivers in NES, that arise from the organs as a fetus develops. Meridian-like channels, called Energetic Integrators in NES, coordinate the information that drives millions of chemical processes, ensuring that the correct information gets to a specific place in the body at the precise time it is needed. Bioenergetic fields, called Energetic Terrains in NES, form environments in tissues to which

---

*The acronym NES is pronounced to rhyme with "Tess," although in the United States many early practitioners and clients pronounced each letter individually, "en ee ess."

pathogens and microbes, such as viruses and bacteria, are attracted if we are exposed to them. Energetic Stars form mini networks of information routes in the body-field that address distortions correlated to specific physiological issues. According to the NES model, everything that means anything in the physical body in terms of health has its energetic and informational counterparts. We can detect, monitor, and change the energetic environment of our body and so can directly influence the state of our health.

Throughout history, mystics and healers have claimed that we are "energy beings." The history of this belief is recounted in countless books and websites, so we will not review it here. Readers who are motivated to review this long history can start with traditional Chinese medicine and the Indian ayurvedic system. There are scores of individual pioneers and visionaries, both ancient and modern, who have devoted themselves to furthering our understanding of the underlying energies of the body. The modern physicians, scientists, and researchers include Edwin Babbitt, Harold Saxon Burr, Albert Szent-Györgyi, Ryke Geerd Hamer, Royal Rife, Samuel Hahnemann, Reinholdt Voll, Helmut Schimmel, Wilhelm Reich, Ida Rolf, Robert O. Becker, Freeman Cope, Herbert Fröhlich, James Oschman, Fritz-Albert Popp, Mae-Wan Ho, Walter Schempp, Peter Marcer, Edgar Mitchell, William Tiller, Candace Pert, and Bruce Lipton, to name only a few. Most of the research into biophysics has been more or less piecemeal, with researchers inquiring into one small aspect or another of the bioenergetics of the body. There have been few attempts to fashion an integrative model of our energetic physiology, which in NES we call the human body-field. The closest model is that of traditional Chinese medicine. However, for all its detail, even the Chinese system does not make clear connections to the modern biochemical understanding of the body. The NES model of the human body-field provides the first truly comprehensive and coherent link between biochemistry and bioenergetics.

NES is a system that is holistic in the best sense of that word. We don't reject the very real biochemical processes of the body. We don't reject the value of allopathic medicine, which is built upon that biochemical framework. However, we are showing that there is more to the body than chemistry. There is a complex energy system that serves as a master control system for the biochemical body. To be truly healthy—to achieve long-lasting wellness—we need to correct distortions and blockages in the complex energy structure that is the human body-field.

The human body-field is a self-organizing, self-directed, intelligent system that directs the information flow of the body, information that is crucial to the genetic, chemical, and physiological processes of the body. To understand the NES model of the body-field you have to unlearn biology, in a sense. You have to put aside your focus on the diagnosis of disease based on symptomology. Symptoms are a consequence of the breakdown of biochemistry. However, chemistry is driven by the interaction of subatomic particles and waves. The root cause of disease, as most complementary practitioners will tell you, is at the level of the energy and information of your body.

NES research to date allows us to describe a model of the human body-field in detail and to determine how it is functioning—how well or poorly it is managing the energy and information that determine the biochemistry of your body. We have created a biotechnology, called the NES–Professional System, that detects problems in the body-field and determines both their severity and their priority for correction. We also have created a line of encoded liquid remedies, which we call Infoceuticals, that can directly influence the body-field, correcting how it processes the information vital to the physical body. The result is a novel system of healing that works in concert with the biochemical system of the body and that directly engages the body's own self-healing capabilities. Although a tremendous amount of research remains to be done, we believe that the NES model of the human body-field represents the dawning of a new era in health care, that our theory details the bioenergetic systems of the body more precisely than any other theory, and that our system for correcting body-field errors is more direct than any other modality, biotechnology, or remedy.

The Foundational Principles of NES

The NES model of the human body-field is based upon the following ten premises. You can use this as a general outline of the main aspects of NES. Please feel free to refer back to this list as you read through the book.

1. The universe is an interconnected network of information and energy. The human body is part of this web of relationships (via feedback loops), and our health is dependent upon the body's correct processing of this information and energy.

2. Although genetics and cellular chemistry are important facets of how the body works, there is a deeper reality to the body, one in which physics, especially the field of quantum electrodynamics, governs physiology. The interaction of quantum waves imparts energy and information that is encoded in what NES calls the human body-field, which serves as a holographic template for the physical body.

3. Information is directed in the body via many kinds of energy, including electromagnetic and vibrational (as phonons, the quantum aspect of sound) energies, and via frequency and phase relationships.

4. As an embryo develops, the organs create Energetic Driver fields, which impart constitutional energy and information to the body-field, and hence to the body.

5. There are at least twelve Energetic Integrator fields, which form a comprehensive communication network in the body-field that directs information to the right place in the body at the right time so that the body functions correctly.

6. Energetic Terrains are energetic disturbances in specific body tissues that create environments hospitable to microorganisms, such as viruses and bacteria, both real and virtual (the microorganism's energy field, rather than the actual microorganism). They can be highly disruptive to the body-field.

7. Symptoms of illness, whether physical or emotional, arise first not

in the physical body but as distortions or blocks in the underlying
energy and information of the human body-field.

8. It is possible to analyze the holographic human body-field to determine if there are distortions in or blocks to the flow of energy and
information that affect the state of our health.

9. Substances and liquids can be encoded or imprinted with information to influence the energetic state of the body-field, and hence of
the physical body. The NES Infoceuticals are created according to
this principle.

10. Correcting distortions in the human body-field can help return the
body to homeostasis, which refers to the body's ability to maintain
equilibrium, a process that is dependent on the body's own self-
healing intelligence.

This book explains the NES model of the human body-field and the
body-field's influence on health in a nontechnical manner that we trust
will be accessible to most readers. We have included a glossary of terms
that might be unfamiliar, both NES-related and scientific, at the end
of the book. Feel free to refer to the glossary as needed while you are
reading. Although we strive in part 2 to preserve the personal narrative
quality of how NES came into being, we understand that most readers
will need the context and background information about physics and
bioenergetics that is provided in part 1. After all, these are not subjects we think about during the course of a normal day, and if you are
interested in the revolution in health care that is already upon us, you
surely will want to know what all the excitement is about. Don't worry:
you don't have to be a physicist or biologist to understand what your
body is really like and how it functions at its deepest energetic level.
You need only an open mind and a healthy curiosity. Although you
could jump ahead to read parts 2 and 3 first, the perspective you will
gain by reading part 1 is bound to alter your perception of yourself and
your place in the world. Beyond providing the framework upon which

NES is built, we hope that the information in part 1 also will inspire you to see yourself as more than your body and foster a greater sense of the wonders of nature.

We understand that some readers may struggle to grasp what is really going on in their bodies at the subatomic level. Believe us when we say that we have shared that struggle! Peter especially wrestled with having to rethink his entire belief system. It was no small feat to grasp some of the strange, although tantalizing, results of his experiments. For most readers, the difficulties will come in believing that so much can take place in their bodies at so infinitesimal a scale. To help readers make the shift from the familiar to the unfamiliar as effortlessly as possible, we will begin our journey by taking you on a tour of your body, into the awe-inspiring interior spaces of yourself. You will see that when we say there is so much more to you than you may imagine, we are speaking quite literally. Then we will introduce you, in nontechnical terms, to the basics of quantum physics, because the human body-field appears to be governed by quantum processes. Finally, we will review some of the intriguing research into the energies of the body and the energetic aspects of health.

Our research—and research the world over—into the human body-field is still very much in its infancy, and yet it reveals a body that is awe-inspiring in its use of the energies of nature. Parts 2 and 3 are devoted exclusively to detailing the NES model of the human body-field and the NES system of health care. We hope that this information will educate you about what health truly is and how NES might help you maintain long-term wellness. We also hope that this new knowledge will help you cultivate a deeper appreciation for the grandeur of your body and body-field. Part 2 recounts how NES grew out of our own needs, for we both were seriously ill and unable to find lasting help from either allopathic or complementary medicine. We then recount Peter's long, and so often perplexing, journey toward understanding the true nature of the human body-field and its role in health. We end part 2 by relating how Harry's vision and Peter's research came together to inspire the creation of Nutri-Energetics. In part 3, we detail the varied aspects of the NES model of bioenergetic health and recount the stories of many of the thousands of people worldwide who have been helped by NES.

We would like to close this introduction by reminding readers that no matter what beliefs they currently hold about what their bodies are made of and how healing works, nature always has the last word! Her truth will eventually be our truth. All that is required is that scientists, researchers, and healers be willing to follow where nature leads. However, as is so often the case in the history of science and medicine, just when scientists and researchers think they have it all figured out—when they think they are on the cusp of that coveted "theory of everything"—nature reveals that she has more secrets waiting to be unveiled. For all of the progress we have made in deciphering the intricacies of the human body-field, we know that we have only gleaned insight into the rudimentary aspects of it. We encourage other researchers to explore the implications of NES and of bioenergetics in general, and we urge health care practitioners and clients to put our system to the test, because we are confident that NES represents a true breakthrough in healing.

A classic hallmark that a theory has hit on a fundamental truth of nature is that it explains how a higher-level order emerges from apparently random and even seemingly chaotic lower-level processes. NES is such a theory. The bioenergetic logic that nature has revealed through Peter's experiments is more than beautiful, it is elegant. It is complex, but that complexity orders itself into a holistic, structured whole that reveals an overarching simplicity. Even though we have grasped only a small part of the larger picture, the implications for health care from what we have uncovered are staggering, and the opportunities for research are rich almost beyond measure.

Most important, however, is the fact that NES works, as thousands of clients can attest. It is not perfect. No health care or wellness system is. However, by using NES, you can directly engage your body's self-healing intelligence in very specific ways. The NES approach to well-being is rooted not in the body but in the various energies and information networks of nature that are expressed in the body. It provides us a novel way to experience the interconnectedness of the cosmos through the medium of our own bodies. The universal energies flow through us. They are not metaphysical energies but appear to be the fields and forces of the real world, of nature. The NES–Professional System provides us the opportunity to quickly and accurately analyze the state of our own body-field and, by using the Infoceuticals, directly change the state of our energy to improve health if we are ill or bolster our ability to stay well if we already are healthy. Thousands of people have discovered NES and are benefiting from it, and we take this opportunity to offer them our gratitude, for without them our research would not have progressed so quickly and our model of the human body-field would not be as fully realized.

PART ONE

◆

The Nature of the Body

1

THE UNIVERSE
OF THE BODY

*Hence this life of yours which you are living is not merely
a piece of the entire existence, but is, in a certain sense, the
whole; only this whole is not so constituted that it can be
surveyed in one single glance.*

PHYSICIST ERWIN SCHRÖDINGER

THE ANNALS OF MEDICINE are filled with anomalies, those cases
that defy rational explanation and baffle even the most brilliant medical minds. For the most part, medical professionals ignore anomalies
such as spontaneous remissions, relegating them, if they report on
them at all, to the footnotes of journal articles. However, we do ourselves a grave disservice by dismissing such anomalies as inexplicable,
for they demonstrate in the most visceral way that hidden deep in the
dim recesses of the body are clues about the mind-body's ability to heal
itself. Consider the following examples of medical anomalies:

▶ A woman suffering from the debilitating effects of decades of
   multiple sclerosis (MS) is confined to a wheelchair, her legs structurally deformed so that she can stand upright or walk a few steps

only while in full leg braces. Her pain worsens until her doctors are forced to sever the tendons to her kneecaps. Over time, some of the tissues and nerves of her legs become irretrievably impaired, her right kneecap slips off center, and her ankles and feet become paralyzed. She suffers with dignity for years, until one night, inexplicably, she hears a voice telling her she can be healed. The next day her legs begin to feel prickly and warm. She is astonished to find she can wiggle her toes. As she examines her legs, she notices that her right knee is no longer deformed. She throws off her braces and stands. In astonishment, she runs through the house, shouting in excitement, and even bounds up a flight of stairs. Her various doctors conduct examinations and tests, which reveal that her brain no longer shows the telltale lesions indicative of MS. Her legs have normal reflexes even though tendons have been severed. Her doctors for the most part are ecstatic at her startling recovery, but they are completely mystified, saying there simply is no medical explanation for it. One of her long-time physicians, however, is so upset, even frightened—because medical science says that MS cannot be reversed or cured—that he dismisses her from his office, calling her a fraud.[1]

▶ A young honors mathematics university student undergoes a brain scan. The doctor is shocked when the scan reveals that the young man has almost no brain! His cortex—the part of the brain that is the seat of intellect, perceptual awareness, and memory—is barely a millimeter thick, having been squashed to almost nothing because of undiagnosed hydrocephalus. However, even without this crucial brain matter, the young man has always functioned normally, with an above-average IQ.[2]

▶ A young girl with lupus, which has no cure and can be controlled only partially by using drugs that have numerous side effects, is conditioned to take her medication while smelling roses and tasting cod-liver oil. Over time, as the conditioning is strengthened, her medications are reduced. Finally, after several years, she is able to stop taking her medications entirely, but she receives all the benefits of those drugs simply by being exposed to the scent of roses or the taste of cod-liver oil.[3]

These stories and others like them are well documented in medical journals and books, and although they are different in detail they share a subtle commonality: the body was able to act to change its physical state. How the body was able to accomplish this is open to question, although this book offers one possible explanation. In the first example, you might be tempted to explain away the remission of MS by citing the mind-body connection, but if the woman's belief system or mind-set was the mechanism for healing, then the healing occurred without any conscious effort on her part. Also, just what do we mean by a mind-body connection? Thoughts, beliefs, hopes, and dreams are intangibles, and to explain how the mind can affect the body we are forced to ask what consciousness is. The most current research tells us that consciousness is a field, perhaps a quantum field. What does such a field do? It conveys energy and information.

In the second example, the young man, by Western medical standards, shouldn't even have a normal, functioning mind, but it is possible to explain his lack of intellectual and behavioral deficits by surmising that other parts of his brain took over the functions normally processed in the cortex. Still, even this explanation leaves us wondering about the plasticity of the brain, about how parts of the brain that may not normally control intellect and awareness can, if necessary, take over these functions. Such plasticity pushes the boundaries of what current biological theory tells us is possible or likely.

The third example can be accounted for as the mind's effect on the biochemistry of the body or by the placebo effect, which involves realizing a deeply held intention or expectation. However, again we are back to asking what the mind is. If it is so powerful that it can change the state of our body and mimic the effects of pharmaceuticals, then why has medicine ignored this natural healing capability for so long, dismissing it derisively as the placebo effect, and why isn't there a Manhattan Project of health care to explore and harness it?

At heart, each of these cases highlights how things as immaterial as mind and thoughts or fields of information play a role in health. The fact that these seemingly miraculous stories are real—and there are hundreds of other such stories in the world's medical literature—assures us that healing is not dependent only on the physical matter of the body. They hint that we should not, as we so often do, relegate to the realm of the metaphysical the mechanisms for interfacing with what appears to be the organizing, quantum-level information fields of nature. At the level of the quantum universe, everything is connected or correlated and so can affect or be affected by everything else, although the robustness of such connections is open to debate. It appears that information fields order the physical world. Because we are part of that physical world, it is not a huge leap to think that our bodies, over the millions of years of our evolutionary development, have inherent links to these underlying energy and information fields. Some scientists have finally taken notice and are marshaling the will and the funding to explore these mysteries.

THE POWER OF INFORMATION

Although we tend to think of information as abstract and insubstantial—not a material *thing* at all—scientists are beginning to view information as something as real as fields, forces, and energy. As science reporter Mark Buchanan wrote in *New Scientist* magazine, an increasing number of physicists and other kinds of scientists "believe that information is a kind of subtle substance that lies behind and beneath physical stuff."[4] The study of information has spawned many new scientific disciplines, starting with cybernetics and advancing through systems theory, complexity theory, chaos theory, fractal geometry, and game theory, to name only a few. Information theory is being applied to create new technologies, from fully realized machines such as those that perform functional magnetic resonance imaging (fMRI) to still theoretical ones such as quantum computers. Information theory has invigorated other disciplines, including ecology, economics, biology, and sociology.

As physicist Jacob D. Bekenstein reminds us, "Ask anybody what the physical world is made of, and you are likely told matter and energy. Yet, if we have learned anything from engineering, biology, and physics, information is just as crucial an ingredient."[5] In the opinion of physicist Anton Zeilinger, information may have a deeper reality than anything else in the universe, so that physics itself might be thought of not as the theory of energy and matter but as the theory of information.[6]

Frontier theorists view information as a guiding and organizing force in nature, a force that creates "systems." In its most general scientific sense, a system is something that organizes and processes information. However, information both drives systems and emerges from them (in effect, information can be either cause or effect). Scale matters in systems theory, with coherent patterns emerging from what might first appear to be chaos or randomness. As one moves down the scale of a system, probing ever deeper into it, one finds patterns within patterns within patterns. A system seems to imprint information about those patterns into itself, so that it can be considered to have "memory."

Gary Schwartz, professor of psychology and medicine, and Linda Russek, assistant professor of medicine, both of the Human Energy Systems Laboratory at the University of Arizona, have outlined the differences between systems concepts and nonsystems concepts. These distinctions, in effect, explain how conventional, reductionist, Newtonian-based science differs from the newest integrative, information-based, and quantum-based sciences.[7]

Nonsystems Concepts: Independent, static, closed, disconnected, linear, random, state-independent, parts, fixed

Systems Concepts: Interdependent, dynamic, open, interactive, nonlinear, emergent, state-dependent, whole, flexible, creative

Those who study the new scientific discipline called "sync," for example, explore the physics of coherent oscillations, which occur when two or more systems resonate together, imparting information to each other.[8] Coherent oscillations explain how individual members of a certain species of firefly synchronize themselves to flash in perfect unison, how a bridge can collapse as the result of the synchronized footfalls of people crossing it, or how electrons can pair up and move in unison to create a phenomenon called superconductivity (the complete loss of electrical resistance).

The systems view of information—as a forcelike entity in its own right that can direct energy and affect matter—is changing the face of biology and medicine. Biology is moving beyond the study of the matter of life and beginning to consider how fields, energies, and information shape and direct life itself. One of the most public debates in medicine currently is the use of embryonic stem cells, which are special because they are precursor cells that can be coaxed into becoming almost any kind of differentiated cell. Scientists don't understand how a stem cell *knows* how to turn itself into a specific kind of cell—a liver, heart, muscle, or nerve cell. From where does it get its information? Biochemistry and DNA cannot provide the full answers, for the processes they either initiate or direct are themselves dependent on information.

Throughout your body, there are trillions of chemical processes that form a tangled web of interconnections to make the enzymes, proteins, hormones, and other substances that your body needs to work properly. All of these processes must be exquisitely timed, and these substances must be produced in specific quantities and delivered with precision to the correct cells. It seems only reasonable to assume that this intricate biological dance must be choreographed by something. That something is information.

One way to gain an appreciation for how crucial information is to the reality of our very lives is to delve into the workings of our own bodies. It is no surprise that most of us are as unfamiliar with the landscapes of our physical selves as we are with the terrain of Mars. So, let us gain an appreciation for how crucial information is by examining the way our own bodies work. Cells are the smallest measure of living things, so that is where we will shift our focus. Because every fiber of our material being is made from cells, our health, or lack of it, depends on how well they function.

EXPLORING THE BIOLOGICAL BODY

No one knows exactly how many cells make up the human body, but the numbers are beyond imagining. At birth, your body has about ten thousand trillion cells. However, because that number decreases radically as you develop, by the time you are an adult your body contains between 50 trillion and 100 trillion cells, which can be grouped into about two hundred different types.[9] It's impossible to make sense of such huge numbers. To get a handle on it, imagine you have a metronome that makes an audible click with each swing of the arm. As the arm swings to the left—click. Back to the right—click. If you heard a click every second, it would take more than 31,546 years to tick off one trillion seconds. If you heard a click once a second for every cell in your body, using the conservative estimate of 50 trillion cells, you would be listening for more than 1.5 million years![10]

However, only about 10 percent of these cells make up the solid aspects of your body, such as your bones and tissues. Approximately 40 percent make up the nonsolid parts of you, such as your blood and lymphatic fluids. You have about 30 trillion red blood cells and 500 million white blood cells circulating through your body. Your lymph system is crowded as well, as it contains roughly one trillion lymphocytes and other immune cells. The other half of the cells in your body are bacterial cells, most of which are beneficial and inhabit your digestive system. To get a true count, you will need to decide if you want to include the cells of the 100 trillion microorganisms that call your eyeballs, mouth, nose, ears, skin, and other areas of your body home. Our bodies are actually vast ecosystems for these organisms, many of which we could not live without because they contribute to the vital functioning of our bodies.[11]

It only makes sense that with so many trillions of cells in our bodies, cells are indeed tiny things. How tiny? About twenty microns wide, on average. To appreciate just how small the average human cell is, imagine marking off one inch on a piece of paper. If you laid average-size cells side by side, you would be able to fit 1,270 into that inch.[12] If you are like most people, you can hardly conceive of anything so small. So it comes as a shock to think that a cell, which seems so incredibly tiny as to be almost nothing, is intricately structured and massively crowded. At the scale of chemistry, it is actually huge: it houses more than a dozen structures inside of itself and more on its surface, and it is host to uncountable numbers of molecules that zip in and out of it every second.

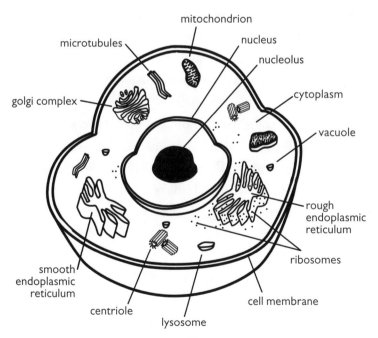

Figure 1.1. Although cells are incredibly tiny, they are intricately constructed, containing dozens of smaller, functioning structures within them that coordinate thousands of processes.

Every cell is the center of a whirlwind of activity, doing everything that is necessary to keep you alive. Science writer Bill Bryson eloquently makes our point:

> If you could visit a cell you wouldn't like it. Blown up to the scale at which atoms were about the size of peas, a cell itself would be a sphere roughly half a mile across, and supported by a complex framework of girders called the cytoskeleton. Within it, millions upon millions of objects—some the size of basketballs, others the size of cars—would whiz around like bullets. There wouldn't be a place you could stand without being pummeled and ripped thousands of times every second from every direction.[13]

What is a cell so busy doing? It depends on what type of cell it is, of course. However, to say that our cells are workhorses is an understatement. Cell biologist Franklin M. Harold calls each cell an "intricate and sophisticated chemical factory." He says, "Even in the simplest cells, this calls for collaborative interactions of many thousands of molecules, large and small, and requires hundreds of concurrent chemical reactions. These break down foodstuffs, extract energy, manufacture precursors, assemble constituents, note and execute genetic instructions and keep all this frantic activity coordinated. The term 'metabolism' designates the sum total of all these chemical processes, derived from the Greek word for 'change.'"[14] Harold's is an elegant way to characterize cells: they manage change. However, the rates of change that a single cell must coordinate are barely fathomable. Which brings us to the subject of the speed of life.

Activities in our body occur at speeds that have no counterpart in our normal, macroscopic world. Every second millions of cells die. They have to be identified and then dismantled and swept from the body, even as new cells are being born to replace them. Take the red blood cells in your body. Every second almost three million red blood cells die, and every second new blood cells are made to replace them.

That's only one type of cell and one set of related activities that takes place in one second. There are millions of other activities taking place in your body during time frames that make seconds feel like forever. In your kidneys, specialized cells are monitoring your salt and water levels, secreting hormones, and removing wastes. Amino acids are arranging themselves into strings that are making up the particular proteins that the body needs at specific times and in exact quantities. The proteins then fold themselves into the intricate three-dimensional structures that determine their function. Each configuration gives a protein a different identity, but somehow proteins know which shape to assume. Ribonucleic acid (RNA) is zipping apart the double helix of DNA, copying the millions of "letters" of the genetic code, proofreading the replication and correcting any mistakes before zipping the new strand of DNA back together again. Messenger RNA is receiving messages from DNA and shuttling those messages around to direct the production of enzymes and other molecules. Your heart is pumping more than a liter of blood a minute. T-cells and other immune cells are tagging, attacking, and destroying foreign organisms such as bacteria and viruses, while leaving harmless microorganisms alone. Adenosine triphosphate (ATP), arguably the busiest molecule in the body, is being broken down to provide energy to power your cells. In fact, every minute millions of cells in your body will each deplete about 500 million ATP molecules, and an equal number of new ATP molecules will be created to rush into those cells to replace them. Neurons are firing, releasing cascades of neurotransmitters, which are fitting like keys into the receptor locks on the surface of cells. Many of the different types of receptors that pepper the surface of cells are themselves active, changing their shape over time and according to different states of the body's internal environment to accept only particular molecular keys, while rejecting others. Thousands upon thousands of other activities and millions upon millions of chemical reactions that are absolutely crucial to your health—and to your life—are going on below the level of your awareness every minute of every day.

Yet this frenzy of activity that is occurring at staggering speeds in spaces too small to imagine is nothing compared with what is going on at the submolecular level of your body. At the quantum level, activity is taking place at speeds that make chemical reactions seem lethargic and in spaces that make cells feel cavernous. Here is where chemistry gives way to physics. Physics is the study of the very small (as in smaller than atoms and therefore "subatomic") and the very fast (as in almost the speed of light, which is slightly more than 186,000 miles per second). As molecular biologist P. W. Atkins wrote of chemistry, "On the one hand it deals with biology and provides explanations for the processes of life. On the other hand it mingles with physics and finds explanations for chemical phenomena in the fundamental processes and particles of the universe."[15] He marveled at the precise nature of the interactions that must take place for chemistry to work at all: "One or two atoms can convert a fuel to a poison, change a color, render an inedible substance edible, or replace a pungent odor with a fragrant one. That changing a single atom can have such consequences is the wonder of the chemical world."[16]

An obvious question is what causes that transformation, that selection of one atom rather than another? What is directing the choice or the need? To answer this kind of question, you have to shift your attention from chemistry to physics. Yet few biologists, or even biochemists, concern themselves much with physics. For all intents and purposes, in the life sciences today, chemistry rules. Even genetics is based on the chemistry of DNA. However, if scientists are not following chemistry down to the level of physics, how can they be sure they are not missing important and fundamental aspects of what is going on in the body? It was not until relatively recently that scientists began to look at the quantum aspects of the body. The young disciplines of quantum biology and biophysics now sanction the study of the quantum processes—the energies and information—that underlie chemistry. Even so, they are still decidedly fringe elements of the conventional scientific world.

Of course, alternative and complementary medicine and science have a rich, and ancient, history of viewing the body in terms of energy, which is fundamentally what physics is about. Traditional Chinese medicine and Indian ayurvedic medicine have long explored the energies of the body. Acupuncture and homeopathy are practiced widely in Asia and Europe (Britain, for example, has at least four exclusively homeopathic hospitals) and are slowly gaining acceptance in the United States and elsewhere. Today, there is growing interest in these unconventional techniques and theories because science is beginning to discover that although chemistry has been wildly successful at explaining many of the mechanisms of the body, it is not adequate by itself to the task of explaining the *integrative* workings of the body. As Deepak Chopra, a physician and prolific writer and speaker, so artfully argues, the body is simply too complex to be ruled by chemistry alone; there is some deeper process involved that keeps everything running at the level of precision the body demands:

> The healing mechanism resides somewhere in this overall complexity, but it is elusive. There is no one organ of healing. How does the body know what to do when it is damaged, then? Medicine has no simple answer. Any one of the processes involved in healing a superficial cut—the clotting of the blood for example—is incredibly complex, so much so that if the mechanism fails, as it does with hemophiliacs, advanced scientific medicine is at a loss to duplicate the impaired function. A doctor can prescribe drugs to replace the missing clotting factor in the blood, but these are temporary, artificial and have numerous side effects. The body's perfect timing will be absent, as well as the superb coordination of a dozen related processes. By comparison, a man-made drug is a stranger in a land where everyone else is blood kin. It can never share the knowledge that everyone else was born with.[17]

Dr. Chopra's assessment of the limits of chemistry is one that is finding grudging acceptance among many biologists. One of the difficulties that confronts scientists in moving from chemistry to physics when analyzing the body is not their intellectual capacities or any inadequacies with their instrumentation, but their method of questioning. To paraphrase Albert Einstein, we can only find answers to the questions we choose to ask. Our questions are limited by our worldview, our paradigm. If scientists believe that chemistry and genetics are all there is to the body, then that is all they will examine. As they shift their perspective from the stuff of life (matter) to the processes of life (energies and information), they are finding a whole new world within the body.

The current trend in mainstream medicine is genetics. Modern research findings about the genetic components of disease have been incredibly enlightening and certainly have improved health care over the last few decades. However, there appears to be a fundamental limit to how much science and, by extension, medicine can achieve by treating the body only as a chemical factory or as being dependent solely, or mostly, on its genetic "blueprint." Eric Landers, who was at the forefront of the Human Genome Project, has called the genome a parts list. Having a parts list alone does not tell you what the pieces are for and how to combine them into something useful.[18] You need an information template for that.

DNA is an alphabet of only four letters, the chemicals (called bases) adenine, thymine, cystosine, and guanine, yet combinations of those four bases, we are told, determine many, if not most, of our core characteristics, from the color of our eyes to our propensity for developing certain diseases. However, for all the progress made in decoding our DNA, scientists still consider 95 percent of it as "junk" DNA because it has no known function. A large portion of this noncoding DNA, as it is called, was at first thought to be a vestige of evolution—bits and pieces of the DNA of other organisms that are our evolutionary ancestors. Recently, however, scientists have begun to glean clues that this "molecular garbage" may have important regulatory functions in the body. In fact, the discovery that junk DNA may have purpose was initially made by scientists who applied linguist theory to analyze the DNA! They found "messages"—a biological grammar and syntax—in the noncoding DNA that may influence how genes function and affect cellular processes.[19] So for all intents and purposes, science still has a long, long way to go even to make sense of how much of our DNA is useful, never mind to tease out its functions in the body.

In terms of current allopathic medicine and biology, manipulating DNA is considered the most promising route to cure disease. However, as genetic research roars ahead, scientists are becoming more sober in their predictions and expectations, for they are finding that there is probably not a one-to-one correspondence between genetics and most of the diseases that kill the majority of people, such as heart disease and cancer. For a few diseases, such as cystic fibrosis and sickle cell anemia, there is an undeniable genetic correlation, but for others the link is tenuous. Most genetic defects occur because you are missing a gene. Others occur because you have a faulty copy of one or more genes. In the latter case, all that genetics can tell you is that you may be *predisposed* toward a particular disease. For the disease to manifest, the associated defective gene or genes have to be "expressed." For example, colon cancer is linked to five different defective genes. Yet, of the 145,000 new cases of colon cancer reported each year in the United States, only 5 percent of the people affected have one of the defective genes. In this case—as confusing as it may seem—having the defective gene gives you a very high probability of getting the disease, yet very few people with the disease actually have the gene.[20] Obviously, something other than mutated genes is causing the cancer in the majority of people with colon cancers.

What is causing the vast majority of cancers and other diseases? One clue comes from the National Institutes of Health. On their Human Genome Project website, they report that environmental factors may be the single most important trigger in whether a genetic mutation is expressed or not: "Scientists estimate that each of us carries between 5 and 50 [gene] mutations that carry some risk for disease or disability. Some of us may not experience negative consequences from the mutations we carry, either because we do not live long enough for it to happen or because we may not be exposed to the relevant environmental triggers."[21]

An intriguing study on twins also revealed a strong correlation between cancer and environmental factors. Identical twins are a unique population for studying the correlation between genes and disease risk because these twins share the same DNA. Yet after taking into account all known risk factors, the researchers for this study found that the single best predictor for why one twin got cancer and the other did not was exposure to environmental toxins and lifestyle choices, such as cigarette smoking.[22] As you will see in part 3, the NES system of health care takes environmental factors—from geomagnetic fields and electromagnetic pollution to chemical toxins and dietary factors—into consideration in the analysis of your body-field, giving you a truly holistic picture of your state of well-being.

EXPLORING THE QUANTUM BODY

For all the strides made in health and medicine—from designer pharmaceuticals to stricter environmental standards to gene therapies—conventional science is falling short of successfully deciphering the complexities of the body. One aspect of the body being overlooked is its quantum nature. However, the NES theory of health is built around what happens in the body at the subatomic level. Physics underlies, even drives, chemistry. So to understand what is really happening in the body, you have to understand something about what is happening at the smallest known scale. This is the scale of electrons, protons, photons, and quarks—the entire "particle zoo" of quantum physics.

It's all relative, as they say, which is why understanding the levels of the body is so important. As physicist Kenneth W. Ford wrote, "By most measures, atoms are small. Yet to some scientists, they are gargantuan. These scientists—nuclear and particle physicists—are concerned with what goes on in bits of space much smaller than atoms, smaller even than the tiny nuclei that sit at the centers of atoms. We call this world the *subatomic world*."[23]

An atom, to use the scientific definition, is a unit of matter that has a central, positively charged nucleus surrounded by a system of electrons. It is very small, about 10^{-8} centimeters.[24] To get a sense of what that number means, imagine ten million atoms arranged side by side. They would cover a distance of less than one-tenth of an inch.[25] However, those are *atoms,* and we are talking about the *sub*atomic world, which is about protons and electrons and other things that can barely be called things, things that are smaller than atoms. Classical physics is fairly straightforward, but the quantum world is outright weird. We discuss quantum physics in the next chapter, but let us point out here that many of the particles of the quantum world are not even really "things" at all.

The fundamental quantum particles—"fundamental" meaning they are not made up of any smaller parts—such as electrons and quarks are not measurable by any normal, macroscopic standards. Scientists have searched for structure in the electron and found none even at distances of less than 10^{-18} meters. They have to set up experiments from which they can *infer* the characteristics of quantum particles, because the "stuff" of the quantum world cannot be apprehended directly. The truth is, the fundamental quantum particles are so infinitesimal that they cannot be considered to have structure at all. Thus they cannot be considered as material things, and the concepts of *measurement* and *observation,* two words often used in science, take on special meanings in quantum mechanics. The point is that quantum entities are not things but are probability waves. That is, an electron is less like a solid object, say a billiard ball, and more like a cloud, a fog of potentiality, with a probability of the electron being anywhere in that fog until it is measured. Only then, upon measurement (or more accurately, upon detection, since these entities are not measureable in terms of length, depth, and other such physical characteristics), can it be said to have a definite location.

Because the quantum domain is so unimaginably tiny, events there occur at equally unimaginable speeds. In conventional biology, although some of the chemical activities of the body occur in nano-seconds, they do not occur at anything approaching quantum speeds. Also, even though the component parts of a single cell are miniscule—400 meters of DNA could be curled up onto the period at the end of any sentence in this book[26]—they are gigantic in comparison with the size of the particles of the quantum world. Yet physicists, such as the late Richard Feynman, have said that quantum theory is necessary to understand the fundamentals of chemistry. One way to begin to clear our possible confusion about the differing rules at the different scales of matter—from the infinitesimal scale of the quantum world to the microscopic world of molecules and cells to the macroscopic world of tissues and organs—is to consider two important properties in biology: emergence and phase change.

Emergence refers to patterns in nature that arise as you move up the scale of reference. To put it in its simplest terms, it means that the whole is greater than the sum of the parts. Emergent proper-ties often border on the miraculous, as seemingly chaotic processes produce order and symmetry at larger scales. For example, the individual ice crystals in a raging snowstorm come together to form a snowflake, or the electrical and chemical impulses of millions of neurons coalesce into a thought. Mathematician Ian Stewart marveled that nature's patterns "emerge from an ocean of complexity like Botticelli's Venus from her half shell—unheralded, transcending their origins."[27] Nobel Prize–winning physicist Robert B. Laughlin explained other qualities of this phenomenon that is so ubiquitous in nature and so fundamental to life: "Emergence means complex organizational structures growing out of simple rules. Emergence means stable inevitability in the way certain things are. Emergence means unpredictability, in the sense of small events causing great and quali-tative changes in larger ones."[28]

Chemical bonding accounts for how atoms group together to form molecules. Then molecules bind to make cells, cells cluster into tissues, which form into organs, and before you know it you have a living organism. Nowhere, at any of those levels, can you find the *one* organ or activity or process that *is* "life." Yet, put all those component parts together—and add in an external environment that supplies nutrients and light and other factors necessary to support life—and you get an *E. coli* bacterium, a mosquito, a salmon, a peacock, a rhinoceros, or a human being. Life is the grandest emergent property of all.

The other property we mentioned was phase change, also called phase transition. We are all familiar with phase changes in the macroscopic world. At room temperature, water is a fluid. Lower the temperature enough, and it forms ice. Raise the temperature enough, and it becomes gaseous and escapes into the air as vapor. Phase changes occur in the subatomic world as well. Beyond certain parameters, atoms lose their individuality and act collectively. Life itself may have emerged from the primordial soup as a phase change of aggregating molecules that catalyzed into a self-organizing, self-replicating organism. You can think of the loss of health or the regaining of it, if you have been ill, as a phase change in the body. Spontaneous regressions from cancer could fall into the class of phase change, as for no reason apparent to conventional science a tumor disappears overnight or within days.

One of the difficulties in pinpointing the cause of disease is that a small input, such as exposure to a toxin from the environment over a long period of time, can build up to a point that pushes the body over a threshold, after which very suddenly the system goes awry. Classical systems, which are governed by the physics of the everyday world, usually follow this pattern of change building up slowly over time and then reaching a breaking point. These are called linear systems, because they tend to follow a steady, sequential course. Nonclassical systems are nonlinear, which means that change often happens suddenly, with a dramatic shift occurring from a tiny, seemingly insignificant cause. (You have no doubt heard the popular metaphor for nonlinearity: a butterfly flapping its wings in Tokyo can affect the weather in Dallas.) The body is a nonlinear, and some would say quantum, system that can experience a rapid shift from a small input. As biophysicist James Oschman reminds us, "In cooperative systems [such as the human body], large transitions can take place sharply and rapidly in response to minute inputs of energy."[29]

We mention emergence and phase change only to provide you with another window into the mystery of the body, for these phenomena provide evidence that what matters in nature is not only matter and energy but also *information*.

A BIOLOGY OF INFORMATION

As an example of how information drives energy and matter, we have only to think of water. One of the most intriguing questions in biology right now is how water works in the body—how an aggregate of water molecules in the body can serve as an information-carrying network that affects almost every physiological function. Water is, of course, crucial to life. Our bodies are more than 70 percent water. However, the water in your body is not like ordinary water. It displays unique characteristics that put the life in living things. For instance, the latest research shows that DNA and genes can carry out their functions only with the help of water. As Felix Franks, of the University of Cambridge, said in a *New Scientist* article, "The Quantum Elixir," "Without water, it is all chemistry, but add water and you get biology."[30]

Water in a living organism is called biological water. Can this type of water imprint and transmit information? Does water have memory? These are among the revolutionary questions facing frontier biologists, and they are finding that the answers are yes and yes. "The Quantum Elixir" article was devoted to water's role in biological activity—its behavior around DNA, in cells, and elsewhere in the body. The research reported on in the article has demonstrated that biological water is governed by a quantum energy called zero-point energy (ZPE), which is the lowest possible energy state of a quantum system. This ZPE energy often is equated with the emptiness of space, with the vacuum. However, what we call empty space is in reality a froth of vibrations at the quantum level. Research into biological water suggests that as a result of the influence of these ZPE vibrations, water molecules in the body take on amazing properties, especially in regard to how hydrogen molecules bond to oxygen and other molecules. The studies also suggest that biological water somehow relays information to proteins so that they connect only to precise sequences of genes and not to others and that water molecules even warn proteins about nearby damaged DNA. To say that scientists are surprised by the strange qualities of biological water as an information-carrying network is an understatement. The author of the article, Robert Matthews, wrote, "Put bluntly, you owe your existence to quantum effects in water that make even the wackiest New Age ideas seem ho-hum."

History records how what was once deemed impossible often turns out to be very possible indeed. For example, at least one of the scientists cited in the article about the quantum nature of biological water thinks that the evidence leads scientists back to homeopathy, which has been dismissed as quackery by much of modern, Western science but has helped millions of ill people the world over. He suggests that homeopathy might be correct in its claim that water can be imprinted with information, that water has a memory.[31] Homeopathic remedies are made from substances, such as minerals or plants, that are placed in a solution, usually mostly water, which is then succussed (vigorously shaken). The solution is then diluted further and the procedure repeated, often until not a single molecule of the original substance remains in the remedy. All that remains is information. In effect, the remedy retains a memory of information about the healing substance that the body can recognize and use. Research conducted by NES extended this theory and resulted in the development of our own type of remedies, called Infoceuticals, which are encoded with information, but in a way wholly unlike the dilution and succussion method of homeopathy. If recent experimental evidence from mainstream scientists continues to mount in homeopathy and NES's favor, conventional scientists might have to revise their opinions—and even their science.

For every question we ask about who we are and how our bodies work, nature teases us with new questions, plants new clues right under our noses, and opens us to new possibilities of how the body regulates itself. Nature's creativity and outright novelty challenge us to remain open to what seemed absurd, and even impossible, to previous generations. Thomas Kuhn, the late professor of the history of science, is famous for his analysis of how scientific thought can be grouped into paradigms, which shift over time. They do so not according to a smooth curve of increasing insight but by abrupt breaks with old philosophies and entrenched ideas. However, history shows us that most truly fundamental leaps forward in scientific understanding are shunned at first. Truly new insights are sometimes too radical an overturning of accepted theory or too threatening to business or academic interests to be evaluated impartially. You have only to think of germ theory, tectonic plate theory, quantum electrodynamics, and string theory to know that even ideas that are accepted widely in our day were dismissed as crackpot ideas by a previous generation of scientists.

Michael Faraday, who developed the first modern theory of electricity in the nineteenth century, was trained as a bookbinder and had no formal scientific training, but his theory became the impetus for all the later breakthroughs in understanding electromagnetism. Academic scientists rejected his theory when he first made it public, more for who he was than for what he was proposing. One critic even suggested smugly that Faraday, who had no university degrees, "ought to return to sixth form mathematics before venturing into Laplacian physics."[32] Similarly, Clair Patterson waged a career-long campaign against the petroleum industry and other corporate and even government interests to prove that lead is toxic to humans. His unrelenting efforts finally resulted in the banning of lead from gasoline, paint, and other consumer products and to stricter standards for airborne lead levels.[33] Physicist George Zweig, who in 1964 was one of the first theorists to propose the reality of quarks—which have since been verified as the most fundamental of all subatomic particles—was denied a post at an American university because a prestigious faculty member claimed his work was that of a charlatan.[34]

The problems of "doing science" persist even today, and perhaps the difficulties are worse than ever. It takes money to pursue science, and it takes publication in peer-reviewed journals to get your science noticed. If you don't fit into the mainstream establishment, you are unlikely to get a hearing for your ideas. Even if you do, science progresses at the proverbial snail's pace. The Institute of Medicine reported in 2001, to the dismay of members of the medical establishment, that it takes an average of "15 to 20 years for new scientific knowledge to percolate down into everyday medical practice."[35]

Theoretical shifts that could change the very understanding of the fundamentals of science can take even longer to become widely known and accepted. Physiologist Gilbert Ling provides a sobering example of how slow science can be to change, even when a radical new theory is backed by impeccable and replicable experiments.[36] For forty years Ling has waged a battle to revise cell theory. Most biologists still view the cell as a bag of liquid enclosed in a semipermeable membrane that has tiny pumps that control what gets through the membrane and into the cell, such as oxygen and nutrients, but Ling has shown that cells cannot possibly work according to the membrane-pump theory. We won't go into the reasons why here, for the explanations are complex. However, as one example, experiments with frog muscle cells proved that to move important ions, such as sodium, in and out of cells via a channel-pump process, cells would need 15 to 30 times *more* energy than is available to them. Ling's research has revealed an alternative mechanism that not only solves the "pump problem," as many researchers call it, but also explains many other processes that have mystified cell biologists. (As an aside, his research also indicates that the water in cells displays unique properties, properties very different from those of regular [nonbiological] water and ones that display the signature of the quantum realm, just as the most current research is confirming.)

Despite the importance of these experiments, Ling's theory, called the association–induction hypothesis, has been slow to find acceptance. You have to wonder why. After all, cells are the very building blocks of life, and how they function has enormous ramifications for health, if for no other reason than because most pharmaceuticals work at the cellular level. Pharmaceuticals often have unintended side effects because they disrupt cells they are not intended to target. Biologists don't understand enough about cell functioning to control those unintended effects. You would think that researchers would welcome a model that better reveals the inner workings of the cell and that can revolutionize the effectiveness of pharmaceuticals. However, as Ling argues, it is not the quality of his or his colleagues' science that is the problem but the threat of their new model to the status quo of the profession of biology in general. Scientists who have built careers on a particular biological model are slow to accept evidence that their model may be flawed.

There are legions of other scientists we could name whose ideas upset the status quo and so were initially rejected, suppressed, or ignored until so much evidence was amassed as to make their theories acceptable or until the cultural climate changed in their favor. We mention the above examples only to remind readers that science, which in an idealistic world is thought of as impartial and objective, is in practice subject to cultural, political, and personal concerns that can mean real breakthroughs can take decades to filter down to the people who pay for and most benefit from them—the public. If history is any guide, progress cannot be stopped, and it is the public itself that propels science forward. One has only to look at the billions of dollars spent annually on complementary health care for evidence that the public wields power over its own destiny, as well it should.

The examples of frontier biology that we have highlighted in this chapter provide evidence that the biologists of the future will need to shift their focus from the purely chemical aspects of biology to its quantum aspects, especially to how information is stored, transmitted, and regulated in the body at the subatomic level. Peter Fraser, whose research led to the creation of the Nutri-Energetics Systems model of the human body-field, independently reached conclusions that are only now coming to light in biology, chemistry, and physics, such as the relevance of zero-point energy to the proper functioning of the body. The NES model grew from a foundation of analyzing the information regulation processes in the body at the quantum level. As Peter says, there is one medicine, but it has two aspects: the biochemical and the bioenergetic. NES represents the first comprehensive synthesis of these two aspects of health.

The truth in the case of biology is that there is a deeper reality to our bodies than conventional science is willing to allow. It is at the quantum level that we find the master control processes that so profoundly influence our health and well-being. In the next two chapters, we take a closer look at these more-fundamental aspects of the body. We first delve into the world of quantum physics and then review research into bioenergetics by pioneering scientists who have followed where nature led. To appreciate the fundamental shift in health care that NES is proposing—and delivering in its clinical system, the NES–Professional System—you have to be grounded in a bit of both physics and bioenergetics. So, let's continue our exploration into the deepest, most elusive aspects of the body—its energy and information.

2

THE MICROWORLD AND THE MACROWORLD

It is quite obvious that there are problems with the Standard Model [of physics]. However, there is nothing particularly unhealthy about such a situation. There are often problems with theories in physics, at least with those that lie on the frontiers of science. If there were no problems, then theoretical speculation and experimental research would come to a halt. Physicists would not know what to do next.

RICHARD MORRIS, *THE EDGES OF SCIENCE*

FOR THE PAST FEW HUNDRED YEARS (and historically as far back as the Greeks), the Western approach to science has been reductionist. Scientists seek to know what something is made of and how it works by probing into and taking apart the object of their study, whether a bacterium, a human cell, or an atom. For example, physicists learn about the characteristics of quantum particles by accelerating streams of atoms or quantum particles to as close to the speed of light as they can and then crashing the particles into each other. The force annihilates the particles, showering detectors with the even smaller particles from which they are made. In this way physicists learn which particles are truly elementary (have no constituent parts) and which are composite particles (e.g., the proton and neutron, which are made of various kinds of smaller particles called quarks). The physicists' tool—the accelerator—is not called an "atom smasher" for nothing! Using this or similar methods, physicists discovered most of the four hundred or so members of the particle zoo of the quantum realm.

The method is not so different in biology. To study a cell, biologists dissolve it in a solution or grind it and then separate out its constituent parts, destroying the cell in order to study it. This is reductionist science at its best. It works beautifully. By taking apart cells, biologists learned that they have a complex and intricate structure. However, this is not *integrative* science. As cell biologist Franklin M. Harold wrote, "We know in our hearts that a cell is far more than an aggregate of individual molecules; it is an organized, structured, purposeful and evolved whole. Unfortunately, analytical practice dictates that we begin our inquiries by grinding the exquisite architecture of the living cell into a pulp. No wonder, then, that the integrative perspective is woefully absent from the molecular view of life as it has developed over the past half-century."[1]

Integrative science strives to understand the whole, in which emergent properties express themselves and so reveal functions and processes that are undecipherable and even undetectable at lower levels. Integrative science is about connections at the systems level, about patterns that are revealed holistically, and about simplicities that arise from a cluster of complexities. *It is a science of synthesis.*

The most recent paradigm in medicine, although it is still in its infancy, is called "integrative medicine," which is a holistic, rather than a reductionist, approach to health. It is a medical mind-set that acknowledges that healing and curing are qualitatively different, that a person is more than his or her disease, and that there is not only a mind-body connection but also a spirit-mind-body connection. Integrative medicine is what author and physician Larry Dossey would classify as Era

III medicine.[2] Dossey views the recent history of medicine as having evolved through three eras. Era I started in the mid-nineteenth century, when medicine was just beginning to become scientific. The physicians of that era considered the body a machine and consciousness an emergent property of the neurophysiology of the brain. By the mid-twentieth century, medicine had begun to enter Era II. Science was studying the placebo effect, which showed clearly that the mind influences the body. Stress, emotions, and other psychological states were recognized as affecting, and in some cases even causing, disease. Lifestyle choices became almost as important a factor in health as genetics or exposure to pathogens or toxins. Attitude, such as the will to live or an optimistic outlook, was identified as an important predictor of who would have a good outcome from a therapy and who might not. We are still in the midst of Era II medicine, of what might be called mind-body medicine. We see only the first glimmers of the dawning of Era III medicine, the hallmark of which is the "nonlocal mind." The term *nonlocal* refers to action at a distance, or how your mind can influence things, people, and events that are spatially separated from you. Era III medicine is built upon the growing body of evidence that consciousness can exist outside of the body and that focused or directed intention can have a healing effect, such that praying for someone could have a positive effect on the state of that person's health. This is truly both an *energy*-based and an *information*-based medicine.

Dossey is not alone in his assessment that the use of focused consciousness and directed energy or intention will be important aspects of the medicine of the future. Cardiac surgeon Mehmet Oz, who combines Eastern and Western medical techniques into his surgical practice, declares that many of his heart surgery patients do better when they also learn how to meditate, use guided imagery, and receive adjunct complementary therapies such as acupuncture and foot reflexology.[3] Acupuncturist Michael Wayne, in his book *Quantum-Integral Medicine,* argues that patients can harness their minds to ramp up their bodies' innate self-healing capabilities, so they can be their own doctors to a much larger extent than ever thought possible.[4] Physicist Amit Goswami, in *The Quantum Doctor: A Physicist's Guide to Health and Healing,* posits that all healing is ultimately dependent upon the proper use of energy, both of the physical body and the conscious mind.[5] Perhaps the best known advocate of Era III medicine is physician and best-selling author Deepak Chopra.[6]

In allopathic medicine—the system of conventional medicine that is taught in most medical schools and that most people use— integrative health care has come to refer to the practice of using both conventional and complementary healing approaches, something that more allopathic physicians have come to accept—or at least tolerate— because millions of their patients are using complementary therapies even while they seek conventional medical care. For complementary physicians and practitioners, however, the term *integrative medicine* takes on a more holistic meaning, implying that the body has heal- ing capabilities that most allopathic doctors would deny. In actuality, there is a deep ideological split between the two groups. Allopathic physicians work within the domain of biochemistry and see them- selves as healers. They have acquired the knowledge to attempt to fix what has gone wrong in the body; their main tools are surgery and the pharmaceuticals and other synthetic compounds that can supply the body with what it lacks. Complementary health professionals, for the most part, would deny that they are healers. They consider the *patient* the healer of his or her own body. Complementary practi- tioners see themselves more as *facilitators,* helping patients to har- ness their bodies' own inner resources. These inner resources are fundamentally consciousness-based and/or energy-based. Moreover, complementary practitioners are not focused only on the body but also on the whole patient, including that person's lifestyle, emotional state, environment, hopes and dreams, relationships, and everything that goes into being a full and productive human being.

Where does Nutri-Energetics fit into this picture? We acknowledge the mind-body connection and even the spirit-mind-body connection, but we have not gone so far as to declare that our physical health is dependent only on the state of our consciousness. It very well may be, and some of our research has hinted at how consciousness influences the body, but we are first and foremost concerned with the *energies* of the body and the *information* that directs those energies. Our model describes a comprehensive energetic physiology of the body and even of the mind, for emotions are not separate from the body, and an energetic pathology for how illness develops and how health can be restored. The NES model is unique, so far as we have been able to determine. It is *integrative* health care in the truest sense of that term; we integrate physics and biology to activate the body's own healing capabilities. Our theory helps explain why complementary modalities, such as acupuncture and homeopathy, work, although our method of health care is as different from those two practices as they are from each other.

NES is concerned with the bioenergetics of the physical body. The term *bioenergetics* has at least two distinct meanings. In conventional biology, it refers to the study of how the cells of the body perform work. In a more general sense, the term describes a relatively recent area of study about the physics of the body, that is, the study of the possible quantum processes of the body. We believe quantum fields—which are fields of information—interact to form a complex system that drives chemistry and influences the deepest mechanisms of biology; they have a structure in the body and also link the body with the environment in complex feedback loops of energy and information. In fact, our research suggests that these energetic systems in the body form a master informational control system for the physiology of the body, directing its biochemistry and physiology. Ours is a theory about the functioning of what we call the human body-field. Peter Fraser has mapped this body-field, and together he and Harry Massey have been able to create a biotechnology, called the NES–Professional System, that can analyze (in a process called a "scan") the relative state of the body-field to determine its level of functioning. The NES Infoceuticals are liquids that are specially imprinted, or encoded, with information that corrects the distortions in the human body-field that were identified via the scan. When distortions are corrected, the body-field then directs the physical body back toward homeostasis, so that it can once again work to keep itself healthy.

That existence of quantum processes and energy fields in the human body is a relatively recent scientific discovery. This area of modern research is still in its infancy, but in actuality the evidence for the energetic reality of the body goes back decades, and even to antiquity if you include spiritual and metaphysical wisdom instead of only laboratory results. We are not going to review that history here, but suffice it to say that most people interested in alternative healing methods have heard of *qi* (also spelled *chi,* and pronounced "chee"), *prana,* the *élan vital,* meridians, chakras, and other terms for the energy of the body from cultures around the world. However, NES is not working with these kinds of energies, which for the most part are cosmic, metaphysical energies that pervade the universe. We repeat that we are dealing with energies that are measurable; they are the energies of matter. We are not seeking to define new energies that have so far escaped the notice of science. We are, instead, finding how the known energies and fields of physics work in the human body. NES falls into the category of biophysics because we are concerned not with metaphysics, but with physics, albeit the physics of physiology.

Most conventional scientists who have expressed an opinion about complementary modalities charge that these therapies have no basis in reality, that complementary practitioners are working with phantom energies that belong more to spirituality than to physiology. They no doubt feel this way because so many complementary models are unable to explain themselves in the language of science. However, NES is different in this respect, too. We have formulated a comprehensive model of how the quantum body-field regulates the processes of the physical body (which is described in parts 2 and 3). Our findings have applications to many complementary practices, especially traditional Chinese medicine, homeopathy, and acupuncture, providing them with an explanation that is based in physics instead of what amounts to metaphysics.

Just what is this quantum physics we keep talking about? It's time we introduced you to the fundamental tenets of quantum theory. Although space limitations require that we cover only a few key concepts of quantum theory, even this abbreviated, layperson's description of the field will orient you enough to understand how bioenergetics is revolutionizing our understanding of the body and what it means to be healthy.

CLASSICAL AND QUANTUM PHYSICS

Physics can be divided into two main theories. Classical theory is built on Newton's laws and applies to the macroscopic world, our everyday world, and the cosmos at large. Quantum theory concerns itself with the subatomic world and also with how matter behaves at extremely high speeds (i.e., near the speed of light, so the theory also has relevance to cosmology).[7] However, it is more accurate to say quantum *theories,* for there are about a half dozen competing theories that attempt to account for the outright weirdness of the quantum world.

The most widely accepted theory is called the Standard Model of quantum mechanics, with its more than four hundred quantum particles (physicists call this the particle zoo). Essentially, the Standard Model is a quantum theory that explains the fundamental particles and their interactions while also accommodating classical theories, such as Einstein's theories of general relativity and special relativity. As with any theory, it can be thought of as an *interpretation* of a body of experimental data, mathematical knowledge, and theoretical speculations. However, it has a number of problems, as we will describe, so physicists keep searching for better interpretations of the quantum facts. Some of the alternatives include the many worlds theory, which tells us that every possible course of action must be taken. In life, for every decision you make, you include certain possibilities and exclude all others. In the many worlds theory, every possibility is being played out; however, these individual realities split off into parallel worlds, or dimensions, that are inaccessible, so you will never run into the uncountable other yous who are living out the consequences of every possible outcome of every possible choice. Then there is string theory, which sees the world as made up of tiny, vibrating packets of energy called strings. This theory holds that the world is multidimensional, although most of the other six dimensions (there are competing theories about how many dimensions there actually are) other than our three physical dimensions (and that of time) are curled up into spaces so small we cannot access them. String theory rose in stature more than twenty years ago to become the prime alternative to the Standard Model, and it has since been extended into brane theory, which is also called M theory. However, string theory is entirely mathematical, and because accelerators (those atom smashers we talked about earlier) cannot achieve the extremely high speeds, and so cannot achieve the extraordinary high energies, needed to test string theory—and may never be able to test it—its star is fading of late.[8] These are only two of the many theories of quantum physics, but we are going to talk mostly about the Standard Model, which is based on the Copenhagen interpretation and the Heisenberg uncertainty principle.

THE BIZARRE QUANTUM WORLD

The quantum world is the realm of matter smaller than atoms. It is an inanimate, nonliving world governed by rules very different from those that govern the classical macroworld. In fact, in a rather mind-numbing philosophical claim, most physicists would call it a "shadow world" that is entirely abstract and mathematical. They posit that although everything in our world is dependent on the quantum nature of the universe, the quantum world is *not* the real world. This philosophical conundrum, however, doesn't stop quantum mechanics from being at the heart of modern science.

At the infinitesimal quantum scale, nature is downright quirky. For example, every particle has an antiparticle, also called a virtual particle. These ghostly particles pop out of nothingness for tiny fractions of a second by borrowing energy from real particles or from the seething energies of the zero-point field (ZPF), which will be described in more detail later but generally can be thought of as a pervasive field that underlies the material universe and contains the lowest possible state of energy, which is the vibrational energy of particles as they pop in and out of existence. The real world exists only because of the interactions between these virtual and real particles: in a whisper of time nothing becomes something and then goes back to being nothing. Yet we, and our world, continue to exist.

We can never directly observe the things of the quantum realm; we can only discover what goes on there indirectly—and what we find is a world that is so counterintuitive, so rife with paradox, that physicists themselves shake their heads in wonder and disbelief. Niels Bohr, one of the fathers of quantum mechanics, once said that anyone who has not been shocked by quantum physics has not understood it. Other physicists, such as Richard Feynman, have claimed that the facts of quantum theory cannot be understood—they are simply too illogical—so we must accept them at face value. In other words, it makes no sense to ask why nature is this way, it just is.

What is so shocking about the quantum realm? Well, for starters, the very act of measuring a particle, say a photon or an electron, changes it. Thus, we can never know everything there is to know about the state of quantum matter, which is the gist of the Heisenberg uncertainty principle. There are fundamental limits about what we can know about a quantum entity, say a particle, at any one time, which is a very different state of affairs from how science functions in our classical macroworld. If you throw a softball, you can, according to classical rules, know precisely both how fast it is going and where it is at every point in its trajectory. With a quantum softball, however, the more you know about the ball's speed, the less you can know about its location. There are limits in the quantum world to how accurately you can determine multiple parameters of an object at the same time. To use an amusing example, if you were driving a quantum car, when you looked at the speedometer to check your speed, you would suddenly be unable to know precisely where you were!

To reiterate, the Heisenberg uncertainty principle says that by measuring information about one property of a quantum particle or system, you sacrifice accurate knowledge about other properties. However, the problem is not a matter of the quantum system being too complex to understand or of not having tools sophisticated enough to examine the object properly: it is *fundamentally impossible* to know simultaneously everything that is going on with a particle at the quantum level. Our level of accuracy in measuring, and by extension in knowing, has a definite limit because conducting an experiment to find out about this world actually *changes* the world.

One of the reasons the quantum realm is an uncertain world is that particles are not discrete, individual objects. Forget what you were taught in high school physics: atoms are not like little solar systems, with electrons orbiting a nucleus like tiny planets orbiting a sun.[9] Particles are waves, too! This is what the Copenhagen interpretation is all about. Named in honor of Danish physicist Niels Bohr, who first offered it as an explanation for the quirky nature of the quantum world, the Copenhagen interpretation says, basically, that matter has two complementary aspects: matter is both wave and particle *at the same time*. However, you can "see" a quantum entity in only one form or the other—either as a wave or a particle—when you study it. When you are not measuring a subatomic particle, it coalesces back into being *both* wave and particle. Therefore, it makes no logical sense to ask what a quantum entity is when you are not measuring it or otherwise "collapsing" it from the world of probability into the world of actuality.

SHEDDING SOME LIGHT ON QUANTUM WEIRDNESS

This peculiar view of reality started with light. It is a no-brainer that light is a wave. After all, sunlight streams to Earth, a shaft of light breaks apart to its constituent colors in a prism, and a flashlight sends out a beam of light. However, in 1905 Albert Einstein, following in the footsteps of some earlier physicists, posited that light also has a particle nature—it comes in discrete "packets." He was eventually proved to be correct, and another physicist, Max Planck, called these packets of light "quanta," the word from which quantum theory gets its name. Because a packet of light was thought of as a particle, the new particle needed a name—the photon.

What was so alarming about the strange new nature of light was that when you probed it to see what it was like—is light a particle or is it a wave?—the answer you got depended *only* on what kind of experiment you performed. One of the most famous experiments in quantum physics, called the double-slit experiment, proved that light seemed to "know" what researchers were doing! If they were seeking the wave nature of light, light accommodated them and revealed itself as a wave, but if they were trying to find photons, light would reveal itself as a stream of discrete particles. The only interpretation of the experiment that made sense was that light is both a wave and a particle at the same time. Some scientists even coined a new term for this strange state of matter—*wavicles*—but it never caught on. The stunning conclusion scientists reached from various forms of the double-slit experiment is that the fundamental nature of light is unknowable (neither purely wavelike nor purely particle-like) unless it is constrained in some way, such as by how we choose to study it. Quantum entities are said to be in a superposition of states: when they are not being detected in some way, which scientists often refer to as measuring a particle, they occupy all possible states at the same time.

Let's take a moment to visit the double-slit experiment, for it is an experiment that shattered much of the certainty of classical science and first revealed the weirdness of the quantum world. This experiment not only revealed wave-particle duality but also suggested that the observer or the act of measuring affects the state of the quantum world. Modern versions of the original experiment continue to intrigue and even astound scientists because they reveal a bizarre phenomenon called nonlocality (also called entanglement and action at a distance), which we will discuss later in this chapter and elsewhere in this book. What follows is, by necessity, a simplified description of the double-slit experiment.

In the classic double-slit experiment, scientists send a stream of photons (or other type of particle) from a single source through their apparatus, forcing the photons to go through one of two tiny holes or slits along the path, call them slit A and slit B, before arriving at a detector. Let's imagine that for the first experiment the scientists close slit A and leave slit B open. They let loose the stream of photons. As expected, many of the photons will pass through the open slit B to hit a detector. They build up as a scattering of points across a region of the detector, thereby indicating that the photons are discrete particles. Think of shooting a gun at a target set up across a field. There will be a random pattern or, depending on your aim, a cluster of hits as the individual bullets contact the target.

Then the scientists conduct a second experiment, in which they leave both slits open. They fire a stream of photons toward the detector. You might think that some of the photons would go through slit A and some through slit B and that as a result there would be two sets of bulletlike patterns at the detector. You would be wrong! Instead, what happens is that over time the strikes at the detector add up in a strange way, creating alternating dark and light bands. (See figure 2.1.) This banded or fringed pattern is a classic interference pattern, and it is created *only* by waves. The photons are now showing their wave nature. Yet why should they? The only difference in the experiment was that two slits were left open instead of one.

This is where the quantum strangeness takes over. As we said, it is as though the photons know the experimental setup. If one slit is open—meaning that there is only one path the photons can take—then they act like particles, firing through the open slitlike bullets, but if both slits are open, meaning that there is more than one path the photons can take, then they spread out like a wave and take all possible paths. Think of water rushing through a seawall that has been breached in several places. The water will flow through wherever it can. With two slits open, the photons act sort of like water: they go wherever they can, by every possible path. They display their wave nature.

The really strange thing is that even if you leave both slits open but slow down the flow of photons so that you can verify that only one photon at a time goes through a particular slit, you still will get the wave interference pattern. This result makes no (common) sense at all, because you just tracked *individual* photons, like bullets, going through one slit or the other. What this experiment shows is that when presented with more than one path, *a single photon goes through both holes at once*, so the pattern at the detector builds up over time as an interference pattern, which is a wave phenomenon. How can a single photon go through two holes simultaneously? Well, it can't if it is behaving like a particle, but it can if it is spread out and acting like a wave. Somehow the photons "know" the state of the experiment. One hole open, behave like a particle. Two holes open, behave like a wave. The manner in which a quantum entity presents itself to us is determined by how the experiment is conducted, which, philosophically at least, suggests that the subatomic world is somehow connected at a very deep level with living, conscious observers.

One consequence of wave-particle duality is that when you are not looking at a particle, say a photon or an electron, you cannot say it is anywhere in particular. Until you measure it, the photon or electron has an equal probability of being here or there. You have to assume that it is *everywhere* at the same time. An unobserved particle is not a point-like thing but is more cloudlike, smeared out, a fog of possibility that cannot be pinned down until you observe it. The act of measurement or observation is said to collapse the wavefunction, turning one possibility among many into an actuality. ("Wavefunction" is the mathematical expression that describes the quantum entity, determining its position in time.) Hence, probability and statistics entered the world of quantum

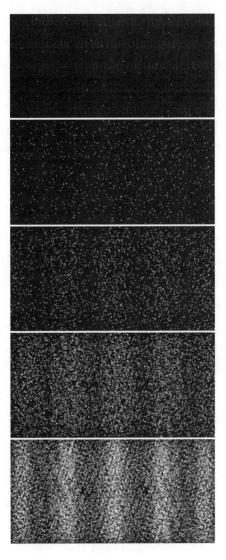

Figure 2.1. In the double-slit experiment, when particles have only one possible path to follow, they hit the detector in a random strike pattern, although clustered in alignment with the slit they went through (first two boxes). This is the classic particle pattern. When particles have more than one path, they take every possible path at once, so the pattern at the detector builds over time to form an interference pattern, which looks like bands of alternating dark and light areas (last three boxes). An interference pattern is created only by waves. The double-slit experiment confirmed what physicists call the wave-particle duality of fundamental quantum entities.

physics, which represented an enormous shift from the certainty that defines measurements in the classical macroworld. (For a more in-depth discussion on waves, including illustrations, see chapter 13.)

No matter where they turned in the quantum world, scientists found equally strange properties of matter. They discovered not only that photons displayed a dual wave-particle nature but also that a host of other particles did, too. In fact, back in the early 1920s, Louis de Broglie, a young Ph.D. student (who, incidentally, was also a prince), argued in his dissertation that there are such things as "matter waves." Basically, he said, *all* matter, not just subatomic particles, has not only a particle nature but a wave nature as well. His was a radical idea, and his dissertation committee thought that perhaps it was too radical to be remotely realistic and so considered rejecting his thesis, but after much deliberation, they finally passed him and awarded him a doctorate in physics. Their good judgment was rewarded in 1927, when experiments proved de Broglie correct. In 1929 he was awarded the Nobel Prize for this theory. The de Broglie matter wave (also called a pilot wave) will play a part in our story later, but for now it is only important for you to realize that at the subatomic level all matter has both wavelike properties and particle-like properties. How quantum entities show themselves depends on our method of observation or measurement.

The wave-particle duality paradox has been minutely examined in many variations of the original double-slit experiment and in many other kinds of experiments over the years, and one interpretation of the results is a theory of quantum physics that says consciousness affects the nature of reality. If something exists only when it is measured, then a logical conclusion, which some physicists have indeed reached, is that *nothing* exists with any certainty unless we observe it, for the conscious human mind is the ultimate measuring instrument. As a consequence, modern quantum physics shape-shifts into metaphysics. For the most part, though, physicists simply prefer not to think about these kinds of philosophical implications.

The double-slit experiment and both its practical and its philosophical implications rattled physicists back in the early days of the young quantum science. Physicist Richard Feynman once claimed that the double-slit experiment is the deepest mystery of quantum science. Over the years, as physicists explored wave-particle duality, the study of quantum physics developed into several distinct disciplines. For example, quantum mechanics is the study of particles and their behaviors, whereas quantum electrodynamics (QED) is the study of the interaction of matter and light, and more generally concerns itself with the wave (or field) aspects of nature. At the level of the quantum realm, QED demonstrates that everything is connected. The world is a vast web of relationships, with everything affecting everything else. Theoretically, because of the wave (or field) nature of the quantum world—and the phenomenon of entanglement, which we will discuss later in this chapter—a particle in my body "knows" what is going on with all the other particles in the universe. Every particle is correlated with or may even causally affect every other particle across the expansive fabric of space-time. Theoretically, at least, ours could be a participatory universe, in which each conscious being affects the expression of the material world.

TROUBLE IN QUANTUMLAND

Despite its mind-stretching implications, the Standard Model of quantum theory grew in stature because it could make precise predictions and experiments kept confirming those predictions to exquisite levels of accuracy. Quantum theory was a huge success, so much so that physicists heralded quantum theory—and QED in particular—as the ultimate answer. They considered it a theory capable of explaining everything. Quite literally, they expected that most of the deepest questions about the universe would be answered by the middle of the twentieth century. Soon they would have a grand unification theory, which would unite all the known forces and particles of nature, and it would be based on the Standard Model.

As we write, at the start of the twenty-first century, those high hopes have been dashed, for scientists in many disciplines have begun grumbling that something is wrong in Quantumland. They are correct, but we have space in this chapter to highlight only a few of those problems.

We can turn to Gordon Kane and his article "The Dawn of Physics Beyond the Standard Model" to review a few of the ten great mysteries of quantum theory as it now stands.[10] One of the biggest problems is that the Standard Model has no place for gravity. A grand unification theory must unite the four fundamental forces of nature: electromagnetic force, weak force, strong force, and gravity. So far, quantum theory has been able to unify all of these forces except for gravity. The more scientists study gravity—and it has been the focus of intense study not only by physicists but also by cosmologists—the more mysterious it appears to be. That is a whole other story, but suffice it to say that the Standard Model's complete lack of success in integrating gravity with the three other fundamental forces is, as Joseph Chilton Pearce once wrote in another context, a huge crack in the cosmic egg!

Another inadequacy that Kane lists is that the Standard Model cannot account for cold, dark matter—a type of matter that scientists believe makes up at least a quarter of the material universe but cannot be directly observed because it does not emit or reflect electromagnetic energy. No known particles in the particle zoo of the Standard Model can account for this matter. Worse, the Standard Model cannot explain fundamental aspects of the big bang theory, the predominant theory of the creation of the universe. The Standard Model's fatal flaw, however, may be that it cannot account for the origin of mass. There are different kinds of mass, such as inertial mass (how resistant something is to a change of its direction or speed, which refers to kinetic energy) and gravitational mass (what we commonly think of as something's weight in a gravitational field). Einstein's famous formula, $E = mc^2$ expresses the equivalence of energy and mass, so physicists often talk about a subatomic particle's mass by referring to its kinetic energy, which they measure in a unit of energy called an electronvolt. To explain the mass of subatomic particles, physicists have proposed a new field, called a Higgs field, which is still only theoretical as it has not been detected. They propose that particles gain mass through their interactions with this Higgs field, but, as Kane says, "the Standard Model cannot explain the very special forms that the Higgs interactions must take" to account for particle mass.[11]

Many physicists now are willing to admit that if the Standard Model is to survive, it must be radically altered. However, even altering the theory may not be enough. As Kane asserts, "In expressing these mysteries, when I say the Standard Model *cannot* explain a given phenomenon, I do not mean that the theory has not yet explained it but might do so one day. The Standard Model is a highly constrained theory, and it cannot *ever* explain the phenomena [listed in his article]."[12]

A growing number of maverick scientists agree with Kane and so are searching for alternatives to the Standard Model of quantum theory. We call these scientists "mavericks" because they truly are going against the status quo. Despite the profound flaws of the Standard Model, it is one of the most experimentally well-verified theories in the history of science. Most scientists choose not to shine a light into the shadowy areas where things are not working so well—or not at all. It's simply better to ignore the problems or to hope that someone, some day, will come up with a fix. Unfortunately for them, most of the fixes are radically overturning what have become almost sacred tenets of the Standard Model.

NONLOCALITY: SPOOKY ACTION AT A DISTANCE

Experiments into one particular area of quantum physics—called quantum entanglement—are yielding surprising results that are overturning long-held beliefs. Entanglement is a curious property of some particles that yokes them together forever. When two particles—or atoms or molecules—are entangled, you no longer can think of them as separate entities, but rather as a holistic system. They become more like a single object, even when the two individual particles are separated by vast distances.

The history of entanglement is immensely fascinating, and if you are interested you can read about it on the Internet and in most physics books. Basically, the theory proposes and experiments have verified that if two particles were ever connected—if they were created together, interacted during the course of their existence, or share certain inherent properties—then they are *forever* entwined. Measuring a property of one particle of the pair means you know something specific about the other particle, even if that second particle is separated from the first by light-years. Entanglement shows how the quantum realm is based on nonlocality, which means basically that local causes can have distant effects, even when there is no possible way a signal or force could travel between two objects fast enough to form a cause-and-effect relationship.

As an example, imagine a pair of particles, A and B. We want to measure a quantum property called spin, which can take one of two states, which for the sake of simplicity we will call spin up and spin down. Each quantum particle is in a superposition of states, so it is both spin up and spin down at the same time, until it is measured and "chooses" one state or the other. (It's true! That's quantum physics for you!) At the moment of measurement, if particle A shows itself as having spin up, then the other particle, particle B, *must* have the opposite spin, down. What's more, particle B must remain correlated to particle A no matter how far apart the two particles are. Say, for instance, that before they measure particle A, scientists send particle B flying off to the outer reaches of the Milky Way. When they measure particle A, they will instantly know the state of particle B (it will have the opposite spin of particle A). What happens to one particle in the pair *instantaneously* affects what happens to the other particle. How can that be? Particle B is at the edge of our galaxy. For information to reach particle B instantaneously, it would have to violate the law that nothing can travel faster than the speed of light.[13]

There actually is no causal explanation for entanglement, and by extension nonlocality, within the domain of the Standard Model, but the phenomenon is real. It has been experimentally verified beyond a doubt. Einstein famously called nonlocality "spooky action at a distance," and for him this phenomenon meant that something was seriously wrong with quantum theory. However, as we have said, the phenomenon is well tested, and by using it scientists have explored the teleportation of entangled quantum particles. However, until only a few years ago, they thought entanglement was a strictly quantum phenomenon, that it could not occur in the macroworld, at the level of atoms, never mind anything larger. Then, in 1998, scientists managed to deal a severe blow to that belief by entangling relatively complex macroscopic particles called fullerenes and other, even larger molecules, as discussed in the following section.

WHERE QUANTUM AND CLASSICAL PHYSICS MEET

Scientists have always assumed that there is some boundary at which the quantum rules give way to the classical rules of our everyday world, and that the Heisenberg uncertainty principle and the Copenhagen interpretation's measurement problem are not applicable in the macroworld. Our normal, everyday world shows itself only via classical physics rules, not quantum ones. An apple, person, or mountain is not a probability that coalesces into matter only when we observe it. During a hike, while you are gazing up at the beauty of the trees around you, you can stub your toe on an unseen rock on the trail. Scientists were sure that somewhere, at some level, there was a clear boundary that separated the quantum world from the classical world. The shift across that hypothetical boundary represents the greatest "phase change" of them all, but until very recently no one had been able to detect where and how it happens.

It turns out there is no well-defined boundary after all. In 2003, Markus Arndt and Anton Zeilinger, of the Institute for Experimental Physics in Austria, were able to show experimentally the wave nature of molecules, such as the biomolecule tetraphenylprophyrin and the massive (by biological standards) fluorinated "buckyball."[14] Science has always told us that the molecules in the macroworld definitely show properties of being particles, so according to the Standard Model they should not display any quantum wavelike properties. But they do. In fact, as of the writing of this book, the fluorinated buckyball holds "the world record for the most massive single particle to display quantum interference."[15] (Interference, remember, is a wave phenomenon.) The result of these experiments is that the crack in the cosmic egg has widened, for these molecules are huge by quantum standards and so should be affected only by the rules of classical physics. Arndt and Zeilinger's experiments are among the first to indicate that there may be no clear-cut division between the quantum and classical worlds.

The cracks in the cosmic egg widen even more if we take this idea farther by suggesting that subatomic particles themselves may be "appearances" and not "real" things at all. In other words, the universe is dominated by waves, not particles. This idea is not new. It goes back to one of the fathers of quantum physics, Erwin Shrödinger, who called particles *Schaumkommen* (most commonly translated as "appearances") and to de Broglie's matter waves. The NES model of the human body-field agrees with a radical theory of quantum physics called space resonance theory, conceived by physicist Milo Wolff, which posits that most particles are indeed only appearances caused by the interaction (interference) of waves, as will be explained in more detail later in this book. Wolff posits that as two waves (of certain types) interact, the very shape of space itself changes, and that what appear to us as different particles really are the different characteristics of space (differing resonances). A theory by physicist John G. Cramer, called the transactional interpretation, also suggests that waves, not particles, may be primary in nature.

Such wave-dependent theories are gaining wider acceptance in the physics community as it becomes clear that they can explain many of the paradoxes and mysteries of the quantum Standard Model, such as wave-particle duality, nonlocality, and entanglement. In fact, a recent experiment by physicist Shahriar Afshar in part verifies the hypotheses of Wolff and Cramer. This experiment has rocked the world of physics, and its results are extremely controversial, as discussed in the following section.

THE END OF PHOTONS?

Afshar carried out a new version of the double-slit experiment, and his results may overturn the original interpretation of that experiment.[16] Remember that the Standard Model interpretation of the double-slit experiment suggests that subatomic "things" exhibit wave-particle duality. Remember also that a subatomic entity such as an electron or photon exists in a superposition of states. In the quantum realm, particles and waves cannot be said to exist in any specific form when we aren't looking at them (measuring and/or observing them). Until they appear in our real world when we collapse the wavefunction, we can't know anything about them with any certainty—not what they are or where they are. Until it is measured, a quantum "thing" is in every possible state at the same time!

Afshar's recent variation on the double-slit experiment may change that interpretation. He contends that he has been able to capture both the particle and wave signatures of a subatomic particle in a *single experiment*. In fact, he believes that the wave aspect of matter takes precedence and that it is the interference of all the waves of the cosmos that results in the appearance of matter (nature's particle aspect). This experiment seems to confirm Schrödinger's intuition that the wave aspect of matter dominates and that particles are illusions that arise out of the behavior of quantum field interactions. The result from Afshar's initial experiment flies in the face of the Standard Model, meaning, as he says, that "something everyone believed for 80 years may be wrong." That "something" to which he is referring is the particle aspect of the photon, for according to Afshar, light may be *only* a wave. He says that if his results hold up, then "we have no other choice but to declare the idea of Einstein's photon dead." The implications of Afshar's experiment, if independently verified, are enormous. As he said, "if the same results are obtained in analogous experiments using particles other than photons then the debate would cover the whole of quantum mechanics."

Wolff and Cramer, as we earlier indicated, are two of the physicists who have been theoretically championing the idea of a wave-dominant reality, although Afshar is among the first physicists who may have demonstrated this premise experimentally. It goes without saying that Afshar's interpretation of the experiment is extremely controversial among mainstream physicists, for it would overturn the established assumptions of the Standard Model. However, even some of the founders of quantum theory would have been on his side. Along with Shrödinger, other physicists, including Einstein, de Broglie, and David Bohm, felt that wave-particle duality and the resulting probabilistic nature of physics showed that the Standard Model was incomplete. They felt there must be underlying laws that would explain away quantum indeterminacy. Today, there are many who join them in the assessment that the Standard Model needs to be radically amended. As Nobel laureate David Gross admitted, at the close of a physics conference in 2005, physicists today are in a "period of utter confusion."[17] However, paradigms die hard, so much so that physicists such as Wolff, Cramer, Afshar, and others usually have a difficult time getting a fair hearing for their theories or acceptance for their experiments.

Anyone paying attention to the state of the field will likely agree that physics is on the cusp of another revolution, one that could change how we think about reality—and ourselves. That revisioning is likely to be every bit as radical as when quantum theory burst onto the scene in the early twentieth century. One of the most important consequences of this upheaval could be a new way of thinking about the body, for it seems only reasonable to assert that if quantum physics underlies everything, and certainly chemistry, then it is also primary in the human body. Thankfully, the paradigm is shifting, and we are finding such evidence, especially in the human body. Bioenergetics and biophysics are growing disciplines that will eventually make inroads into the staid terrain of conventional medicine. As you are reading this book, biologists and others are dusting off mounds of old research and reexamining the work of many researchers from the early part of last century. These researchers were once dismissed as charlatans at worst or as sadly misguided at best, but now open-minded biologists and biophysicists are realizing what many of them really were—visionaries and pioneers. We humbly acknowledge that we stand on their shoulders, and we turn now to a brief overview of some of their evidence for the biophysics—the quantum nature—of the body.

3

THE INTELLIGENCE
OF THE BODY

*Quantum physicists discovered that physical atoms are
made up of vortices of energy that are constantly spinning
and vibrating; each atom is like a wobbly spinning top
that radiates energy. Because each atom has its own
specific energy signature (wobble), assemblies of atoms
(molecules) collectively radiate their own identifying
energy patterns. So every material structure in the
universe, including you and me, radiates a unique energy
signature.*

CELL BIOLOGIST BRUCE H. LIPTON,
THE BIOLOGY OF BELIEF

THE TWENTY-FIRST CENTURY is being called the century of biology,
but it might better be called the century of quantum biology. Within
the past few decades, scientists have found, among many other startling findings, that the body may be holographic in nature, cells in the
human body emit light, immune cells have neuronlike synapses, the
connective tissue of the body forms a sophisticated information network not unlike a second nervous system, muscles may store memories,

and water can be imprinted with information. As they develop ever more sophisticated tools and ask new kinds of questions, researchers are proving that the body is more of a self-organizing, intelligent network of information than ever thought possible. Their progress largely is the result of applying physics to biology.

It goes without saying that the body is one of the most complex of living systems. However, biophysics is not the physics of traditional scientists; it takes a more creative, and ever daring, approach to understanding the nature of living systems. As Koichiro Matsuno and Raymond C. Paton wrote, "Biology is not about applying quantum mechanics as it is already known through the experiences of traditional physics, but rather about an attempt to extend quantum mechanics in the manner that the physicists have not tried."[1]

The study of possible quantum processes in the body is still in its infancy, but one area of intense interest is the electromagnetic processes in the body—light in the body. Scientists once thought that electric energy and magnetic energy were different, but eventually they were found to be two aspects of one force. The varying lengths and frequencies (energy levels) of electromagnetic waves make up the electromagnetic spectrum. The electromagnetic spectrum ranges from radio waves (long wavelengths and low energies) to X-rays and gamma rays (short wavelengths and high energies), with visible light falling at about the midpoint. Of course, modern science has known for decades that the body contains all kinds of energies, including electromagnetic energy. Because the brain produces different kinds of electromagnetic waves (e.g., alpha, beta, delta, theta), doctors can detect brain states using an electroencephalograph (known as an EEG) and determine the electrical state of the heart using the electrocardiograph (known as an ECG).

Magnetics is big business in medicine, especially in imaging. Most readers will be familiar with the MRI (magnetic resonance imaging) machine, which uses magnetics to create an image of tissue by measuring tissue density. It is a static technology. However, the newer fMRI (functional magnetic resonance imaging) is a dynamic technology that images parts of the body, such as the brain, as they are working. For instance, in the brain, fMRI measures blood flow, volume, and oxygenation and so can see how different parts of the brain become active as the person whose brain is being imaged carries out different tasks. An fMRI machine is able to create three-dimensional images of body tissues by exciting the protons in our cells. Protons have magnetic properties, so they can be thought of as tiny biomagnets. They are part of the nuclei of hydrogen atoms, and hydrogen is part of the trillions of water molecules in our bodies. The fMRI machine creates an extremely strong magnetic field (estimated to be about thirty thousand times the strength of Earth's magnetic field) and then fires radio waves at the patient's body, which affect the orientation of the proton biomagnets, causing them to transmit at a particular frequency. The fMRI machine then uses mathematical calculations and other techniques to construct a hologram of the body part that the machine has scanned.

The fMRI machine may, in fact, be medicine's first holographic instrument. Traditionally, a hologram is a three-dimensional image created on a two-dimensional photographic plate.[2] When coherent light (such as laser light) is shined on the plate, the image leaps off the flat surface into three dimensions, seeming to float in midair. You can rotate the image to see it from all directions. (What you are seeing, really, is a record of wave interference patterns and phase.) A hologram doesn't have to be a photographic image. Some maverick scientists posit that our brains and even our entire universe are holograms or display holographic properties.

A hologram has some curious properties. Let's say we make a hologram of an apple. If you cut up that hologram, instead of getting bits and pieces of the apple image, you get many *complete* apple images, only each apple is smaller and a bit less clear than the original. If you rotate your holographic apple, it would look exactly as though you were turning a real apple in your hand. Move the top of the image toward you, and the apple's stem comes into view; move the top away from you far enough and you'll see the bottom of the apple.

It is important to remember that a hologram is really nothing more than a display of the intensity of the light—a record of the photons—given off by an object or scene. Bioluminescence is the light emitted by living organisms; it is the collective light given off by individual "biophotons." Biophotonic and bioelectromagnetic research dominate the study of energies in the body, so that is where we will begin our review of bioenergetics. Before we do, let us take a moment to comment on two aspects of biophysics research that present special challenges to those who study possible quantum processes in the body.

One of the many difficulties in testing biological systems—human or otherwise—for quantum processes is that the studies must be conducted *in vivo,* which means with living, not dead, tissue. This requirement, of course, presents challenges most other scientists, even conventional biologists, do not face. Biologists usually take cells apart to study them. It is reductionist, not integrative, science. Studying dead or ground up cells can teach us a lot, but it cannot tell us much about the coherent quantum processes that emerge only within the matrix of a living system. So biophysicists, because they ideally must study live human beings or live tissue, have huge methodological challenges to surmount as they work to turn their young science into a thriving, mature science.

The second challenge facing frontier scientists is one more of belief than of methodology. Conventional scientists deny that quantum effects can ever be detected in the body (or in anything much larger than atoms) because of a phenomenon called decoherence, which rests on two pillars: size and environment. The rule is that the larger the mass of an object, the smaller the de Broglie matter wave, which represents the wave aspect of matter and, hence, is its quantum signature. Because the de Broglie matter wave is incredibly small in comparison with the mass of a human body, we cannot detect, and so cannot extract, any quantum information from our bodies. In addition, it is claimed that decoherence cannot be detected because all macroscopic objects are in interaction with complex environments, and there is no way to separate coherent quantum information from the "noise" produced by those interactions. In other words, physical things much larger than atoms are too messy—there are too many intricate and complex interactions going on for scientists to be able to sort out only the quantum signals of the object. The only way to do that, according to the Standard Model of quantum physics, is to isolate the object or system from the environment to keep it from any interaction with light, heat, gas molecules, and other things that could collapse the quantum wavefunction. Because we cannot yet do that, conventional scientists tell us that the quantum-classical boundary can never be breached, decoherence rules, and as a result, macroscopic objects are subject only to the laws of classical physics.

Not so fast! Nature often has a way of one-upping science. Recently researchers have observed quantum interference in the macroworld, detecting the nature of large molecules. As previously stated, they have been able to entangle atoms and large molecules, which means they have coaxed individual particles to pair up to work as a team. At the quantum level, entangled photons make lasers possible, and entangled electrons account for superconductivity. Entanglement was thought to be a quantum-only process. However, recent breakthroughs in macroscopic entanglement are breaching the boundary science had thought was impenetrable.[3]

For example, Brian Juldgaard and his team of researchers have entangled cesium gas molecules. Other scientists have entangled sodium ions and even atoms, which are huge by quantum standards. Scientists have even entangled subatomic particles and then teleported the information carried by the particles, a phenomenon that previously had been only a plot device for science fiction novels. That fabled fixed boundary between the microworld and the macroworld is slipping, and it's slipping faster than ever expected. In fact, more and more physicists and biologists, and especially consciousness researchers, are realizing that the reductionist scientific methods and theories of the past cannot ever adequately explain life and the processes of living systems. They are turning to quantum physics for explanations, and they are detecting its fingerprints almost everywhere they look. What they are finding may change the face of quantum physics, because, as Mark Buchanan wrote, although it may seem as though information arises from quantum particles, the reality may be exactly the opposite: "Quantum particles might be catching their behaviour from the information they contain."[4]

More and more evidence is being amassed in favor of the theory that life, at a level more fundamental than that shown through chemistry, is dependent on fields of information: a cell knows how and when to divide, a protein knows how and when to fold itself into an intricate three-dimensional structure, and a muscle knows how and when to react to the intention someone has of moving her leg. Many, many researchers are teasing out the information processes of the body, and they are finding that those information networks are directed by quantum, not classical, rules.

Information and quantum entanglement are, of course, at the heart of consciousness studies as well. Many researchers are positing that entanglement may explain consciousness—and they are able to show it, macroscopically. For example, in his book *Entangled Minds: Extrasensory Experiences in a Quantum Reality,* Dean Radin, laboratory director at the Institute of Noetic Sciences and former researcher into paranormal phenomenon for the US government, describes an experiment in which researchers not only were able to show entanglement of brain states but also were able to capture the physical, biological effect of entanglement.[5] Two subjects were placed in two widely separated rooms that were specially screened to prevent electromagnetic and other kinds of energies from penetrating. Each subject was hooked up to a machine that could pinpoint his brain activity. A light was pulsed into the eyes of one of the subjects, causing a specific part of his brain to become active. At the time of the light pulsation into the first subject's eyes, the brain of the other subject, who was in the other room and so not exposed to any light pulsation, also became active in the same spot, as indicated by the brain scanning technology. This is a nonlocal, and hence quantum, event. The only plausible explanation is that the brain waves of the two subjects somehow became entangled at the quantum level. What is truly astounding in this experiment and others like it is that there was *a nearly instantaneous transfer of information that caused very real effects in the macroscopic world.* The mechanism for this transfer appears to be a quantum field of *consciousness* that, because of some form of entanglement (a form not currently understood within the parameters of the Standard Model of quantum mechanics), can transmit information about the state of one subject's brain to the brain of another subject instantaneously. The fact that the effect was nearly instantaneous across space and penetrated an electromagnetically screened room means that no electromagnetic energy signal could have been the cause. The change, then, must have been mediated through an *information field,* which is not constrained by relativity theory.

Such experiments mystify even frontier scientists, for they suggest that at some deep, fundamental level we are all connected. The most plausible mechanism for such a web of relationships is the field effect— that fields of information permeate the universe and everything is part of this intricate web of relationships, linking us in ways we have only begun to imagine, never mind explore. In terms of decoherence, such experiments suggest that a fixed boundary between the quantum and the nonquantum worlds is an illusion. Everything in the universe is entangled with everything else, so everything, at some primordial level, affects or correlates with everything else.

A few conventional biologists are beginning to see that isolating the study of life from its environment creates a false dichotomy. They suggest that the way to broach the presumed barrier between the microworld and the macroworld is to learn to measure the particle/mass/object system *and* the environment in which it is entangled. For example, mathematician Chris Clarke reasoned, "Decoherence is the loss of quantum information to the environment; but the universe as a whole *has no environment.* Cosmologically, information is never lost. . . . This suggests . . . that the universe remains coherent;

it was, is and always will be a pure quantum system. The non-coherence of medium scale physics . . . is only an approximate consequence of our worm's-eye view."[6]

Radin and his colleagues in consciousness and paranormal research may be accomplishing what Clarke is suggesting is possible—measuring the object of study in interaction with the environment. It also may be what NES has accomplished in measuring the human body-field. Conventional science tends to isolate objects for study. However, a NES assessment is not a measure of the *isolated* body-field but instead is a measure of the functional integrity of the body-field *in relation to the environment,* both inner and outer. That is, it is a measure of the state of the body-field in relation to everything from the external environment (electromagnetic waves, gravity, exposure to pollutants and toxins, and so on) and from the person's internal state (his or her emotions, diet, cellular metabolism, and the like). You might say it is a measure of the state of the body-field's *feedback loops.* Biologists will tell you that nothing living exists in isolation. Even single-cell organisms need to receive input, such as food, from the environment. The physics of life is the physics of loops of information that provide feedback between the organism and the environment, so that the organism can constantly adjust itself and maintain homeostasis. Biologists even have names for the formal studies of the feedback loops between cells and living organisms and their environments—systems biology and epigenetics (which means "control above genetics").

Cell biologist and former Princeton University professor Bruce Lipton, in his book *The Biology of Belief,* wrote about his own scientific and personal epiphany of how information (in the form of feedback between cells and their environments) constitutes intelligence in the body. He said, as he was trying to keep isolated cell cultures alive for study, "Twenty years after my mentor Irv Konigsberg's advice to first consider the environment when your cells are ailing, I finally got it. DNA does not control biology, and the nucleus of the cell itself is not the brain of the cell. Just like you and me, cells are shaped by where they live. In other words, it's the environment, stupid."[7]

Although much more research needs to be done to prove the following conjecture, NES may be the first biotechnology that can measure the state of a person's health by taking into account the *entanglement* of the environment with the body (via the body-field). A NES–Professional System scan may be measuring whether the information that cells are receiving from the external and internal environments is getting through to them properly, in a state that is coherent and undistorted. A series of NES scans over time may be peeling back the layers of the holographic body-field, the information fields that record everything that has happened to the person over time and the effects of everything to which he or she has been exposed, and accessing the information stored in each layer.

The scientific paradigm is shifting, and bioenergetics and biophysics are blossoming disciplines that could eventually make inroads into the staid terrain of conventional medicine. In fact, we at NES are so bold as to suggest that living, organic systems will turn out to be something like a "third realm" of nature. Classical physics and quantum physics currently are seen as the two primary, but separate, realms of nature. This third realm likely will reveal itself as a fusion or integration of the two. The next great revolution is happening now—and it is about the *integrative* properties of life. The revolution depends on our continuing to discover new methods, both intellectual and technological, for exploring living, breathing human beings (and other organisms) and the special properties that define life. As we do, a new medicine will emerge—a view of health that integrates both our physical and energetic aspects. Let's look now at some of the evidence for this new view of the body.

BIOPHOTONS

German biophysicist Fritz-Albert Popp is widely considered the father of modern bioelectromagnetic research, having coined the term *bio-*

photon in the 1970s.[8] He is a man fascinated by light, especially how light interacts with the body, and his research is largely responsible for spurring scientists from around the world to unlock the secrets of how the body produces and uses ultraweak light and other electromagnetic waves.

Among Popp's early major discoveries was that carcinogenic compounds use light differently than do noncarcinogenic compounds. Many chemicals absorb light and then can be made to re-emit that light. What Popp found was that carcinogenic compounds somehow changed the light signal used by cells, jumbling it before the cells re-emitted it. What's more, to his and others' amazement, Popp found that carcinogens particularly liked to scramble light at a frequency of 380 nanometers. He came to believe that this was a special wavelength in regard to the body, and he soon made a connection to the photo-repair mechanisms by which cells repair the damage done to them by ultraviolet rays from the sun and other sources. Photo-repair is a well verified but little understood process, and Popp made the daring intellectual leap of positing that to conduct photo-repair, cells must themselves be emitting light. As he probed farther, he was shocked to discover that there is one wavelength at which the cellular photo-repair process works most efficiently. You guessed it—at 380 nanometers! Perhaps, he reasoned, compounds that cause cancer do so because they block the precise wavelength of light that the cells need to repair ultraviolet damage.

To further explore light in the body, Popp needed new technology that could detect such light at ultraweak intensities. Bernhard Ruth, one of his graduate students, rose to the challenge, and soon he and Popp were using the new technology to explore whether living cells emit light. They started with cucumber seeds, and they indeed found light, but, they reasoned, perhaps the light was a by-product of photosynthesis. So they grew cucumber seeds in the dark and tested them under conditions that would guarantee that photosynthesis would have no effect. They still found light. What's more, they found *coherent* light.

As previously explained, it is thought that quantum processes give way to classical ones in the hot, wet environment of the body because heat and chaotic influences from the environment lead to decoherence of the quantum signals. That Popp found *coherent* light in the body amounted to an overturning of some of the most deeply entrenched beliefs in physics and biology. What's so special about coherent light? Well, it means that individual photons somehow become connected and cooperative, working together to transmit information about the state of the system. Think of an unruly crowd of fans at a football game suddenly focusing their attention and rising together in groups to do the wave cheer. That's coherence at work. The individuals are still individuals, but for a certain amount of time they come together, acting as one, in a purposeful behavior that has meaning. No one believed quantum particles in the body could cooperate like that. After further research, Popp came to believe that the source of the coherent light in the body is DNA. He believes that DNA uses light signals to coordinate the hundreds of thousands of chemical processes that occur every second in every cell of the body.

Popp eventually tested his theory on both healthy and ill people. What he found was intriguing. The cells of healthy people emitted coherent light, but in ill people, the emitted light was scrambled or their cells emitted either too much or too little coherent light. Journalist Lynne McTaggart, in recounting the results of those early tests, wrote:

> In every instance, the cancer patients had lost these natural periodic rhythms and also their coherence. The lines of internal communication were scrambled. They had lost their connection with the world. In effect, their light was going out.
>
> Just the opposite occurred with multiple sclerosis. MS was a state of too much order. Individuals with this disease were taking in too much light, and this was inhibiting the ability of cells to do their job. . . . MS patients were drowning in light.[9]

The results of Popp's experiments have not yet led to any viable therapies, but they pointed researchers in directions they had never thought to go. Indeed, many researchers around the world followed Popp's lead, studying bioluminescence in the body and the role of biophotons in health and disease. As one example, a team led by Korean scientists confirmed what other researchers in Germany, Japan, Russia, Poland, Italy, China, and the United States have found—that the body does indeed emit ultraweak coherent light. In their article "Biophoton Emission from the Hands," the Korean-led team reported that they detected 34 percent more biophotons (in the range of 300–650 nanometers) coming from the hands of their twenty healthy volunteers than could be expected if the photons were simply a result of natural background emissions. They also confirmed that the biophotons were not created as a consequence of thermal radiation or body heat.[10]

THE CELL

In chapter 1, we briefly mentioned Gilbert Ling's revamping of cell membrane theory.[11] He and many other molecular and cell biologists do not believe that the sodium-potassium, membrane-pump theory of the cell can be correct. Their reasons include that cells do not have enough energy to keep the pumps working and that the cell membrane sac by itself does not allow sodium ions to pass through it, as the pump-channel theory predicts. Whereas conventional biologists identify the cell nucleus, which contains DNA, as the command center of the cell, Ling raises the cell protoplasm to primary status in cell functioning. This protoplasm, a kind of internal cellular matrix, has been the focus of intense study by frontier scientists, for it appears that the most vital functioning of the cell takes place here. In fact, the cellular protoplasm matrix may be more important than the DNA that is curled up in the nucleus of every cell. However, Ling is not the only scientist overturning established wisdom about cell functioning.

Lipton sees the cell membrane as primary and, like Ling, views the cell nucleus, and DNA, as less important. He has recounted experiments with enucleated cells, which are cells from which the nucleus has been removed. DNA is supposed to program everything vital to the life of a cell, to be the cell's "brain." However, cells in which the nucleus, and hence the DNA, had been removed survived, and functioned, for more than two months! Lipton wrote, "Viable enucleated cells do not lie about like brain-dead lumps of cytoplasm on life-support systems. These cells actively ingest and metabolize food, maintain coordinated operation of their physiologic systems (respiration, digestion, excretion, motility, etc.), retain an ability to communicate with other cells, and are able to engage in appropriate responses to growth and protection-requiring environmental stimuli."[12]

Although these enucleated cells cannot divide or reproduce parts of proteins they need for long-term survival, Lipton's experiments demonstrate, nonetheless, that the nucleus is not the control center of the cell. The enucleated cells can function normally, they just can't reproduce, which leads Lipton to suggest that biologists who believe a cell's intelligence is in the nucleus are confusing a cell's gonads for its brain! Instead, he believes the cell membrane is the primary information control-and-command center. The cell membrane receives signals from the outside world, interprets those signals in relation to its condition and that of all the other cells of the body, and then transmits the appropriate information into the interior of the cell. Those environmental signals, for instance, can cause cells to spur protein shape changes, and the changes in turn pass information on to the DNA in the cell nucleus. Lipton wrote, "Studies of protein synthesis reveal that epigenetic [above the level of genes] 'dials' can create 2000 or more variations of [regulatory] proteins from the same gene blueprint."[13]

The blueprint of life, then, may not be DNA, but rather our cells' ability (intelligence) to communicate with the environment. Cells are not isolated bags of fluid that are containers for life's engine (DNA) but rather are the receiver-antenna systems—the broadcast stations—

for sending instructions to DNA by monitoring environments both internal to the body and external to it. These feedback loops then coordinate life's essential functions.

Other researchers are conducting experiments that are confirming that the cell's primacy as a communication center for the body is at least partly dependent on its ability to serve as the receiver of environmental input. W. R. Adey, a researcher of bio-electromagnetism, reviewed what he called the "growing scientific consensus" among cell and molecular biologists that cells are sensitive to external fields, such as environmental electromagnetic fields, and that these fields impart information that cells use at the atomic level to coordinate physiological activity.[14] Physicist Herbert Fröhlich, whose work we will discuss in more detail later in this chapter, found that cells oscillate, or vibrate, in a collective way that allows a kind of cooperative information network, or field, to be set up in the body. (These oscillations have come to be known as Fröhlich oscillations.) Information can travel almost instantaneously to every nook and cranny of the body via such a field. Fröhlich also postulates that the collection of cells that makes up the living matrix of the body form a crystalline array by which the body becomes extremely sensitive to environmental signals. We could cite many, many other studies that show how the boundaries between the cell's interior (and our genetic material) and the external environment are less rigid than conventional biologists would have us believe. However, we trust that our point has been made: cells may be thought of as having a kind of intelligence, actively cooperating in vast communication networks within the body and between the body and its environment.

THE CONNECTIVE TISSUE MATRIX

The body is abuzz with signals and messages that keep the complex machinery of its biology functioning. We tend to think of the brain as the generator of the body's intelligence, but information is being sent and received continuously to and by the nervous and muscular systems, the network of connective tissue, the circulatory and immune systems, and many other biological structures and systems. Recent studies have revealed that this communication is coordinated not only by the brain but also by the connective tissue that forms a far-reaching network in the body.

Bioenergetics research is showing that many types of biological molecules are configured in a crystalline lattice that allows the molecules to be packed together tightly, so that signals are able to race through the lattice network of molecules at nearly instantaneous speeds. The connective tissue in the body, in particular, appears to be an efficient transmitter of information. This matrix is composed of several different kinds of tissues, generally called fascial tissue, that run through the body at varying depths. The Langer's lines, or tension lines, are a network of superficial fascia that lies just under the skin, and the perineural system is a web of connective tissue that spreads throughout the body around nerves, allowing neural waves from the brain to propagate through the entire body. The digestive and lymphatic systems are formed from a type of connective tissue called collagen, and the muscular system is made of still another kind of connective tissue, myofascia. As Oschman wrote in *Energy Medicine in Therapeutics and Human Performance*:

> All movements, of the body as a whole and of its smallest parts, are created by tensions carried through the connective tissue fabric. It is a liquid crystal material and its components are semiconductors. . . . One of the semiconductor properties of connective tissue is *piezo-electricity*, from the Greek, meaning "pressure electricity." Because of piezoelectricity, every movement of the body, every pressure and every tension anywhere, generates a variety of oscillating bioelectrical signals or microcurrents and other kinds of signals. . . .[15]

Because cells are surrounded by and embedded in connective tissue, they can communicate via this piezoelectrical network, turning the body into one vast electromagnetic signaling system so that every cell knows what every other cell is doing.

Other studies show that connective tissue—as a major information network—may be crucial to many of the body's other critical functions. It may mediate the body's emotional state (because memory, especially traumatic memory, may be stored in muscles and other tissues), its ability to deal with toxins, and the capacity of cells to efficiently process energy (in the form of ATP). The connective tissue matrix may be the most unexplored territory of the body when it comes to information processing, and discovering its riches is bound to drastically change the way we think of health and treat illness.

MICROTUBULES

Cells themselves contain their own type of connective tissue—the cytoskeleton. Among other structures, a cell's cytoskeleton contains microtubules—miniscule hollow tubes—that have become a focus of study in biophysics because quantum processes in the microtubules of the brain may explain the mechanisms of memory and even account for consciousness itself. In fact, one of the most promising theories for explaining consciousness comes from biophysics researchers who postulate that consciousness is holographic. Whereas conventional brain researchers describe consciousness as arising from the electrochemical processes that occur across synapses and being dependent on neurons, biophysics researchers postulate that microtubules may actually be the structures from which consciousness, in whole or in part, arises, for within them occurs the strange process of quantum tunneling.[16] This is a well-verified process in physics in which particles, such as electrons, can travel from one place (inside the microtubules) to another (outside the microtubules) without having to travel the distance in between! In other words, quantum particles can go through walls without actually going through the walls. They just appear on the other side. Scientists speculate that the quantum nature of this process allows information to be distributed in the body almost instantaneously.

Other researchers suggest that memory is found not just in the brain but is distributed throughout the body, with the implication that the microtubules in the cytoskeleton of cells play a crucial role in body-memory storage and distribution. As you will see later in this book, the NES model of health recognizes that microtubules, and cavities of all shapes and sizes, are vital to the health of the body, for one of their most important functions appears to be as collectors of zero-point energy, which is vital to the constitution of the body and its well-being.

THE PERINEURAL SYSTEM

Dr. Robert O. Becker is a pioneer in the study of the effects of electromagnetic waves on health.[17] The area of his research that most intrigues us in this chapter is his insight into the workings of the perineural system, that web of connective tissue that surrounds nerves and that can be thought of as a separate nervous system. The central nervous system, which is brain-dependent, is known for its speed. When you are in danger, you can't think, you have to react. The sympathetic division of your autonomic nervous system provides the rush of energy that helps you respond quickly when you are threatened.

However, for most of the day-to-day physiological functions that keep you alive, precision is preferable to speed. Your cells, tissues, and organs have to perform work that is exacting, such as producing a specific hormone in just the right amount and at just the right time. When they don't, illness, especially chronic illnesses, can result. The brain-based system is more skilled in getting messages where they need to go quickly rather than getting every detail of the message correct. Becker describes the perineural system as the perfect system to transmit this kind of precise information because it transfers information via very slow waves. He views the perineural system as an analog system, whereas the brain-based nervous system is a fast-pulse, digital system.

Peter's research supports and confirms aspects of Becker's work. In part 2 of this book, we describe how NES grew out of Peter's initial search for a deeper understanding of the acupuncture meridians. These medians are thought to be energy channels in the body, but what kind of energy runs through them and how that energy affects the body is largely unexplained. In traditional Chinese medicine there is a belief that a life-force energy, called qi, flows through these meridian channels, many of which lie just under the skin. Deeper inner channels branch from the main channels, but these inner meridians do not have acupuncture points at the skin level as do the surface meridians. Qi must flow properly through the meridians to all parts of the body for a person to be healthy and emotionally balanced.

Many Chinese and other texts suggest that the meridians are in fact linked intimately (from an informational perspective) with the skin, which is, after all, the largest organ of the body. It is widely believed that acupuncture needles, which are inserted through the skin, may be stimulating energy channels that travel through the body. These channels appear to be connected to the Langer's lines, the superficial connective tissue that lies just beneath the skin, but Peter did not find that this was case. In his experiments, he found that the meridians, especially the liver meridian, are linked tightly to the deeper layers of connective tissue and barely "talk" to the skin or upper layers at all. It is likely that the NES Integrators, as Peter came to call the information "route maps" of the body, are connected not to the Langer's lines but rather to the perineural system. This surprising result tallies with the work of Becker and other scientists who view the connective tissue as an information network that is critical to the proper functioning of the body and the maintenance of health. These findings also corroborate the theories of Ida Rolf, the developer of the deep-tissue therapy, Rolfing, that is named after her, and the developers of the various forms of myofascial release therapy, who believe that the condition of a person's deep-layer connective tissue reflects the state of their overall health.

THE IMMUNE SYSTEM

That the matrix of connective tissue carries information as a kind of second brain—or another type of nervous system—in the body is not the stuff of science fiction. Also, more than the connective tissue network may be involved in forming this information highway. One recent study, reported in *Scientific American* in 2006, shows that synapses, which until now have been found only in the neural network of the brain, have been discovered in the immune system. Researchers have found immune cells that grow structured but adaptable connections that look like and appear to work like the synapses in the brain.[18] They speculate that these immune cells may "form an information-sharing network to fight disease."

Although their findings are controversial, these immunologists posit that the functions of these immune system synapses "could include initiating communication, or terminating it, or serving to modulate the volume, so to speak, of signals between two cells." They also have discovered that viruses may be able to exploit these immune cell synapses. One research team mentioned in the article reported seeing "'viral synapse' phenomena, and so it seems that viruses, which are known for hijacking cellular machinery to copy their genetic material, may also be able to co-opt cellular mechanisms for communication to propel themselves from one cell to another."

COHERENT FIELDS

The history of vibrational medicine is too long and complex to properly review in this chapter, but several aspects of this discipline are crucial to our investigation of the bioenergetic and quantum processes in the body. Resonance in particular is turning out to be an important method of intercellular communication. The term *resonance* refers to shared frequencies within a system. It takes two forms: destructive or constructive. A classic example of the destructive force of resonance is a platoon of soldiers marching across a bridge. Because they are marching in step, their boots strike the bridge at the same time, which sets up a shared frequency, or resonance. The combined vibrations cause a ramping up of energy. As the resonance from the soldiers' footfalls travels through the structure of the bridge, the bridge begins to vibrate at the same energy level as the footfalls, and the resonance between the two can actually cause the structural integrity of the bridge to give way, causing a collapse. In a more familiar example, the resonance set up between a singer and a crystal wine goblet can cause the goblet to shatter.

Resonance also can be constructive, as when it takes the form of coupled oscillators, which form coherent fields. Individual systems, which each might be chaotic on their own, can take on new qualities or characteristics as the individual elements coalesce into an ordered whole. Visible light is a stream of freewheeling photons, but focus that stream of light, making it supercoherent, and you have a laser. In the body, coherent resonant fields may enable individual molecules, cells, and even organ systems to share information.

Albert Szent-Györgyi, a Nobel prize–winning biochemist who made major discoveries in the 1940s about how certain cell molecules (specifically mysoin) control muscle functioning, is considered by many to be among the leading figures in the history of bioenergetics.[19] Many of his speculations about how the body works have been verified by a later generation of biophysics researchers. One of Szent-Györgyi's ideas was that energy transfer in the body is mediated by coupled oscillators, which are two separate things that link up, often through resonance, to work together as a single system. Think of two pendulums connected by a rod. Set one of the pendulums swinging and through resonance it will cause the other pendulum to begin to swing as well. What's more, the two pendulums will become synchronized, with their motion perfectly matched. That motion is transferred through resonance, making a coupled harmonic oscillator. Szent-Györgyi surmised that cells in the body might work according to a similar process.

Research has since shown that amino acids, proteins, and many types of molecules act as coupled oscillators in the body if they are close enough together. Information travels through the network via resonance that is caused by the movements of the body and of the molecules within the body. These motions can even create electromagnetic fields that, because they are networked together like a giant web, send energy and information to every part of the body. Confirmation of this theory has come from many fronts, but a representative study is one that was carried out in 1991 by K. J. Pienta and D. S. Coffey.[20] They suggest that the cytoskeleton of cells may act as coupled harmonic oscillators, allowing information from the outside of cells to be sent deep into the interior of cells, and even into DNA itself. Their work supports the work of Ling and Lipton, who both propose that the cell membrane (or protoplasm), not DNA, is the command-and-control center of cells.

Herbert Fröhlich also was a major contributor to unlocking the secrets of biological information processing.[21] Among his most intriguing ideas is that of quantum coherence in the body. Whereas Popp found *coherent light* being emitted by living organisms, Fröhlich postulated that, based on the principles of quantum physics, biological systems must produce *coherent vibrations* (in the form of oscillations), and because they are coherent, these oscillations may have laserlike properties.

Fröhlich's intellectual curiosity was legendary, and he made important contributions in areas as diverse as solid-state physics and biology. His work generally is highly technical, but his creative ideas stimulated biophysical research on many fronts. Among his many fascinations in biology was the electrical properties of cells. In proportion to their size, cells set up huge electrical fields across their membranes, with a negative polarity inside the cell and a positive one outside the cell. Connective tissues, made up of collagen arrays, also set up electrical fields that, in part, are generated by movements—the contractions and extensions of muscles and tendons for example. Nerves and glands also produce electrical fields as they conduct signals and secrete fluids, respectively. Everywhere within the body there are electrical fields interacting. In addition, the trillions of molecules in the body, because they, like all matter, are made of subatomic particles, are themselves in motion, producing tiny vibrations that together add up to create enormous energy potentials and oscillating fields. Fröhlich thought that these myriad individual fields must also act collectively, in a cooperative and coherent manner, and he understood that because of their very coherence they must be exquisitely sensitive to the external fields of nature.

Fröhlich's theories about coherent vibrations and oscillating fields spurred many other researchers to seek out quantum processes in the body. His and their work has led to the first inkling of understanding of how coherent fields communicate information to the body to influence a host of physiological functions, from the growth of organisms to the vigor of the immune system.

———◆———

In this brief overview, we have selected a sampling of the kinds of work being done by scientists that suggest there is a deep and pervasive energetic reality to the body and that biology works with quantum processes and not only according to classical rules. There are dozens of other exciting new areas of inquiry that are pushing the boundaries of what we know about the body, one of the most exciting being neurocardiology. In this new discipline, researchers are finding that the heart is not just a pump but also a sensory organ! It contains neural cells, can direct the brain and other body processes (including regulating hormones), and appears to be a center of emotion and memory.[22] All of these areas of research are increasing our understanding of the most fundamental processes of biology and have direct implications in our understanding of illness and health. The body's emission of ultraweak coherent light can indicate the presence of disease before it may even be evident to us. Electromagnetic fields can act as carriers of information. Molecules and cells can "talk" via coupled oscillating fields. With only these few examples as our guides, we can make theoretical inroads to a new kind of health care, a system that seeks to understand quantum biological processes, measure them, and create new ways to address the body at the quantum level.

Now, enough background and context. We trust that you have gained a sufficient understanding of the issues and controversies swirling through the disciplines of biology, physics, and bioenergetics to be able to appreciate the information we will present in the rest of this book. We will show not only how NES is pushing the boundaries of bioenergetics but also how we are staking out entirely new territory.

When we began our individual journeys, we had no idea we would be pioneering a new kind of health care. Our goals were humble—to find help for our own chronic illnesses. However, not unlike the scientists we have discussed in this first part of the book, because we were not afraid to explore ideas that others warned us would be fruitless, or even mad, we were able to advance, bit by bit, toward a new vision of how the body works. So we move now to part 2, in which we recount our personal journeys from illness to health and the subsequent unfolding of our collaborative vision, which led to the development of Nutri-Energetics Systems.

PART TWO

---◆---

The Birth of
Nutri-Energetics Systems

4

Descent into Illness

HARRY MASSEY WAS ILL, and getting sicker by the month. Over four years, his health had deteriorated steadily, until he was nearly bedridden. The likely cause: chronic fatigue syndrome (CFS). This is an uncertain diagnosis, not a clear-cut disease but more an identifiable constellation of symptoms with no known cause. It was designated a specific medical condition only in the early 1990s. Although the actual symptoms vary from patient to patient, a CFS diagnosis usually results when a patient has suffered with several of the following symptoms and there is no other cause to account for them: unrelenting fatigue for at least six consecutive months, short-term memory problems, aching joints and muscles, tender lymph nodes, chronic sleeplessness, headaches, generally impaired thinking, and more. There are several hypotheses about what causes CFS. Some researchers feel that CFS is the result of a cascade of things gone wrong in the body and will never be pinned down to one identifiable cause. Other research points toward specific breakdowns, such as a cortisol insufficiency in the central nervous system, a general immune system dysfunction, or side effects of multiple infectious agents in the body. Because there is no identifiable cause, there is no cure, and, perhaps worse, there is no effective, long-term treatment.

For CFS patients, the syndrome can be devastating. For months they can feel relatively well and function fairly normally, and then the crushing fatigue hits like a storm, forming a black cloud over their lives and usually driving them into bed. For the most part, however, the decline is slow, worsening over months or years until many CFS patients are unable to carry on with their normal activities. The other symptoms can come and go as well, but they, too, generally worsen over time. All that most CFS patients can do is hope for the best, but prepare for the worst.

Harry's illness began innocently enough. It was 1994, and he had decided to leave his native England for a "gap year" in Australia to teach teenagers sailing and kayaking. An enthusiastic and skilled athlete, he looked forward to an enjoyable respite before buckling down and meeting the demands of university life. While in Australia, Harry spent his free time exploring the country, and during one of his travels he developed a serious fever. He felt feverish for two weeks, and although he recovered, he never fully regained his strength. Two months later, his lips began to swell and he developed chest pains. His breathing became labored. Every breath was sharp and painful, as though he were inhaling shards of glass. He finally checked into a hospital in Cairns, but the doctors could find nothing medically to account for his symptoms. They assumed that he had developed allergies as a result of whatever had caused his previous fever.

When he returned to England later that year to begin studying at the university, Harry felt fairly well. He resumed doing the things he loved: hiking, sailing, and especially rock climbing. He was fine as long as he did not overexert himself. He knew immediately when he had, for the labored breathing and chest pains would return and then a general malaise overtook him from which it took longer and longer to recover. Still, Harry was not one to hold back. He used willpower to overcome the pain and fatigue. It was either 100 percent or nothing! His climbing and paragliding styles spoke volumes about his stamina and fearlessness. Although he is a skilled climber, and one not given to recklessness, the sport is not without its dangers. During one ice climb up Ben Nevis, a piton came loose and Harry fell thirty feet. Despite being shaken and in pain, he continued the climb. It was not until five years later, during an X-ray examination, that he discovered he had fractured his back, probably during that fall. Another time, while paragliding, his wing partially collapsed and he was in free fall over the rugged English coast. A classic English castle was perched halfway up the cliff, and Harry was headed straight for it. Fighting for control while free-falling almost 500 feet, he maneuvered the lines until he finally managed to partially reinflate the wing. He was within feet of the castle's stone walls and the cliff before he managed to swing himself wide and land safely. Although shaken, he knew he had to launch again immediately, for if he didn't he might never paraglide again.

So Harry carried on, pushing himself, going full out, using willpower to maintain his rigorous academic and recreational pursuits. It was not until his final year of university that his serious health problems began. Overwork and too much hard exercise had taken their toll, and Harry was continually suffering from colds and other viral infections. His chest was in a constant squeeze and his breathing labored. His lymph glands were in a perpetual state of swelling. Even his thinking seemed to be getting foggier and foggier.

He had managed to finish school, but looking back, Harry describes the next several years as an "encompassing black cloud, a dreamland that I hoped one day I would get out of. As I got more and more ill, I clung to the thought that my life had been good before this illness and it would one day be good again."

Although Harry soldiered on, even taking a summer climbing trip in the Alps, he could no longer deny that he was getting sicker. After each climb, it would take longer and longer to recover his strength. At one point, after climbing Dent du Géant, a 13,000-foot peak in the French Alps, it was all he could do to drag himself to his tent. He did not have the energy to break camp, load his car, and drive home. He ended up staying in his tent for a week, almost all of that time spent lying in his sleeping bag. He survived on the food he had with him: bread, tuna, and dried fruit. When he finally summoned the strength to head home, he had to take breaks from driving every thirty minutes to rest.

The time had come to get serious about seeking medical care. Over the next several years, Harry made the rounds of physicians and specialists, but he was never given a definitive diagnosis, and none of the treatments or pharmaceuticals he was given helped for very long. At one point, his doctors thought he might have pancreatic cancer, but, thankfully, he didn't. No one seemed to know how to help him, and the continual cycle of hope and disappointment was among the greatest frustrations of this period.

Despite the medical ups and downs, Harry refused to allow the mysterious illness to derail his life. He applied to and was accepted into the master's of business degree program at a British university, but only one week into the program, he knew he did not have the strength or clarity of thought to continue. Instead of quitting, he received approval to split the one-year course over two years. Most days he could not get out of bed to attend lectures, so friends would take notes for him. With their help, he managed to make it through his first year. He says now, "Looking back, I should never have done that. I should have concentrated on getting well, instead of pushing myself harder." He could no longer deny that not only was he ill but he also was *seriously* ill. For all intents and purposes, his world had shrunk to the size of his apartment. He decided he needed to put as much attention into getting well as he had put into his schoolwork and sports in the past.

So Harry took stock, and what he found startled him. He was much worse off than he had allowed himself to believe. Going through his medical records, he discovered that he had had one of the lowest magnesium blood counts ever recorded in England. He suffered from unrelenting chest pain, gallbladder tenderness, and swollen glands. His memory had deteriorated, and it took enormous effort to apply himself to any focused mental exercise. He was horrified to realize that for the past year he had been unable on most days to walk more than 100 yards before collapsing in exhaustion. He was essentially bedridden, and he was not prepared to live like that any longer.

Having received little relief from conventional medicine, Harry turned to alternative measures. He knew next to nothing about them, so he applied every ounce of spare energy he had to educating himself and evaluating his options. Lying in bed, he read dozens of books about everything from fasting to homeopathy to macrobiotics. It was confusing trying to sort out all the competing claims about what causes the loss of health and what can best restore it. He says, "Different groups gave different solutions to my health problems. I read about everything: nutrition, raw food, juicing, kombucha tea, herbal medicine, yoga, Hulda Clark and Max Gerson and other alternative healers, ozone therapy, chelation, hypnotism, psychotherapy, the I Ching, and countless other therapies and schools of thought. For the most part, each group presented persuasive arguments to support their point of view. The raw foods people said that because we evolved from apes we should be eating only raw vegetables and fruits. The blood-type people said that your diet should be designed to work with and support the characteristics of your blood group. Dr. Max Gerson claimed you have to load your body with vitamins from organic fruits and vegetables and detoxify your body with enemas. Acupuncturists declared that your governor meridian had excess yin. Psychologists thought you are refusing to let go of your past. None of them gives you a clear explanation of what is going on, and, anyway, how could they all be right? But there had to be a system. I was sure that there was some way to know what was really going on in my body and that there was something I could do to help my body fix itself. If such a system existed, I was determined to find it."

Harry gave the most promising therapies a fair trial. He already had changed his diet, eating only raw foods, but he now tried Gerson's vitamin and mineral therapy and used homeopathy for seven months. Each seemed to help a bit, but none restored his health. Of all the systems he had read about, the one that made the most sense to him was detoxification. His descent into illness had started in Australia with a fever; obviously something foreign had entered his body. That something had initiated the process of losing his health, and maybe by removing it the process could be reversed. So, before the start of the second year of his master's program, Harry traveled to a South African clinic to undertake a cleansing fast and detoxifying enema regime. A friend of his who had suffered from CFS had claimed to be cured by following the program.

The program did seem to work, at least in cleansing Harry's body. Over the month he was there, his body released masses of white, jelly-like parasites, but otherwise, the fasting was making him sicker. His weight dropped from 154 pounds to just over 111 pounds. The weight loss added to his feelings of fatigue, and Harry returned to England considerably worse off than when he had left. "I was by now," he said, "properly disabled." By the time he returned home, he discovered that the friend who had recommended the clinic was, in fact, relapsing and was back at the clinic herself.

Harry was resolved to complete the master's program, so he returned to school, and with the help of friends attending class for him and taking notes, he managed to graduate, a significant achievement considering that he was nearly bedridden for the entire year. With school behind him, Harry devoted himself to trying other alternative approaches to restore his health. He moved home, swallowed his pride, and allowed his mother to care for him for the next year. Not wanting to be financially dependent, Harry started a small Internet business, for he could work easily enough off a laptop computer from bed. He tried many different therapies, but nothing helped. He especially concentrated his efforts on nutrition, even studying from home for a nutrition degree. He also sought the assistance of the physicians at the Dove Clinic, where doctors integrate allopathic and alternative methods. It was there that Harry first heard about Peter Fraser.

One day, while hooked up to an IV that was dripping vitamins into his system, Harry saw Dr. Julian Kenyon, one of the founders of the clinic and a respected researcher of alternative health care. During their conversation, Harry asked Kenyon who he thought were the best researchers into alternative health care in the world. He named Peter Fraser among a few others, and on Harry's request, he provided Peter's contact information. A few months later, Harry actually wrote to Peter, an Australian, telling him of his interest in alternative therapies and asking about his work. Peter replied, sending Harry a paper on his bioenergetic theory. Although Harry did not understand much of Peter's theory, he posted the paper on his website.

By September 2000, Harry had succeeded in building his Internet business, and he decided to go to the United States. He would combine business in California with personal research, for he had heard there was a thriving alternative health care community there and was hopeful he would find someone or some method that would help him. Over the previous few years, Harry had been educating himself about bioenergetics and biophysics—about the energies of the body. He even explored subjects as varied as electronics, computers, chaos theory, and information theory. He felt there was something promising in this bioenergetic approach to healing, but none of the makers of the biotechnologies he knew about or had tried could provide a coherent theory of how they worked. They seemed to be missing something important, but Harry could not yet figure out what that something was.

Harry spent more than a year in the United States, and while there he got the education he was seeking. He made dozens of contacts with alternative healers and bioenergetics scientists, and he began to apply himself to bioenergetics as rigorously as he had to every other endeavor he had undertaken. Although he was still so ill that he could work only a few hours a day before collapsing into bed, he made the most of both his work time and downtime.

During that downtime, while resting in bed, Harry thought for hours at a time about the subtle energies of the body, the role of consciousness in health, how energy-based biotechnologies work to connect the real world with the virtual world, and just about every other aspect of health and healing. He dreamed very big dreams: one day, he hoped, he would play a part in bringing a leading-edge biotechnology to every person's home. Why should ill people, he reasoned, who don't even feel like getting out of bed, have to drag themselves from office to office, clinic to clinic, in search of someone who could figure out what is going on in their bodies? Why couldn't someone devise a way to let the body tell us what was going on with it and how it could best correct itself? If there were a subtle, quantum, or some other kind of organizing energy that underlies physiology, driving biochemistry and the workings of our cells and organs, then he felt there ought to be a way to detect and decipher the messages of this energy system.

The hours Harry spent thinking while curled up in bed or on a couch began to pay off. A theory was forming in his imagination. The problem with current energy-based biotechnologies, Harry speculated, was first and foremost the switch. The switch is the point of connection between the real and the virtual, between the realm of pure information and pulling that information (or some of it) into the physical world, so that we can detect and use it. In Harry's view, you could call those organizing virtual forces quantum forces, consciousness, or whatever you wanted—the name didn't matter—but the mechanics of how these forces worked mattered very much.

Information—the virtual part—is always carried on the back of a wave, say a frequency wave, which is the real part. This wave—as the real carrier or matter wave—and the virtual information carried on it would have to exhibit certain properties, such as being self-organizing and self-correcting. So there would be patterns, some kind of overarching order to the whole arrangement, although that order would be changing all the time because any living system would be dynamic, not static. A real-to-virtual switch would somehow allow a machine to capture information about the state of a system, what Peter calls a picture of it, that reveals how that information is configured or stored at one moment in time. It would never be the entire picture, but it would provide a snapshot in time, from which information could then be extracted.

Harry had read about remote viewing, and this phenomenon interested him and also seemed to have application to the real-versus-virtual paradox. Remote viewing is a process by which a person, using only his mind, is able to describe a scene, building, or object that is far distant from him and from which he cannot possibly have any sensory data input. The United States government, and many of the governments of other major world powers, had run covert programs to train remote viewers, and they had developed protocols that allowed just about anyone to develop remote viewing skills. By intending to connect with their target, and writing down the images and impressions they received about it, remote viewers had achieved astonishing success in identifying and describing their target in detail. No one was able to determine the mechanism of that information transfer, but scientific protocols had been developed for getting that information with an often high degree of accuracy.

The key was intention. Remote viewers would be given targets "blind," that is, they would not know what the target (the place or thing they were seeking information about) was when they began a session. Yet somehow a remote viewer's mind was able to "find" the target, to pick it out of all the possible targets. For all practical purposes, the number of possible targets was nearly infinite, because the target could be anything: a planet in the solar system, a person, an exotic new technology, a secret document, a building, or a location. Setting up an intention seemed to connect a remote viewer to an energy web in the universe over which information could be imparted. However, Harry reasoned, "intention seems to be more of a *link* to information; it doesn't tell us much about how the information is transferred or captured." Intention got remote viewers there—to wherever the target was in a remote viewing exercise—but it wasn't the mechanism by which they actually extracted the information from the target. The US government's remote viewing team did not concern itself much with the "how" of remote viewing. They only knew that it worked, so they used it. Harry was concerned with the "how," and it did not appear to be intention—or, at least, *only* intention.

Intention is a decidedly slippery term, one that can mean just about anything. No matter how Harry thought about it, it appeared to be a *linking* process, not an *extracting* process. The same seemed to be true of many of the current health biotechnologies. For example, many of the biotechnologies on the market allow you to perform "healing at a distance" because they function through the use of focused intention. You intend to connect with a person who is physically distant from you to do something, perhaps send a corrective healing frequency or pick up useful information about the state of that person's health, but intention still is only the connection point. Something more is going on that is allowing information transfer to take place. Although remote viewing and other parapsychology experiments had shown evidence that intention actually worked to connect people and things, it was a decidedly imprecise and hit-or-miss approach. The biggest problem for health biotechnologies, from a quantum physics perspective, was how the operator of the system could disentangle his or her own body-field from the field of the person who was to receive the healing or whose sample was being tested. Without a way to decouple the fields, contamination, or "noise," would be a problem, and everything important about the process would depend on the skill of the operator. The ambiguity of using intention as a primary switch between the real and the virtual presented myriad problems, and if you came right down to it, from a physics perspective, would even make any machine unnecessary!

Another part of the equation in building a better biotechnology was how to measure the energies of the body-field at all. The range of energies at play in the body goes far beyond the narrow range of the electromagnetic spectrum, especially that of frequency, which is what most biotechnologies measure. What was missing was a comprehensive understanding not only of how the body-field itself functions but also of how it influences the physical body. Even as Harry continued to work out a way to devise a better switch so that a computer could more reliably, objectively, and accurately detect and transfer energy and information, he realized that no technological advance would matter if there wasn't a *theory* of the body-field (and, by extension, of energetic healing) that was worth applying his ideas to. He had not yet found a sufficiently comprehensive theory—until he remembered Peter's work. Put in this new context, the ideas Peter had outlined in his paper made a lot more sense to Harry.

Harry placed a call to Peter in Australia and explained some of his ideas to him. Peter immediately sensed their validity in regard to his own theory of healing and the body-field map he had devised but didn't quite know what to do with. At Harry's invitation, Peter flew to California. For a week, they did little else but talk. The rush of ideas between them was like flint to steel: they set off sparks that soon grew into a bonfire of more daring ideas and even deeper insights. Peter's more than twenty years of data-gathering and theorizing were catalyzed by Harry's philosophical and technological insights, and by the time Peter prepared to return to Australia, the plan was laid to attempt to marry Harry's technological ideas with Peter's theory of the human body-field.

Despite his excitement at the new venture, Harry's first priority remained his health. Peter was a man with a radical theory of healing and Harry wanted to put it to the test, so he asked Peter to take him on as a client. Peter agreed. After all, Peter's entire life's work had grown out of his own battle with illness. He, too, had suffered from CFS—for more than ten years—and what would come to be the NES system of health care had been birthed out of his own journey toward regaining health.

5

GLIMPSES INTO THE
VIRTUAL BODY

IN 1983, PETER FRASER HAD BEEN TEACHING acupuncture for nearly thirteen years at a school he had founded. He had earned a four-year degree in acupuncture from a school in the Netherlands, and over the years his interest in nontraditional healing methods had prompted him to learn classical homeopathy and travel around Southeast Asia, Taiwan, and China to study traditional Chinese medicine (TCM). He had been instrumental in creating clinical and ethical standards for the acupuncture profession in Australia, and now his school was about to be folded into Melbourne's Victoria University as the first degreed acupuncture program in the state of Victoria. Peter had been invited to join the program as a professor and administrator, but he decided he had spent enough time in academia. Although only in his midforties, he was not feeling well, so he decided to retire, reduce his stress level, take better care of himself, and set up a private practice. During the next year he married, moved to the country, and opened a practice that combined acupuncture, homeopathy, and herbalism.

As his health declined, Peter sought the assistance of several alternative practitioners he knew, and they agreed his symptoms could be lumped into that most vague of diagnoses, CFS. Despite his own considerable healing knowledge and that of the circle of experts who treated him, Peter's health continued to fail. He described the down-turn of events as the CFS worsened:

"Gradually it takes hold and despite trying all manner of treatments, your life falls apart. You don't have the energy or stamina, and everything begins to go. Over the years, I lost my marriage and most of my practice. I managed to work, to earn the barest of livings. I moved to a small house by the sea and saw only enough clients to keep food on the table and a roof over my head. I would have to go to bed at three or four o'clock in the afternoon, and some days I slept fourteen or fifteen hours. My little cottage was less than one hundred meters from the sea, but I often could not even get to the shore. I would reserve all my energy to go to the grocery store to get the things I needed to live. CFS also fogs your brain and impairs your memory. I remember going to Melbourne, a city I lived in for nearly thirty years, and I would get lost. I didn't know where I was or how to get about! It was humiliating!

"So I tried everything I could think of to help myself. I did all the things I knew how to do, and other things I learned. I used Royal Jelly, a bee product rich in the B vitamins. I took all the right vitamins and herbs in megadoses. I tried many different treatments. You do feel better for a little while, but then you relapse. Sometimes the relapses are quite severe. Finally, it got to the point where I had just enough energy to see people, make a pittance of a living, answer the phone, and do what I had to do to survive. I was turning into a vegetable at what should have been the peak of my life."

Like Harry, Peter searched outside of his known world and his comfort zone for help. Eventually, he emulated Edward Bach, creator of the Bach Flower Remedies, which are herbal medicinals said to capture the healing essence of plants. Peter was a nature lover and herbalist, so he decided to see if there were plants from the Australian environment that might help treat his symptoms. Peter had an early version of an electronic imprinting device, so he could, if he needed to, make homeopathic-like remedies from any flowers or plants that seemed promising in treating his symptoms.[1] He had devised a way to test plants for their "energetic signatures" by using an electrodermal-type testing machine, which is an electronic machine that is said to detect the distinct energy of a substance.[2] Traditionally, electrodermal machines have been used to detect changes in electrical resistance at the acupuncture points on skin, indicating where there might be a blockage. However, you also can use such a machine to detect whether there is an energetic imprint in one sample that is similar to—or sets up a like-like response to—a different substance. Peter was quite skeptical of such claims, particularly because the operator can heavily influence the machine's results and has to be quite careful to screen out interfering signals. He also knew that conventional science discredited the machines, but he had toyed with electronic devices since he was a teenager and enjoyed playing around with them. As much as he respected conventional science, Peter knew that energy (in the nonbiochemical sense) had no place in its theory of how the body worked. For the most part, Western scientists ignore or dismiss acupuncture and TCM, despite the fact that they are the primary medical systems in much of Asia and have a track record of impressive results when administered by well-trained practitioners. However, for Peter the bottom line was that "when you are desperate, you welcome relief from wherever you can find it!"

So out into nature Peter went. Considering the state of his health and lack of energy, it took him more than a year to gather and test various native Australian plants against samples of his own blood and saliva for any efficacy in fighting the constellation of symptoms labeled CFS. Friends from around the country, and even a few from other countries, sent him additional plants and flowers to test. However, as he readily admits, "I did not really know what I was looking for, and so nothing I did made much sense! But I kept at it."

Finally, after testing 112 plants and flowers, Peter found three that had energetically matched, or as he calls it "talked to," his own blood or saliva samples. Somehow these three plants matched the energy signature of his blood and saliva. That is, there was some kind of energetic link or communication between Peter's body-field (via his blood or saliva samples) and the unique energy imprint of the plants. Being ever the curious mind, Peter decided to extend his search. He wanted to test blood and saliva samples from other CFS patients against the herbal medicinals he was making to see if the energetic response would be different from that of his own samples. He also wondered if the samples from CFS patients in general showed any energetic peculiarities when they were matched against each other, blood sample against blood sample or saliva sample against saliva sample. "No one had ever thought to ask that question as far as I knew," he said, "and I thought it a most interesting question!" He put out the word, and soon practitioners he knew from several countries were sending him saliva samples from their CFS clients.[3] What he found intrigued him.

When Peter tested the various saliva samples from all of these different people, they did not talk to each other, so there seemed to be no general CFS "tag" in the samples that was common to these patients. (A tag in this respect is any common aspect of the samples that would link them all to a specific condition, in this case CFS.) He was in contact at the time with a microbiologist, and they would have long conversations in which she would challenge Peter to think more deeply and ask more questions. She, of course, questioned his testing method. Even though she would eventually leave the field of microbiology to become an herbalist herself, she kept Peter on his toes about using such unconventional methods, checking his results, and keeping a skeptical, more scientific frame of reference. Under her tutelage, Peter learned a great deal about microbiology, especially about virology.

What surprised Peter about his test results was that many of the flower nectars contained the energetic imprint of various viruses, especially the Flaviviridae family of viruses, which are associated with encephalitis. Peter decided to test the CFS patients' saliva samples he had been sent for the energetic signature of that family of viruses: he found that almost all of them contained a tag to the Flaviviridae family of viruses in general or at least the energetic signature of them. In addition, one of the three flowers that had matched Peter's blood sample also matched the Flaviviridae virus imprint, so using the homeopathic logic that like treats like, Peter thought that the flower might provide a remedy in treating the disease. Following that lead, Peter concocted a medicinal using that flower extract and began taking it.

Within ten days, he developed a flulike response to the remedy. He knew that was a good thing. As many homeopaths and other complementary health care professionals recognize, when the immune system starts to kick in after not working effectively for a long time, it causes a flulike episode. His immune system was recognizing an invader organism, or to put it more accurately, although his immune system had initially failed to mount an attack on the real virus, it was now responding to it via the virtual imprint of the virus. Peter admits that despite his years of training in acupuncture, homeopathy, and TCM, he didn't have a clue about the mechanisms underlying the effect with the virtual virus. However, he couldn't deny that taking the flower medicinal was helping him. He would have long stretches in which he felt healthy and had ample energy, but then, as is common with CFS, he would relapse. Eventually, much later, when he had worked out the structure of the human body-field, he would realize that the relapses were most likely an effect of the virus mutating, moving from one compartment of the body-field to another.

Compartment was Peter's early term for what would later become known in NES as an Energetic Integrator, an information pathway in the body that has a particular structure and regulates specific physiological processes at the energetic level. According to the Nutri-Energetics model, there are twelve Energetic Integrators in the human body-field. The virus was jumping from one Energetic Integrator to another, in effect going into hiding; each time it jumped, the patient was likely to have a relapse. Peter later would come to the conjecture that some kinds of changes that scientists call mutations are caused not by a microbe actually changing its genetic structure but by it shifting from Integrator to Integrator. Because each Energetic Integrator functions at a different frequency range, Peter's would eventually come to define a mutation, from an energetic perspective, as a microbe changing its carrier frequency. Much later, when Peter developed the Infoceuticals, he would create one called Field Stabilizer that prevented, or at least slowed, this kind of Integrator-shifting mutation. However, at that time, Peter was a long way from having even the first inklings of the system that would be called Nutri-Energetics.

Over the next several years, Peter continued experimenting with energetic imprinting and expended most of his energy in managing his relapses. It would take many more years, until 1998, before Peter considered himself cured of CFS. Yet his early research had led to one major breakthrough in his understanding and his experimental technique: he had learned to make energetic matches between a client's body-field and a substance that could effect a healing response. He wrote to several researchers about this method, in particular to Kenyon, who had written a treatise on acupuncture.[4] Kenyon had been encouraging, but for the most part Peter was on his own, exploring largely uncharted territory.

His apparatus appeared to be making consistent matches between a client's body-field (via saliva samples if the client wasn't there in person) and ampoules of therapeutic substances that were placed on plates on the machine. The matching was demonstrated by a sudden change in skin conductivity at certain acupuncture points. This change registered on the machine as a drop in the indicator needle. However, what more, if anything, was going on, Peter did not know. He began to read about physics and biophysics, but most of his time was spent continuing the matching experiments and gathering data.

During the late 1980s and into the early 1990s, Peter plunged more deeply into questions he had about acupuncture. Despite his credentials and achievements in that field, he had never been satisfied with acupuncture's explanations of the meridian system. Nor, for that matter, was he satisfied with the explanations provided by TCM, the system from which the theory of the meridians and the practice of acupuncture had emerged. Those explanations were too metaphoric; they relied too heavily on philosophy and metaphysics.

Peter said, "Despite my training in the field of acupuncture and traditional Chinese medicine, I realized that the explanations for the meridians were just so much talk. I wanted to define the acupuncture points and meridians in a more practical way. So that's when I decided to play around with them with the machines I had. I didn't expect to get very far, especially since I did not know what these machines were really doing. In fact, no traditional scientist trusted these machines. So I knew I was out in left field, so to speak. But that's where I like to be! Left alone and able to explore with no one telling me how mad I might be!"

As Peter said, no one knows what acupuncture meridians actually are. Although many researchers have looked for it, the qi that is said to flow through the meridians has never been detected in the body, although evidence has been found for electrical changes in the body at the acupuncture points and along the meridians. Peter was not surprised that so far no one had discovered qi, for he did not believe it existed. He saw no need to invoke an unknown cosmic force to explain the energies of the body. It made better sense, at least from a scientific perspective, to assume that if the body used energy to regulate health, it would be using one of the known energies of physics. In addition, Peter was of the mind that just knowing about or detecting energy in the body was of little clinical value. Of greater interest to him was trying to decipher how the body *uses* information. The traditional Chinese medical view of energy and information was mostly philosophical and explained through metaphors and analogies. Peter was interested in teasing the science from that poetry.

To complicate matters, most acupuncturists believe that the energy that flows through the meridians is, at least in part, electromagnetic in nature, although no one really knows for sure. Peter was growing more and more certain that whatever the imprinting and electrodermal-type measurement machines he had been using were doing, they were picking up more than electromagnetic energies. There may be a change in the electrical conductivity at the skin, he surmised, but this was only a consequence of what was happening at a deeper energetic level in the body. What was happening at that deeper level remained unknown, but Peter began to suspect that he was exploring a quantum field process of some kind.

Peter also understood that if there were quantum processes in the body, he faced another thorny issue: sorting the real from the virtual. Biology and chemistry are real, but any quantum processes underlying them are dependent on particles and waves, the mostly abstract, although fundamental, energies of the subatomic world. At this point in his research, however, Peter understood that speculating about the meaning of the data he was gathering was less productive than simply gathering more of that data. He concentrated his efforts on his experiments to see where, if anywhere, they led him in his quest for answers.

In the late 1980s, Peter had begun to amass homeopathic tissue samples, getting many from companies in Australia and importing others. He gathered thousands of ampoules, which contained the homeopathic, or energetic, imprints of just about everything of importance in the body.[5] He had ampoules representing nearly two hundred different kinds of cells and various kinds of tissues, from skin to gut to brain samples, and blood, enzymes, hormones, and the like. He had amassed droves of minerals and elements from calcium to potassium to zinc, and he had samples of environmental chemicals and toxins. He then attempted to match energetic aspects of the contents of each ampoule to various acupuncture points on the body, using himself as the guinea pig. All acupuncture points are connected via channels of energy, called meridians, which can zigzag around the body connecting to various organs and body tissues. In TCM, there are twelve main meridians and 365 acupuncture points along those meridians.[6]

To get a feel for what a meridian is, consider the kidney meridian, which is one of the twelve major meridians. This bilateral energy channel starts at the soles of the feet, flows up the inside of the legs, moves across the abdomen and along the chest, continues to the back of the throat, and ends at the root of the tongue. Inner branching channels run from the main kidney meridian to the root of the tongue and on to the inner ears and brain tissue. Traditionally, there are twenty-seven acupuncture points along the kidney meridian.

There are myriad health-related associations for each of the twelve main meridians and the deeper, inner meridians that branch from them. To continue with our example, an imbalance of the kidney meridian may result in eating disorders, changes in complexion, weakened vision, feelings of anxiety or fear, or other symptoms that from a commonsense, cause-and-effect perspective have nothing to do with kidney function. For instance, by stimulating an acupuncture point at one end of the kidney meridian, in the foot, an acupuncturist can seek to alleviate a headache, because the other end of the channel affects the head and brain.

Peter explored the meridians by doggedly testing the contents of thousands of ampoules against the acupuncture points for energetic matches. A match suggested that the substance in the test ampoule was important to the proper functioning of that meridian or to the organs and body processes correlated to that meridian. A match meant there was an energy connection, a communication between the two. Peter methodically went through the thousands of combinations of possible matches. He tested each kind of tissue against each of the acupuncture points to see if they matched. He tested individual elements, such as calcium, one by one to see which acupuncture points, and by extension, which meridians, connected with it, suggesting that those channels of energy might be involved in the proper use of that element in the body. The work was slow and repetitious, for when he found a match, he tested and retested it to verify the results.

By the early 1990s, Peter had recorded the results of those thousands of initial matching experiments and had begun to graphically represent the matches as a web of relationships. The drawing was a series of concentric circles intersected by lines of varying lengths and orientations that radiated outward from the center. The rings and lines were peppered with dots representing various acupuncture points. He called his drawing the "spiderweb diagram."

In addition to mapping out the energy matches between the substances in the ampoules and the meridians, Peter had been gathering data about how each of the various samples in the thousands of ampoules matched with each other. He asked all manner of questions, looking at which cells, tissues, or organs would communicate with—or as he liked to phrase it, talk to—each other. Would heart tissue talk to brain tissue more readily than to liver tissue? Which elements would or wouldn't chromium talk to? How did muscle tissue react when matched with a known toxin, such as lead? Matches indicated that there might be some common information network that energetically linked those items.

Peter was continually amazed at his findings. Some of them confirmed the ancient Chinese system of medicine. For example, TCM views the heart meridian as the master connector, holding all the energies of the body together and linking them to the brain. Peter found that was the case, but he also was able to bring an amazing level of anatomical specificity to the matches. According to his tests, the only part of the brain that the heart talked to was the midbrain. It did not set up an energetic match with the higher-level, more integrative parts of the brain. This finding was of immense interest because the midbrain controls many of the regulatory functions of the body, such as blood pressure, blood sugar levels, and body temperature. The ancient Chinese had their energetic anatomy partly right, and now Peter was able to show why at the anatomical level.

Another surprising result involved the liver meridian. In TCM, the liver meridian has an internal channel that connects to the eye and the top of the head. Peter found in his matching experiments that the liver meridian did indeed talk to the eye, but only to the retina and iris. He was documenting what amounted to the first detailed bioenergetic anatomical model.

The matching tests validated or extended aspects of TCM in still other ways. The energy that flows through the twelve main meridians does so just under the skin, so the meridians, particularly the liver meridian, are connected to all types of tissues, especially skin tissue. However, the inner meridians, sometimes called the horizontal meridians or *luo,* are said to extend throughout the body's connective tissue and deep into the body. Peter's tests confirmed this, not only for the inner meridians but for the main ones as well. He found, in fact, that the meridians, did not talk to the skin, but they did connect strongly to connective tissue, which forms a massive network in our bodies. It is a web of tough, fibrous fascia and branching tissue that serves as a soft framework (in contrast to the solid scaffolding of bone) for the body, reaching every cell in the body.

As stated in part 1, connective tissue's role is seen primarily in motor functions, such as muscle contraction and extension. Beyond that, most conventional biologists pay it little attention. Biophysicists, in contrast, are concentrating much of their study on this massive inner structure. They believe that the connective tissue matrix is vitally important to our overall health, serving as a kind of second nervous system through which information is transmitted instantly across our entire body. They have even provided tantalizing evidence of quantum processes at work in the body via the crystalline lattice network of connective tissue.[7] What Peter found through his matching experiments was that *every* meridian, not just the liver meridian, communicated with at least one kind of connective tissue, and many talked to several different kinds simultaneously. This was evidence that there was indeed a massive information network in the body that conventional biology knew next to nothing about. His experiments were unintentionally bringing a level of specificity to the ancient Chinese system that helped explain the biology of the body from both physiological and energetic perspectives.

Another of Peter's important early findings showed how elements communicate in the body. He found, for example, that calcium talked to most cells and tissues of the body, which is not surprising because calcium is involved in thousands of critical biochemical activities and at least partially makes up the cytoskeleton of many kinds of cells. Other, more complex elements, such as deuterium, made next to no matches, which again is not surprising because this element is not important to health. Peter discovered that, generally, the elements that come earliest in the periodic table—hydrogen, carbon, boron, oxygen, nitrogen, sodium, magnesium, potassium, and calcium—match most vigorously with the body. Most of the elements that come later in the periodic table, with a few exceptions, do not talk much or at all to the body. This is exactly what you find in the biochemistry of the body: the elements early in the periodic table are ubiquitous in the body and are important to its proper functioning. Although the findings themselves were not new or unexpected, their importance lies in the fact that Peter, using unconventional testing procedures, was replicating on an entirely energetic level many well-known facts of biochemistry. This was evidence that this testing method was viable.

By the mid-1990s, Peter had gained enough confidence in his testing method—although he was still unable to explain it theoretically—to attempt a rather outrageous experiment. He had toyed with the idea that he could make an imprint of the energy at an acupuncture point *directly* into a liquid. Until now he only had imprinted actual substances, or matter. Now he was thinking of trying to capture the energy signature of an acupuncture point—in effect capturing the energy flow of a meridian—in liquid. Peter modified the two machines he was using—the electrodermal-type measurement device and the imprinting machine—and conducted the experiment. It took many tries before he perfected his technique and actually succeeded. The liquid was active; it was imprinted with energy directly from an acupuncture point! Peter was more convinced than ever that whatever signal was being imprinted into the liquid, it was not entirely, or even mostly, electromagnetic in nature.

No one was more surprised with this result or mystified by its implications than Peter. He said, "I had no idea what on earth was going on!

It was mad, I admit it! But repeated testing showed that something was going on, and it could not be electronic! So I was left wondering what was it that was being detected and even transferred. It took me a while to realize it could only be information. I had somehow been able to imprint information from the body, via an acupuncture point or perhaps even the entire meridian channel, into a liquid. I had no idea how that could actually happen."

Homeopaths claim to be able to imprint liquids with the energetic signature of a substance, using a method involving cycles of dilution and succussion, but Peter was doing it electronically. He found, as the homeopaths did, that a liquid could retain the memory of the biological activity of a substance. What's more, he found liquid could hold the memory of information culled directly from the body, via the meridians! However, he had no good scientific explanation for how he was able to do that. Although the theoretical issues continued to mystify Peter, he pressed on with his matching experiments. He had found a reliable method of measuring an acupuncture point on the body and making an energetic imprint of it, and he wanted to explore the implications of this new technique. The matching experiments were revealing what kinds of information were being carried by which meridian, and as he slowly but methodically built up his spiderweb diagram, Peter began to realize that he was creating what amounted to a map of the information pathways of the body, or more correctly, of some kind of structured energy body, which he would come to call the human bodyfield. However, he still had no idea what this map was good for. How would it be useful in clinical practice? Knowing where information flowed in the body and even what that information was did nothing to help a clinician affect that flow. How could one reliably detect energy that was impeded or distorted? How exactly would such an energetic problem affect the physical body? Could a person actually correct physical problems only by manipulating the energies and information of the body? These were the kinds of questions that motivated Peter to continue what seemed to be endless rounds of matching experiments.

Peter's persistence paid off handsomely on the day he realized that the ninety-six internal meridians he had been mapping could be ordered into twelve groups. In TCM, there are twelve main meridians. However, Peter had never made the assumption that there were *only* twelve major information pathways in the body, so he had been experimenting with nearly one hundred primary and secondary meridians. He had spent innumerable hours organizing his voluminous data, trying to find order and connections, applying different mathematical schemas to the data. For more than twenty years he had been studying the ancient Chinese transformational mathematics that had been formalized metaphorically in the I Ching. On that particular day, using that method, he found the key that unlocked a pattern.

Peter explained, "After I finally realized there was an *order* to how the ninety-six inner meridians matched, they logically grouped themselves into twelve categories. There are twelve groups in Chinese medicine as well. That fact *alone* does not mean it has any relevance in the reality of the body. It could simply be a coincidence, but I suspected otherwise. By matching and measuring and trying to find a sound reason for a pattern, I found that the ninety-six individual inner meridians could be transformed into twelve main groups. This was marvelous, as the ninety-six-meridian system was much too complicated to ever do anything practical with, at least from a health perspective, but reducing them to a pattern of only twelve groups simplified things, made things more workable.

"That was a great moment because when a complex system begins to simplify itself, it means you can begin to understand it. A structure starts to emerge, and structure means information! Nature likes to organize complexity into larger but simpler and higher-order patterns. I was just beginning to catch a glimpse of this emergent higher order and the information it might contain.

"For practical purposes," he continued, "I still couldn't work out what on earth it was exactly that I was capturing in the tests and how I could use it. I thought it must be some sort of imprint of those meridians, but I was still left with huge questions. What is it? Is it a signal of some kind? No, no one can detect a signal as a fixed charge. Lots of people have tried, but they have never reliably detected a charge at the acupuncture points. Maybe it was some kind of *potential* charge? I thought that, yes, you can modulate a charge, but it doesn't make any sense, because to have a charge you have to have a field, some energy moving through the body. No one had ever proved that there was energy in the body, although there was plenty of anecdotal evidence for it and a long healing tradition behind it. Although I had been think-ing about fields and learning a little about quantum physics, I couldn't work out at all how you could possibly get information transfer—which there had to be for the body to work properly—just because you had a charge. I had what amounted to a structure and a space—a geometry of the body-field—emerging. What I did not have at that time was any theory that could make sense of it. That theory is, in all probability, quantum electrodynamics. I didn't have much of that yet, but it was a great moment when the system simplified itself! This meant I was uncovering some kind of inner structure, some order and pattern. You can figure out the meaning behind an order and a pattern if you work hard enough at it!"

Soon after this breakthrough, Peter was able to make another signifi-cant advance in his work. He figured out that there was a sequence to the twelve main channels or, as Peter called them at first, compartments of the body-field. Each of these compartments differed in significant ways, theoretically and practically, from the Chinese meridians, starting with the fact that they were not simply passive conduits for life-force energy, or qi. The compartments themselves were somehow *actively* involved in the movement of the very specific kinds of information that the body needs to function correctly. As he explored the relationships among the various compartments, Peter discovered that they had a preferred sequence, an order of importance in their role in the body. *If the sequence was not fol-lowed, then the compartments did not talk to each other as easily or at all.* This sequence obviously had profound implications for healing because it indicated that there was a preferred order for how the body might best be returned from a state of imbalance (in which its self-regulation systems are not working correctly) to homeostasis (in which its self-regulating systems are restored).

It turned out that the body-field compartments, the Energetic Integrators, are noncommutative. In mathematics, you can add 1 + 2 + 3 to get 6. If you reorder the numbers, 2 + 1 + 3, they still add up to 6. Addition is commutative—order doesn't matter—but this is not how the energy or information of the body-field works. Peter found out that the order of the Integrators was noncommutative—order mattered in how well the different Integrators communicated with each other. If they were addressed out of order, the efficiency of the communication links suffered. The implications were potentially enormous for healing.

This turn of events brought back memories of Peter's own training in Chinese medicine. He remembered that during his studies he had been told that there are two systems for ordering the main meridians and that the one that was most widely known contained errors. The errors had been inserted into the system intentionally by the ancient teachers. The mark of mastery of the practice, he was told, was when a student recognized the errors and so could, on his or her own, discover the proper order. That old story, which he had once thought was apocryphal, was now turning out to have truth to it, and it motivated Peter to continue exploring the body-field for order and pattern. Once he had the order of the energetic compartments fairly well set, Peter was able to modify his spiderweb diagram even further, adding another level of detail to what would eventually become a map, or template, of the human body-field.

———◆———

Peter was now more than ten years into his matching experiments. He had amassed mounds of notes and data, and his spiderweb diagram was sufficiently detailed to show that there was directionality to the flow of energy and information he had found in the matching experiments. A structure was emerging that suggested that the human body-field had order, or sequencing, to it and that energy flowed through this field in specific ways. Many ancient cultures had models of how energy flows according to specific parameters, including direction, along pathways in the body's energy field. If those pathways become distorted or blocked, the energy flow slows or even stops entirely. As the energy flow becomes less efficient, the body loses homeostasis and displays the symptoms of illness. However, Peter's work took him far beyond the commonly accepted models of chakras, auras, or other generalized kinds of body-field structures.

Peter by now was fairly certain that he was detecting fields, which meant that, like it or not, he had entered the realm of quantum electrodynamics (QED). There are always two aspects to a quantum system: the real and the virtual. The field is the real part of the system, whereas the information is the virtual part of it. That much made sense to Peter, but he knew that if there are fields in the body, they have to be able to offload information in very specific ways. Information has to be delivered to the right place in the body at the proper time, often within incredibly fine-tuned parameters. Electromagnetism by itself, Peter suspected, could not account for such a system.

Peter said, "In the mid-1990s, my brain just got stuck. I had reached a new stage in the development of the spiderweb diagram, of what I thought could be a map of the human body-field, but I couldn't talk with anyone about it. There were no words for it. Not even any science for it, at least that I knew much about. I didn't know what it all meant. During the day, I would make an amazing discovery about how parts of the body-field matched, and at night I would go home with a bottle of champagne and celebrate by myself, but a few hours later I would collapse in doubt, saying 'This can't possibly be correct. This is absurd!' I was on a roller coaster mentally, but ideas kept flooding in. I would make a connection that could explain something about the body beautifully, something that biochemistry couldn't explain very well or at all, but because mine was a bioenergetic explanation, I figured no one would believe me. But that connection suggested others, and I couldn't stop testing these ideas. I was driven at the same time that I was questioning everything. I would think if X is so, then Y must be so, and in the middle of the night I would leap out of bed and go test that idea. I did that thousands of times over those years. At one moment I would be overcome with excitement and curiosity, and at the next I would collapse in devastation and doubt.

"It was a trying time, and that mental stress is why it took more than ten years for me to trust the map I was creating," Peter continued. "The real problem was wrapping my mind around my extremely unconventional methods. By then I knew that electromagnetism wasn't the main thing with these electrodermal-type machines. It appeared to be the photon. You have to have an electron to get the photon mediation, but it was the photon that seemed to be most important, to carry the information—or at least that is what I surmised at that time. I even wrote to the creators of many of these machines with my speculations about how they must really be working, but I never heard anything back.

"One thing was for sure. I knew I needed to learn more about physics," Peter said. "I was beginning to find patterns in my work. I knew the matching tests showed that things connected in the body in specific order and according to a preferred sequence. The heart talks to the kidneys, but the kidneys don't necessarily talk *back* to the heart. There seemed to be a direction to how this energy flowed. This was of critical importance. It could have huge ramifications on healing. Maybe the errors in so many of these electrodermal screening measurements and maybe the lack of consistent results with so many complementary modalities, like acupuncture and homeopathy, occurred because the body was not being tested or treated in the *correct order*. I was still in the very early stages of figuring out the complexities of the compartments, what would become the Energetic Integrator system. The Integrators are about how information is transferred and regulated in the body, but at that time I had no real theory, and I knew that whatever theory was accountable for this data had to be grounded in physics. An Australian biologist and oncologist, by the name of Dr. Bevan Reid, who was also very involved at that point in his career in alternative science, became my first real mentor in that regard. Meeting him was the start of a whole new period in my work."[8]

◆

Peter had met Reid in the early 1990s, but Reid had not seemed particularly interested in his work. Although Peter had set up a correspondence with a few researchers into alternative therapies, such as Kenyon in England, it would be more convenient to discuss his ideas with someone in Australia, which narrowed the field considerably. Reid was in his own backyard so Peter decided to contact him again. This time Reid invited Peter to meet with him, and they spent many hours discussing Peter's work. Reid was considerably more interested now, and a few days after their initial meeting, when they met again, Peter showed Reid his spiderweb diagram, which was turning out to be essentially a wiring diagram of the energy compartments of the body-field. Reid was immediately struck by the system of connections Peter had worked out and by the structure or geometry that was emerging from his data, but he was unimpressed with the metaphysical language by which Peter was still attempting to explain it. Reid felt that for Western scientists to take alternative medicine seriously, alternative practitioners had better start using the language of science. Reid was not being condescending as much as practical. He insisted that Peter talk in terms that scientists could understand. Without a common language, it was unlikely the two groups could ever establish a fruitful collaboration. He also urged Peter to increase his efforts to see how the anomalies he was finding in how the body works could answer some of the unsolved mysteries of biology. He urged Peter to look at the cracks in biology, for there he might find useful avenues of exploration in his own work.

For hours most mornings, Reid coached Peter by telephone in biology, oncology, quantum physics, bioenergetics, and more. The conversations stimulated Peter to think in ways he never had before, and they gave him hope that his work was leading somewhere useful. Reid was a maverick. He was secure enough in his own intellect to be unapologetic about his belief that it was only a matter of time before medicine acknowledged that energy and information were at least as important as biochemistry in the workings of the body and the regulation of health. However, Reid's real value to Peter lay in his willingness to give Peter's offbeat testing methods a fair appraisal. Together, they repeated many of Peter's matching experiments and devised new ones. One experiment in particular was of enormous importance—an experiment that appeared to take the electron out of the testing procedure!

After conversations with Reid, Peter had begun to think more seriously about directionality and the flow of information under various spatial constraints. He would spend hours thinking about structures in space—energetic geometry, if you will. Reid was in agreement that Peter was somehow making measurements that had relevance at the level of QED. If that were so, then perhaps it was not the physical substances in the ampoules that were matching, but the space, or the field, around the ampoules that was being modified. Peter had originally thought that a match could only occur if the energies of or information in the two ampoules—or the substances in them— were complementary to each other. Now Reid was suggesting that it might be the "shape of space" that matched, a kind of space resonance. Perhaps when the configurations of space matched, they took on some kind of energetic—and, in the body, biological—utilitarianism.

In physics, energy shapes space. Something has to excite or perturb the QED field. It could be sound (phonons), photons, or any number of other things or causes. All fields in one way or another are shaped by a force. Gravity alters the orbit of planets. Einstein's space-time warps under the influence of the mass of objects. The rush of air through our vocal cords vibrates air molecules and carves bursts of air into distinct words. When a metal plate across which sand has been spread is subjected to sound waves, the sand rearranges itself from a shapeless mass into intricate geometric patterns (refer to figure 8.2 on page 157). Nature appears to favor an energetic geometry, so it was not a huge stretch to think the body might as well.

Peter and Reid set to work to test some of these ideas. Among their first experiments was one that would attempt to detect any spatial structures or fields that might be important to the energetic matching process. The experiment also would explore whether electrons or photons were the dominant carriers of information during the matching process. Peter and Reid modified the electrodermal-type measurement machine Peter had been using so that they could add extra ampoules to the testing platform. Instead of one plate, they now had two connected plates on which to place ampoules. They set up the electrical field and put an ampoule onto each of the plates. These were ampoules they knew should show a matching response, and, indeed, they got a matching response, as evidenced by the drop in the indicator needle. Then they withdrew the ampoules, Reid disconnected the wires from the machine, and they replaced the ampoules on the two plates. The matching response reappeared, as the indicator revealed, even though the machine was not plugged in! They tested this effect over the next hours and days. They always got the same results. After the initial match had been made in an electrostatic field (the real field), the energy match held over time, even when the electrostatic field was withdrawn (by unplugging the machine) and only the virtual field remained. This residual virtual field seemed to affect physical matter.

Reid helped Peter formulate a possible explanation. They knew that a virtual field (or, more specifically, the information contained within that field) must be carried by a real field. In the same way that virtual particles pop out of the vacuum because they borrow energy from real particles or the vacuum itself, the virtual always piggybacks on the real. By initially setting up the matching response in a real electrostatic field, they were able then to get the virtual matching response. After that virtual field response had been established, it persisted for a time, even when the real field was withdrawn.[9] Reid was as astonished as Peter at the outcome of the experiments. They also realized that this result suggested that the effect was photon dependent, not electron dependent.

They decided to test the theory further. They got a lead plate and placed it between the two matching ampoules in a virtual field. Immediately the match indication disappeared. As they took the lead plate away, the response returned to show a match. As Peter told it, "Reid nearly fell over!" Over time, they tested various metals, but only lead, tin, tantalum, and ytterbium plates blocked the virtual field.

In one further set of experiments, Reid had the idea to rotate the second plate, to see if there was any directionality to the virtual field effect. In test after test, they adjusted the plates so they were positioned 90 degrees to each other (perpendicular) and then rotated the second plate a few degrees at a time away from 90 degrees. What they found intrigued them. The matching effect held only when the fields were in 90-degree alignment. The match weakened for 2 or 3 degrees in either direction of 90 degrees, then disappeared altogether at any deviation greater than 5 degrees. The test was suggesting that orientation was important, which could hold true only if there were indeed some kind of geometry—some structure in space, as Peter now called it—at play in the effect.

They didn't know if this result would apply to living organisms, but as a conventionally trained physician, Reid immediately saw its possible relevance to the body. Certain types of cells are spatially and geometrically aligned. For example, epithelial cells, which generally are flat, cuboidal, or columnar in shape, line the major cavities and organs of the body. They are sheets of *polarized* cells, which means they have a preferred orientation.[10] Some epithelial cells tend to form at perpendicular, that is, 90 degree, angles to the base membrane. So do the cells of the cornea and intestines. Reid and Peter speculated that these precisely oriented cells might have a quantum-level function, some bioenergetic purpose that had to do with carrying the virtual information of the body, the information that works below the level of chemistry and DNA. Skin cells are epithelial cells, and skin is the largest organ in our body and is what connects us directly to our environment. Reid and

Peter speculated that the sheets of polarized epithelial cells in our body are somehow defining space and connecting us to the energies of the environment and even to the virtual energies of the cosmos.

Cultures from around the world and throughout history speak of pervasive natural energy, calling it qi, prana, and other names. NES would later come to call this pervasive, universal energy the Source energy, and Peter and Harry feel that it is not some unknown cosmic energy but a real energy of physics, what is called zero-point energy (ZPE), the energy of the zero-point field (ZPF). As briefly explained previously, the ZPF in quantum field theory is associated with the vacuum, which is erroneously thought of as empty space, but quantum physics tells us there can be no such thing as empty space. It has shown that the vacuum—space that is at the lowest possible temperature of absolute zero on the Kelvin scale—is awash in the energy of micro-scopic vibrations produced by the interaction of subatomic particles. In fact, physicists metaphorically describe the ZPF as a sea of cosmic foam because it is seething with energy as virtual quantum particles zip in and out of existence. They estimate that there is more energy in the ZPF than there is in all the matter in the universe. As Peter would show later, cavities (more or less hollow structures) are important as structures for collecting and storing Source energy, ZPE, or whatever name you want to call it.[11] It is no surprise that all the major organs of the body are cavities themselves and that they are composed of smaller structures that are called microtubules, which are tiny cavities. Cells also are cavities and contain within them many other tubular-shaped structures. Cavities are efficient structures in which to store, amplify, and even tune energy, as will be discussed later in chapter 10.

Reid's tutelage gave Peter the confidence to move ahead with his research and supplied the first general outlines of a theory. Although Reid had provided Peter with a foundation of physics knowledge, and they had come up with the barest outlines of a tentative theory involving photons and quantum entanglement to explain what Peter was finding, they both knew that they were exploring areas totally outside the domain of conventional science. However, wasn't that true of many, if not most, truly revolutionary theories and discoveries? Peter finally accepted that he might always be an outsider and decided not to worry about acceptance by "the academy." What was most important to him was to continue exploring the body-field and refining his map. He undertook his research with renewed enthusiasm, and as the 1990s drew to a close he began an explosive period of experimentation. In the next few years, he would meet Harry Massey, who would initiate the development of the computer software that would put Peter's testing of body-field energies on more stable experimental ground. Together they would solidify a comprehensive theory of body-field structure and dynamics, and begin to develop the remedies, which would come to be called Infoceuticals, that would provide information directly to the body-field to correct any distortions in it.

6

CALIFORNIA
COLLABORATION

IN THE FALL OF 2001, Peter arrived in California to meet with Harry. Their phone conversations had been long and intense, filled with rambling theoretical and technical musings punctuated by bursts of insights that further illuminated Peter's experimental work into the human body-field. When they finally met, the fervor of their creative collaboration only heightened. For ten days, they talked all day and long into the night about everything from biology to quantum theory to the politics and practicalities of health care. Peter described his years of experiments to Harry, recounted his efforts to make sense of his data, and generally outlined his understanding of the human body-field. They discussed how the body-field could be the underlying control mechanism for health.

For example, Peter had by now thought deeply about the sequence of the compartments, the meridian-like information routes in the body that would come to be called Energetic Integrators. He realized there was a big body-field (see chapter 9), but that it was made up of several subfield structures (the aggregation of all of the Energetic Drivers, Energetic Integrators, and so on). All of these subfields appeared to be connected in a single large feedback loop that could be thought of as a big body-field wave. In terms of the Integrators, compartment 12 appeared to be at the end of the full body-field wave and compartment 1 at the beginning of the wave. If information was distorted along this sequence from compartment 1 to 12, then corrupted information would be fed from the end of the wave, at compartment 12, back into the beginning of the wave, at compartment 1. The continual feeding back of distorted information into the full body-field wave would gradually cause the body to lose homeostasis.

Peter, like Harry, also had spent hours thinking about the real versus the virtual worlds. Over the years in Australia, he had spent hours walking with his dog in the mountains, thinking about how to integrate the two realms. Most of the research being done in bioenergetics was focusing on electromagnetism and the biophotons emitted by cells in living things, but by now Peter did not think they played significant roles in information exchange in the body-field.

Peter said, "I had been puzzling about this ever since the Reid days: how do the real and virtual link? How do they talk to each other? That question occupied me for more than five years. Obviously you can't have two worlds. There is one world, perhaps with two linked aspects to it. The awful duality! We don't want it! We want to live in one world! There must be a physical link, an energetic link, and once we had the link, then we could read the human body-field.

"Scientists and medical doctors could already read the physical with various instruments, electronic and photonic," Peter added. "There were all kinds of machines, such as ECGs and fMRI machines, for reading the electromagnetic and other known energies of the physical body, but when it came to the virtual, we had no real way to measure it because we didn't know what it was! I thought there must be some kind of mathematical projection to capture it.

"One of the thoughts that occurred to me during this time," he continued, "was that the great real-versus-virtual debate might be nothing more than a construction created by a faulty model of physics. My mentor, Dr. Reid, had once said that visible photons—light, electromagnetism—do not play a crucial part in the quantum *informa-*

tion field effect. Light plays a role in *energy* exchange but has little to do with transferring information. I had finally been able to verify this through my matching experiments, but I was still uncertain about the role of the electron versus photon.

"I described to Harry how during those walks and then back in my lab, where I did the matching experiments day and night, I had tried to work that problem out," Peter explained. "Harry was the first person, apart from Dr. Reid, who was willing to lower expectations about the usefulness of the visible photon in information exchange. Of course, now we know visible photons *energize* the QED field—and we use them in certain ways in our Infoceutical imprinting process—but they are not crucial as a mechanism of the *information exchange* process in the body-field. They may not even be discrete particles at all, if you take into account the latest frontier physics experiments. It is the electron, after all, that is paramount in that process. It wasn't until late 2005 that we found a physicist with a theory that matched our own research and intuition—Milo Wolff and his space resonance theory. That is a theory in which an electron is an oscillating spherical standing wave. When two electrons, or spherical standing waves, interact, there is a change in the resonance of space at the point of intersection. If Wolff's model turns out to be correct, then the idea of matching as I perfected it stands on firmer ground. To put it simply, a match can be thought of as the change of the resistance or permittivity—what can be thought of as the shape or structure—of space, but I am not talking in terms of electromagnetic fields, although I use the words *resistance* and *permittivity*. Those are just convenient terms to help describe this change in what Milo Wolff calls space resonance. The change in the structure of space affects the expression of matter, with different space resonances representing different arrangements of electrons, which results, for example, in the periodic table of elements. Perhaps the de Broglie matter wave is actually a space resonance. What's more, perhaps this change in space resonance is what drives chemistry, at the sub-atomic level, thereby directing the body's physiology. Space resonance is an illuminating way to explain what I had been measuring in all my ampoule matching experiments for more than twenty years.

"But that physics model came years later," Peter noted. "My time talking with Harry during that first visit was marvelous in that he really got what I was talking about! What's more—and this was his really important contribution at that time—he offered creative ideas about how we could represent my data and program it into a computer. That was the real breakthrough that made my wild ideas possible for clinical application."

One of the theoretical discussions that Harry and Peter had, which grew out of their past individual speculations about the real versus the virtual, was about matching. They were back to discussing the fundamental question: What is happening when the virtual gets pulled into the physical, real world? Physicists talked about measurement and the collapse of the wavefunction, which makes a probability in the quantum realm into a certainty in the physical world. Before a measurement is taken, an electron or photon is a fog of potentiality, with probabilities of the quantum particle being here or there. However, after you make the measurement, you can pinpoint a particle's location. One way to talk about such an occurrence is to describe it as nature making matches, as sorting through all potentials and finding the best match for the situation (the experimental setup). Harry filled Peter in on his thoughts about a real-to-virtual switch and a way that such a connection point between the real and the virtual could be made using a computer. He explained that intention was a part of matching, a link between things, but not a *mechanism* for extracting information. Something else was going on.

That something must be a process or mechanism in nature that allows the various energies of the cosmos and the almost unlimited kinds of information to communicate in useful, organized, and coherent ways. Somehow, there was a way that nature allowed disparate things to come together and then to form meaningful patterns. There was a way things matched to each other to create something out of nothing, bring order to chaos, make the improbable possible, and make creative yet practical use of almost infinite variables. Intention might capitalize on this process, but the process itself went beyond merely linking things. It must be responsible for *ordering* things as well.

Peter shared his ideas about matching with Harry, having realized that almost everything at the heart of quantum physics could be considered as a matching process. According to the Standard Model, an electron is both a wave and a particle at the same time. How you see an electron—or any particle for that matter—depends on what kind of experiment you set up. So, Peter reasoned, another way to describe this wave-particle duality, and by extension much of what must be going on in the realm of the virtual—the realm of the fundamental energies of matter—is matching.

In the virtual, or quantum, world, all possible states coexist. This is called a superposition in quantum mechanics. However, when someone or something makes a measurement, some underlying process of matching goes on in the web of information that tests all possible states and selects the one that most closely matches the state under investigation. The act of measuring—which is a process of matching—collapses the wavefunction, which turns something virtual (neither measurable nor even knowable in either a quantitative or qualitative way) into something real (measurable, with identifiable characteristics) according to the context of the measurement. From the realm of the superposition of all possibilities, the entity under consideration displays one aspect of itself, which just happens to be the aspect that meets the conditions of the investigation.

Harry had spent years musing about the idea of matching information holograms at a distance, whereas Peter's focus had been more on how and where the information holograms were "located" in a wavefunction. As they meshed their ideas, a new understanding dawned. They envisioned another aspect of reality underlying the world of matter, in which information is continually weaving itself into a web of relationships. Perhaps, as the mystics say, consciousness is the ultimate "matchmaker." There was no way to know for sure, but one thing was certain to them: where there is order, there are rules or processes, and these could be useful for objectifying the process of measuring the energy and information of the body-field.

For example, they realized that nature does not decree that there be only one correct answer to a question. This insight has enormous implications for any healing biotechnology. Allopathic medicine recognizes this in its testing by denoting certain normal ranges for things, such as aspects of blood chemistry. The body has flexibility. It can handle fluctuations within certain parameters. Your cholesterol level should be below 200, so 175 is in the safe range, as is 183 and 167. It is not necessary to detect the one right answer when dealing with many of the parameters of the body, for the body at the systems level often doesn't need a single correct answer. The same is true of nature at large.

As Harry explained, "Nature seems to seek out the *best possible answer* from the many possibilities that fit the circumstances. This is different from the statistical probability that rules the quantum world. This is not about chance or randomness. It is more about emergence, ordering, pattern forming."

Nature as we know it, they reasoned, is the result of the information and energies of the universe making better and better matches. The result is an ever-increasing level of organization of nature over time, despite the reality of entropy (the tendency toward disorder or equilibrium). The self-organized, complex reality we live in may be an emergent property of nature's penchant for matching, and nature appears to be expert at finding the *best possible* matches. In a very real sense, the process of matching is an evolutionary one, with the best answers leaving their mark in the world of matter and the less efficient or suitable matches falling away. All of Peter's matching experiments could be explained according to this process, with the degree of indicator drop in the machine signaling the strength of the match between the energetic signature of two items being tested.

Peter had been startled at some of his findings in the early testing, back in the mid-1980s, for he discovered that some matches seemed to disappear when a better or more appropriate match was made. He said, "This was curiously unscientific! Science demands repeatability. Yet in biochemistry, things are different. We know that when the body manufactures the complex molecules of a hormone or an enzyme and it doesn't have access to a key ingredient during that process, it can make a substitution. Some enzymes, for example, can substitute copper for zinc. The body, in effect, is choosing the best solution to the problem at hand. This kind of inquiry led me to the idea of context. A match is made in context, and a best match is relative to that context. That idea describes how medicine works."

The notion of scale also was important, with larger matching patterns forming from the many smaller, previous matches, which would partly explain emergence and phase changes. In nature, there are finely tuned constants that are necessary for life. At the largest scales, there are the finely tuned cosmological constants that make our universe possible. At the other end of the scale, there are the precise parameters that make life possible, such as the precisely ordered sequences of amino acids that must form to create the proteins that do the most crucial work in the body. If you change any of these constants by even a tiny bit, there is no universe as we know it and no amino acids stringing themselves together in useful ways.

However, it also is true that most of life persists not because of precision, but because of flexibility. Life is characterized by its amazing ability to adapt and change, to continually interact with its environment. This adaptability means that the range of possible matches that information and energy can make for life to gain hold and flourish are quite wide indeed. A match can only be considered the best match within the context of the circumstances. Hence, biologists have found microbes thriving in the most inhospitable of places, from the hottest or most barren deserts to the coldest expanses of the polar regions. What works under one set of circumstances (or at one scale) can be deadly under another, and life, obviously, has figured out how to use the energy and information of a particular environment to its own benefit. At a theoretical level, it appeared to Harry and Peter that the deepest, most potent creative processes of life were dependent on this continual matching process.

So, what exactly is a best-possible match? The answer is that it all depends on the question or context. Consider the following example: A man, Jim, was born on January 12, 1978. On January 13, 2008, you are asked, "How old is Jim?" You could give several answers that would be more or less accurate and informative: Jim is thirty years old, Jim is between twenty-nine and thirty-one years old, Jim is less than forty years old, and so on. The most factually accurate answer of the choices mentioned above is that Jim is thirty years old, but any of these answers would be a fairly accurate assessment of Jim's age depending on what you need the information for. As you refine the context of your question (your question can be thought of as a measurement parameter), *the less desirable answers drop out first, and the matches get better and better.*

How might matching work in the natural world? What might be the mechanisms? Former professor of philosophy Ervin Laszlo tackles this question in his book *Science and the Akashic Field: An Integral Theory of Everything.* His Akashic Field, or as he more colloquially calls it, the A-field, is similar to, if indeed not equivalent to, the zero-point field. He wrote, "that the A-field informs all things with all other things follows as the simplest and most meaningful explanation of the nonlocality and entanglement we have encountered in physics and in cosmology, as well as in biology and in consciousness research."[1] He explained that although the A-field cannot be perceived directly, just as the gravitational field cannot, its effects can be perceived in the real world, and these effects are a result of how the A-field conveys information between things that match, or correlate. He wrote:

> The A-field conveys the most direct, intense, and therefore evident information between things that are closely similar to one another

(i.e., that are "isomorphic"—have the same basic form). This is because A-field information is carried by superposed vacuum wave-interference patterns that are equivalent to holograms. We know that in a hologram every element meshes with isomorphic elements: with those that are similar to it. Scientists call such meshing "conjugation"—a holographic pattern is *conjugate* with similar patterns in any assortment of patterns, however vast.[2]

Edgar Mitchell, former astronaut and founder of the Institute of Noetic Sciences, and his collaborators have applied similar ideas to the study of consciousness, which he believes is holographic and claims arises as a result of "phase-conjugate-adaptive-resonance."[3] This is a mathematics term that describes how resonance takes place: entities in the universe—including consciousness and other nonmaterial things—meet or move into union when they resonate because they share a similar (conjugate) energetic relationship through their wave phase relationships. Those phase relationships carry information. Both Laszlo and Mitchell, and others, describe mechanisms that so far have not been measured explicitly—or have they? Peter's matching experiments seem to indicate that he has in fact found a way to measure the effects of the holographic resonances of the human body-field and the structures in space that are created by these resonances. His matches reveal the conjugate systems between the body-field and physical body.

In NES terms, matching might best be described as a process by which similarities and differences become describable. Matching occurs between what we call "structures of information." Information is as real as energy, and like energy it can be ordered and disordered. The massive amounts of information that underlie the human body aggregate and so structure themselves in specific ways to form a larger, ordered, self-organizing structure that we call the human body-field. The body-field is like a set of nested systems within systems, and aggregation—the process by which larger and more ordered information systems emerge from interconnections among smaller, underlying subsystems—is a dynamic process whereby various kinds of structured information combine, interact, and inform each other to form the big body-field.

Harry had thought a lot about how these ideas could be refined to construct a better biotechnology. Many biotechnologies try to determine the one correct answer to a question. They might determine, for instance, that an organ or organism had a specific vibration or frequency. They test the body for this signature message, and if they do not find it or find a distorted message, then they try to give the body the corrective vibration or frequency. Depending on the machine, the corrective message might be sent via an auditory tone, electrical pulse, or colored light. Theoretically, this kind of approach would work, but—and this was the big "but" for Harry and Peter—it would deal largely, or even only, with the electromagnetic aspects of the body. Peter was convinced there was a deeper reality to the body-field and body. Plus, even if a distorted frequency is reset to the correct one, the process is a reactive approach to health, not unlike that of allopathic medicine, rather than a proactive one, because the *consequence* (or symptom) of the underlying energetic problem is what is addressed, not the *underlying process itself.* In other words, if the liver "goes out," such biotechnologies would attempt to reset the liver's natural vibration, but they wouldn't deal with the reason why that organ lost its natural frequency in the first place.

Peter and Harry wanted to approach energetic healing from an entirely different perspective. The human body operates within a range of parameters, so any test would have to be sensitive to the *relative* nature of how it functions. It might be more useful, they reasoned, to design a biotechnology that could test for the functional integrity of the body-field—how all the processes were functioning relative to one another and to the environment, instead of in isolation. Peter had a theoretical model of the body-field that explained these underlying matching processes. Peter's understanding of the human body-field was that it is dynamic, ever changing, so any corrections to it would be relative. There is a complex interconnectedness among the thousands of body functions, and the body, ultimately, is regulated by the body-field. Therefore, at the systems level—that of the full body-field—there would be more than one way for the body-field to make corrections to return the body to homeostasis. The process, of course, works in both constructive (as in increasing organization and well-being) and destructive (as in deterioration or illness) ways. In the body, there is a sensitivity to scale: the body can accommodate many small distortions, but when the changes aggregate, these small errors create larger, more serious problems at the systems level, degrading the system's function over time if the errors are left uncorrected. Peter was growing more and more interested in the idea of aggregation, because the big body-field, as a field of information that is structured in specific ways, is composed of systems and subsystems. Aggregation could be thought of as a dynamic process whereby various kinds of structured, conjugate information combine, interact, and inform each other to form the big body-field.

The uniqueness and power of Peter's approach was that it got to the heart of how energy fields are organized—how the matching is taking place in the body. Instead of trying to impress a fix on the body, which is a static approach to healing, the biotechnology he and Harry would create would determine how best to match the *dynamic* processes of the body-field. If they could interpret the *relationships* among dynamic matching patterns—and all of Peter's research had been leading in that direction—then they could better determine how the underlying distortions of the body-field were affecting biochemistry and, hence, physiology. In this way, clinicians could work with, rather than in spite of, the body's own self-healing control mechanisms.

Harry had a sense of how to make a match to a client's dynamic body-field using a QED field, which is put out by the computer processor itself, and software programmed with certain kinds of algorithms (a process that remains NES proprietary, intellectual property). The software would analyze the body-field scan to determine the relative best match from a range of many possible matches. Peter had a theory of the body-field that was comprehensive enough to be of real value clinically because it was not grounded in metaphysical energies but was, instead, relating quantum fields to the actual anatomy and physiology of the body. His esoteric matching experiments had yielded a plethora of connections to hard biological data so that any quantum-field matches (space resonances) made in a scan of a person's body-field could be tagged to the biochemistry and physiology of the physical body.

As they continued talking during this first face-to-face meeting, Peter's more than twenty years of data-gathering and theory were catalyzed by Harry's philosophical and technological insights. They formulated a plan to create a biotechnology based on Peter's model of an energetic biology of the human body-field and an energetic pathology of illness and health. However, Harry also wanted to experience Peter's remedies for himself. He would test the remedies to see if they helped his CFS. So that work, too, began during this visit.

———◆———

Peter began treating Harry by giving him a remedy he made for the Flaviviridae virus, which Peter believed was largely responsible for CFS. The remedies he was using at that time were meridian complexes, that is, they were modeled after Peter's earlier work exploring the meridians, although his spiderweb diagram had revealed that the group of twelve compartments had a specific sequence that deviated from the order specified in traditional Chinese medicine. The liquid remedies were taken, as the new Infoceuticals are now, as drops in a small glass of water. Harry reacted within a few days of taking the general Flaviviridae remedy, experiencing a detoxification episode in the form of severe flulike symptoms.

As previously stated, a flulike episode is a common, although by no means universal, reaction when the body moves from being compromised energetically, and hence physically, to becoming functional again. As the body's immune systems begin to fully function again, the person may experience muscle aches, fever, headache, fatigue, and the other symptoms of an actual flu. In complementary medicine circles, this initial reaction to a treatment is often referred to as a healing reaction.[4] Although a patient may initially feel as though he or she is getting sicker for a short time, the flulike episode actually indicates that the body is finally doing what it is supposed to be doing—responding to an imbalance, perhaps caused by a foreign invader such as a virus or bacteria. Usually, a healing reaction passes within a few days to a week.

Harry was forced back into bed for part of the time Peter was visiting, but by the end of Peter's stay, Harry was feeling much better. Peter warned Harry that correcting the root problem would take longer than a few weeks, for Peter knew that relapses are common with CFS. He had worked out a theory of the mutation of the virus through different energetic compartments of the body-field to explain the relapses, and he knew that there were many aspects of Harry's body-field that would require correction. It had taken Peter nearly ten years to recover from CFS himself, so he warned Harry that his own recovery would take time. Peter impressed on Harry that he would continue treating him only if he agreed to follow his instructions to the letter. Harry agreed. So before he returned to Australia, Peter left Harry with several remedies, which they would eventually develop into some of the Energetic Integrator Infoceuticals, to correct distortions in specific compartments of his body-field.

As Harry took these remedies and his body began to work more efficiently, he experienced additional healing reactions. Harry explained that "Peter's system of testing showed correlations to environmental toxins, particularly cadmium, dioxin, radiation, organochlorides, and organophosphates. Immunity is heavily affected by energy compartments 4, 10, and 11, and these showed significant damage in me. . . . The main distortions in compartments 4, 10, and 11 are energetically related to hormones (compartment 11, correlating to the male hormones), causing severe stress, which in turn affected compartments 1, 7, and 12. Compartment 7 especially links with the cerebral cortex and, as such, was the probable correlation to the decline previously of my mental functioning, which ran the gamut from a growing phobia about driving and dyslexia to more physical things like tremors in my hands. I knew it would take many, many months of using the remedies to clean up my body and bring it back to normal."

Harry experienced unexpected emotional responses to the remedies, including vivid dreams. He said, "The combination of remedies for compartments 1, 7, and 12 began unblocking years of bottled up emotions. I began to get amazing flashbacks and realizations, mostly in dreams, into the significant events that had shaped my life. I had what I can only describe as a sort of peace or feelings of resolution."

Harry precisely followed Peter's instructions, and after a few months on the remedies, he felt much better. In fact, he thought he was back to normal, if not cured, but Peter knew better. He had worked with scores of CFS clients, and he knew from their and his own experience that relapses are a problem. Getting better took time, often a year or longer, and if clients stopped the program after their first "feeling like myself again" period, they were bound to slip back into suffering because the body-field was not yet fully functional.

Despite the relief his clients had experienced over time, and even their complete remission from their conditions, Peter had never been happy with the remedies, which were still not much more than energetic meridian complexes. He felt they did not work as well—or as predictably—as his theory suggested they could. As he explained his reservations about the remedies to Harry, they began to discuss Peter's ideas of the energetic compartments of the body-field as structures in space. He and Harry discussed how frequency plays a part in the compartments because each compartment seems to work within a specific frequency range. However, frequency is about electromagnetism and time. Peter knew by then, even if he couldn't prove it, that the human body-field is dependent more on ultrahigh-frequency quantum waves than on electromagnetic ones, and time, he knew, is not well understood in quantum mechanics. Many of the quantum mathematical equations work just as well if you are plotting a particle's motion backward in time as if you are plotting it forward

in time, as was evident in the revolutionary work in quantum electrodynamics done by Feynman in his path integrals work and the
technique called "sum over histories."

The twelve compartments of the body-field are, as Peter stated, "structures that are specific to frequency ranges, but they are more than just
those frequency ranges." What Peter felt he was doing was tied directly
to how those structures—the holographic channels of linked information
in the body-field that drive biochemistry in the body—become distorted,
so that information becomes degraded or misdirected. Peter was not sure
exactly what he could do to make the remedies better, and his discussions
with Harry about the compartments as structures—or more accurately as
arrangements—in space had been rather abstract, to say the least. At one
point in their conversation about this topic during their California visit,
Harry, ever the one to get directly to the point, had simply said, "Well,
why don't you just correct the structures in space instead of trying to
correct energetic copies of meridians?"

Peter remembers the shock he felt when he understood what Harry
was saying: that he should move from the real to the virtual, from the
actual ampoules containing imprinted information of meridians, which
carry only a small portion of the information flowing through the
body, to the way the space resonances actually carry information. "It
just sort of hit me, when he said that. I had tried to do something like
that back in 1998, but I hadn't gotten anywhere. I didn't really know
what to do, but when Harry said that, so point blank, I knew he got
what I was trying to say. By that one comment, I knew that he believed
in what I was doing. That was huge for me! I was used to being dismissed as some kind of crank, but he believed I could do it. So when I
returned home, I tried again to measure the compartment structures as
if they were space resonances, and I did it! I figured it out. Of course,
it took years of me and Harry working together to perfect the range of
remedies, but that comment started me on the right road again."

7

THE DREAM IS
REALIZED

WHEN PETER RETURNED TO AUSTRALIA, he immediately began to explore the ways he could improve on the remedies to help Harry get over his relapse more quickly and make a lasting recovery. Peter had expected Harry's relapse, and he also knew that he had a lot riding on helping Harry get better. If he did, then they would collaborate in making a clinical system a reality, meaning that his years of painstaking work might finally see the light of day in a broader health care setting. Otherwise, he knew he might continue toiling in the dank backwaters of subtropical Australia forever.

Peter said, "Harry had a typical problem that occurs with CFS patients. They don't want to eat, which further weakens them. He had terrible nutritional problems. From my knowledge of traditional Chinese medicine, I knew his stomach meridian was a problem, but I wondered where to start. I knew from homeopathy and other traditions about all the things that can go wrong with the stomach, that it is a place where toxins such as cadmium end up, but I was not about to treat 'like with like,' which is a law of homeopathy. I vowed early on never to give any toxin to the body, even in an energetic form. I didn't then, and we still don't now with our fully developed NES Infoceuticals. Instead I went back to the matching idea and my matching experiments. I needed to find out more about what talks to what in the stomach, what is energetically linked, what is pushing what in terms of energy and information regulation processes. I was looking for what drives the system, and that is how the Driver Infoceuticals came about and where they got their name. If Dr. Reid had taught me anything, it was to look for what powers things."

In traditional Chinese medicine, there is the idea of the "orbs" of the body as major energetic functional units. *Orbs* is an archaic term for the organs, such as the pancreas or lungs. Peter said, "I knew about the orbs, and I also knew that you can't get energy from nowhere, and I reasoned that some parts of the stomach must be contributing energy to the field, while other parts might not. I did many, many matching experiments to see what talked to what, what aspects of the stomach's cellular anatomy were pushing energy in the big body-field, and I worked it out. My technique, as I have said, is proprietary, but when I made that first Driver remedy—Stomach Driver—and Harry took it, it worked! Although two days after taking it, he experienced a major stomach detox!"

Harry indeed had experienced the effects of the Stomach Driver remedy. Since he became ill with CFS, he had experienced stomach pains, sometimes so severe that he would double over. Allopathic tests had shown a negative result for any physical problems, and no conventional treatments had helped, but after only two days of taking the Stomach Driver, Harry began experiencing a healing reaction, mainly in the area of his intestines and colon. For a few days his stools became especially odorous, and he felt mild stomach pain. His digestive system quickly recovered, and as he continued to take Stomach Driver he noticed he was no longer bloated, which had been a chronic condition throughout his years of CFS, and he no longer had stomach pains.

As Peter explained to Harry, the Stomach Driver remedy had provided information to his body-field that it needed to direct the proper functioning of his physical body, in this case the stomach and intestines. After his organs started working correctly, there was no longer a hospitable environment in which pathogens could thrive, so his body was able to shed them. In effect, his bowel flora balance had shifted. His body was doing what it was designed to do—after the information it needed had been restored.

Over the next several months, Peter worked out the dynamics of how the nervous system, heart, and lungs each worked as "drivers," or generators, of energy for the full body-field. He made Driver remedies for these systems and sent them to Harry, who experienced varied healing reactions as he took them. For example, he had been a smoker, and the Lung Driver remedy had an immediate effect on his lung system. For a few days he coughed up thick mucus, perhaps from the cadmium and other tobacco-based toxins that had accumulated over the years from smoking. Soon, however, he felt that he could breathe freely and deeply again, something he had not felt in nearly a decade.

The energetic correction to his nervous system resulted in subtler kinds of reactions. Harry said, "I noticed a really peculiar change. I went from a pattern of being permanently wired and then being completely drained to feeling more balanced. I had always tended to overdo things and then would collapse as a result. Now I was actually feeling quite relaxed. I had the most normal sleep I had had in years. I was still tired, but it was a relaxed sort of tired, almost as if my body was finally catching up on years' worth of rest. It was like all those years of driving myself dropped away. My body knew it was time to recuperate. I was, of course, at that time still trying to get a business off the ground, but I was suddenly very much more relaxed about it and, as a result, produced a higher quality of work even while recovering from illness. I am convinced I would have healed even more quickly if I had not had the pressure of starting a business."

Peter also was further developing early versions of what would become the Energetic Integrator Infoceuticals. As Harry took those, he soon noticed that he was regaining his coordination and balance. The improvements continued, and within five months Harry was actually rock climbing again. As he resumed climbing, he noticed other changes.

Chronic pain from an old shoulder injury had disappeared. The muscles around his left forearm, which had atrophied slightly and so were less developed compared with those around his other forearm, started to fill out. His hands and feet were no longer perpetually cold, his allergies disappeared, and his mental clarity returned. In fact, Harry felt he was in better shape than he had been even in his healthy, pre-CFS days.

Today, Harry likes to caution people that he and Peter often took much larger doses of those prototype Infoceuticals than are recommended with the new, more refined, and hence more effective Infoceuticals. Healing reactions are not universal, especially not to the severity of those Harry experienced. Furthermore, Peter's research over the past three years has significantly furthered their knowledge about both specific energy arrangements in the body-field and the sequence in which the body-field is best corrected, so a NES protocol today would differ significantly from what Harry experienced only a few years ago.

While Harry was recovering, he and Peter kept in constant contact, and Peter even flew to the United States to see Harry again. During that second visit, they formalized their collaboration. They would call their business Nutri-Energetics Systems, because of their view that information was like a life-sustaining nutrient for the human body-field and that there was a system to healing that involved many facets that had to be coordinated into an integrated whole. The liquid remedies would be called Infoceuticals, because they input quantum-field information directly into the body-field. The Energetic Drivers had already been named, but a new term was coined for the twelve meridian-like compartments—Energetic Integrators. (For a more detailed discussion of Integrators, Drivers, and other body-field components, see chapter 9 and the specific sections in part 3.) These are the routes for information in the body-field that are arranged in a precise order according to frequency. (After additional research, Peter and Harry realized they were organized according to phase as well, as discussed in chapter 13.) The Energetic Integrators turned out to be much more than traditional meridians, for they are linked to specific biochemical and physiological processes. They also have a specific sequence, or order, that when followed leads to better clinical results.

Peter and Harry also started talking seriously about the technical end of things. Harry flew a computer programmer over from England to start the process of turning Peter's data into a workable software program. Peter had been refining and reorganizing his data all along, but before the actual computer programming was to begin, he wanted to check and recheck his data. (It would take almost a year to get the program written and tested, but, amazingly, the system worked the first time they tried it.)

Peter had brought some of his equipment with him on this second trip, and he carried out various preliminary experiments based on his and Harry's brainstorming sessions. He had been mulling over Harry's advice about the Energetic Integrators—to try to directly correct the structures in space of these channels, rather than try to correct energetic copies of meridians. Each Energetic Integrator covered dozens of specific kinds of information, from how elements are used in the body to specific cellular functions to data on particular parts of organs or body systems. Peter's tests had become so specific that he was able to pinpoint energetic-physical links to a very fine degree. For example, the paranasal sinuses are found in Energetic Integrator 1, but the frontal sinus is in Energetic Integrator 5 and the maxillary sinuses are in 11. It would be much too complex to try to pinpoint the actual distortion in the body-field for every part of the body. Instead, Harry and Peter reasoned, they could deal with the distortion of the larger structure—the *entire* Integrator—within which that specific information flowed. So instead of trying to fix any errors in the hundreds of discrete pieces of information that flowed through a single Integrator, Peter instead would optimize the Integrator structure itself.

What are these Integrator structures? There are various ways to describe them, all of them rather abstract. Peter explained, "They are compartments within quantum fields, but as a group they are much broader than that in nature. They can be most easily grasped by thinking about them as arrangements of information in space. All information exchange takes place via the interaction of energized electrons, which changes the resonance, or as I like to call it, the permittivity, of space."

Peter further explained, "These Integrators, these arrangements of information or self-organizing informational structures, can be represented by mathematical data sets. Through the matching experiments, I got all sorts of data, sets of numbers. Language really is a problem here. What are numbers? Abstract things, but they explain nature, as all of physics demonstrates. You can think of them as representing arrangements not of energy, but of information. All of physics, in the Standard Model, is about energy transfer, but what I am focused on is *information* transfer. That is a huge shift in focus! I am talking about the holographic information that rides on top of the physical, energetic waves, be they electromagnetic or otherwise. In NES we are interested in the arrangement of information, not the energy, which is why we are doing something completely different from all others, such as those researchers who are looking into biophotons, or light in the body.

"To get a structure in space," he continued, "you have to get repeated locations or arrangements of data. The structure represents the *repeatability* of that same arrangement in space. We are talking about quantum space here, not the ether or the air or any physical, classical space. You have to get past geometry, so you can't really visualize any of this. It's hard to wrap your mind around it!

"This field structure, this holographic arrangement of information, can be so strong that it is self-organizing—it returns to its original configuration or sequence or whatever you want to call it even after it is disturbed. Normal physics, even quantum physics, except perhaps in the case of Richard Feynman's work, says it is not possible to find such things, locations of quantum things in time, but I did! I am saying there are more rules in nature than current quantum mechanics has so far found. That's a huge statement, I know. I admit I was off on my own, doing my own thing, and coming up with sets of data that could actually *do* things. Conventional science would say, 'No, you can't do that, it's not possible,' but it is! Then when talking to Harry during those two visits, I suddenly realized that with the Integrators all we had to do was to measure *how space was behaving when it was affected by different frequencies.* I thought to myself, 'Of course! It is the different frequencies that are the trouble!' but then I remembered that they are the frequencies of quantum physics, which are supposed to be impossible to measure.

"That thought did not stop me. I went straight away and tried the impossible. I used the apparatus I had first created in Australia and simply began to measure nothingness! Of course, what I was really measuring was the permittivity of space that I had termed an Energetic Integrator, but I surmised that there may be ranges of frequencies in the decadary scale that affected those structures, and, to my great surprise, sets of data appeared where, of course, there was supposed to be nothing. I was measuring space and how it was structured at different frequencies! I have to give Harry the credit, really, as the discovery was made at his prompting, when he suggested I try to make the Infoeculicals work to change the structure of space instead of sticking with the meridian complex idea.

"I have to admit that my brain just about collapsed under the weight of it all. It's like a Zen koan. There are answers, but they are not really answers as we expect answers to appear. They are not logical, or even explainable in some cases. That's why physicists say that the only way to truly grasp nature is to know the equations that support the concept.

"I had originally started with meridians, and in acupuncture there is an agreed-on sequence to how energy flows, but what I was finding went beyond that. Meridians are thought to be channels that work largely through connective tissue, which is only doing part of the work that needs to be done. They go deep, but not deep enough to really affect the whole big body-field, the full wave. When Harry suggested that I correct the structures in space and not the meridian complexes,

I ran with that idea. I dropped all my old data and sort of started from scratch. I dropped a lot of the Reid information and theory, too. The experiments I did to measure these things I call structures in space are proprietary, but I can tell you I got data. Lots of data!

"When space gets distorted, the electrons don't end up where they are supposed to be. It wasn't until then that I figured out that each Integrator had a sort of signature of the correct movement of electrons within a certain frequency range. Still another breakthrough came with the realization that there are 'constants' for each Integrator, which are data sets related to spin, frequency, and phase. Each Energetic Integrator covers a wide frequency range, from less than 1 hertz to about 10^{12} hertz. Today, we know phase also plays a major role in pathology. With this new data, things really started to work with the Integrator Infoceuticals, and we were able to imprint that data into the Infoceuticals. There is really no comparison between those early prototype remedies and the new range of Infoceuticals. They started out based mostly on the acupuncture meridians, but now they contain representations of *entire* meridians within them, but even that meridian information is only a tiny piece of the information imprinted into an Infoceutical, for they have become much broader than that."

As Peter and Harry worked to bring their biotechnology to life, and to market, they realized that education was going to be a big part of helping people understand their approach to health care. NES is based on a set of principles and concepts that is quite foreign to allopathic medicine. Because Peter was dealing with energetic structures, albeit quantum ones, and not the specific parts of the physical body per se, the clinical emphasis of the NES health care system is focused at the *energetic systems* level, not the *physical symptoms* level. The Infoceuticals do not directly affect anything physical in the body, for all of the organs and physiological processes and such are subsystems of the larger body, which itself is under the control, energetically, of the full bodyfield. So the NES–Professional System, the biotechnology that puts Peter's theory into clinical practice, is not designed to be diagnostic or to

treat or even to prevent disease in the allopathic sense. Unlike allopathic doctors, NES health care professionals do not need to determine
exactly what has gone wrong in the body or even what specific organ
or part of an organ is malfunctioning. Instead, the NES scan reveals
where the body-field is losing power (Energetic Drivers) and where
information is being degraded or misdirected (Energetic Integrators).
NES is concerned with the functional integrity of the body-field—with
how well aspects of it are working in comparison to the whole. By correcting a specific Energetic Integrator, any physiological function that
falls within that Ingegrator can be corrected. The body-field feeds that
information to the body, which knows what it needs and so uses only
what is useful to it at that time.

To use an analogy, NES is focused on the conductor of the orches-
tra (the big body-field), not on the individual musicians (the physical
aspects of the body). The fact is that everything in the body is so interconnected that trying to pinpoint a specific fix is nearly impossible or
causes other unintended problems, which is why pharmaceuticals so
often have unintended side effects. With NES, you are simply providing your body, via the body-field, with information that allows it once
again to do what it was originally designed to do, so that everything
works together smoothly and efficiently. In this way, NES does not
treat the body at all but instead simply provides information to jump-
start the body's own self-healing mechanisms and capabilities.

As Peter said, "With NES, we have a new theory of pathology, partly
based on Feynman's path integrals theory, as incredible as that may seem,
and more recently on Milo Wolff's space resonance theory, but, really,
pathology is as simple as this: electrons do what they should or they don't!
When they don't, we get problems in the body-field, and with time they
show up in the body. Of course, devising a system to fix what goes wrong
is amazingly complex. It took me nearly twenty years to get to the point
where I felt I had even the first real inkling of what was going in the body-
field. We have done an enormous amount of work, but much remains to
be done. The body-field is so marvelously intricate that it will take life-

times to figure it all out, but we have a good sense of how it is working at the holistic, systems level, and we are getting great clinical results just from correcting the body-field at that level."

Peter's refinement of the Infoceuticals took a considerable amount of time and involved the synthesis of many different types of information. For instance, during this explosive period of developmental research, he was able to tag the Infoceuticals to cells, organs, and other aspects of body structure and physiology. He explained, "I had made remedies with most everything in them except the constant. Harry and I made up some remedies that added the constant, but they were much too strong. That drove me back to the lab and more experiments. I found that if we added the constants as well as data about different types of cells associated with the organs for that Integrator or Driver, then we could get a good and tolerable effect. Some people could feel the effect of an Infoceutical in ten minutes! So that's how I really got into tagging the Infoceuticals, to further link the information—the virtual part of the body-field—to the real physiology of the body. It's only in this way that the Infoceuticals can be said to be directed toward the physical body at all, but it is really an energetic connection.

"There were some amazing results. The Infoceuticals can't hurt you, because they are simply information, and the body will only use what it needs or wants, but some of the ways they help can be unexpected, because everything is so connected in the body and we can't know all of those connections. The body is a vast network of communication pathways, and we certainly don't have them all mapped down to very fine levels. That will take lifetimes. I worked from the information back to what it matched in the body, but we can learn from things happening the other way around, too! Here is one story that demonstrates how we can work back from the real to the virtual:

"One lady who agreed to try the new Stomach Driver came to me and said, 'Did you know that I got a chiropractic adjustment from that Infoceutical?' I just said, 'What?' because I had no idea what she was talking about. So she went on, 'Yes, I took Stomach Driver and my back clicked!' Apparently she had a chronic disc problem in her lower back, and it resolved itself in only a matter of minutes from the effects of the Stomach Driver Infoceutical. The information—what we might call the virtual aspect of things—activated energetic connections that also helped correct a very real back problem. From that clue, I could go back to the lab and do a matching experiment to see if there actually was an energetic connection between the Stomach Driver and the spine.

"I never dismiss strange stories like this," Peter stated. "I am always curious enough to follow up on them. That particular result was pretty strange, and it sent me back into the lab to see what that could be about. I found through my matching tests that the segment of the spine she was talking about actually was related energetically to the stomach! I had never thought to test the two for a match, but it turns out that they are connected, they match, they 'talk' to each other—whatever you want to call it. You could say NES links with osteopathy and chiropractic!

"It doesn't always work out that way," Peter continued. "Sometimes people say that this or that happened, and I go to the lab and check, and the match cannot be verified. So perhaps it is just placebo, or something too complex for me to work out as yet, but many times it does work out, and we get a new piece of the body-field puzzle. Things like that happened all the time. There is so much to know, so many energetic links to know about this wonderful, complex thing we call the body that we don't even have the sense to know what questions to ask. We at NES are only doing a small piece of it all. We have done loads of testing and keep refining our understanding. NES practitioners have to be the kind of people who not only like being on the cutting edge of healing but want to constantly stay there because there is always more to know! We are only taking the first steps to a truly comprehensive energy medicine, a new view of energetic pathology."

———◆———

By 2004, Harry and the computer programmer had succeeded in finding a way to codify Peter's data and encode it in software. The next challenge was finding a way to standardize and automate the Infoceutical imprinting process. Imprinting by hand was a slow process, and the first several machines they built did not work well. It took six tries to finally engineer and build a machine that could reliably and accurately imprint the Infoceuticals with specific quantum information. Today, the bottles are filled at a commercial plant, which follows the latest safety and health quality-control standards. The energetic imprinting, however, is done by specially trained NES personnel. The process of imprinting is complex, but it involves converting the holographic information into data sets, creating large electrostatic fields, injecting photons of certain colors, and managing other physics and engineering parameters that are proprietary to NES.

Beyond figuring out how to represent the holographic information, Peter and Harry had to find a carrier substance for this information in the Infoceuticals. The liquid in the Infoceuticals is purified water, but the quantum data must be energized, or imprinted, onto a physical medium, called the carrier, in that water, and not into the water itself. Although nature seems to be able to imprint information into biological water, no one has figured out how to mimic nature, at least not for complex data sets. The dilution–succussion method of homeopathy works but is not a very efficient system, and the water has to be imprinted using actual physical substances that are believed to stimulate a healing response, which severely limits the kinds of information that can be imprinted. Peter and Harry were not seeking to give the body the imprint of a corrective physical substance; they were seeking to directly imprint abstract information, the data sets derived from Peter's matching experiments. They spent months testing dozens of substances until they found that the most stable and reliable carrier material was a collection of plant-derived minerals. When you take an Infoceutical as drops in water, these micronutrients carry the information into your body, where the information is made available to your body-field. Every bottle of NES Infoceuticals carries the same few physical ingredients, so you can't tell them apart by the ingredients list. The differences are in the information encoded into them, so that Liver Driver, for example, is encoded with different information than Source Driver or Muscle Driver.

Peter and Harry's collaboration quickly bore fruit, and in July 2004 Peter relocated from Australia to England to work with Harry, who had returned home after more than a year in the United States. The first NES clinical system was introduced that same summer, although because of continuing research the software has undergone several updates and the NES clinical protocol has changed over time. As Peter continued his research, he developed more and more Infoceuticals (which are discussed in detail in part 3). For example, in the early days of NES there was only one Big Field Infoceutical, which dealt with the body-field's alignment with Earth energies such as the magnetic polar and equatorial axes.* A related Infoceutical—the Polarity Infoceutical—has since been added to deal with the body-field's relation to electrostatic fields. Originally there were only eleven Energetic Drivers, but more have been added, for a total of sixteen as of this writing. In the early days, there also were more than two dozen other kinds of Infoceuticals, called Shock Adjusters, each of which addressed a specific type of information distortion, such as for emotional stress, audio or visual acuity, female cycle, electromagnetic fields, nerve detoxification, and body-field collapse. All of these, except for the Emotional Stress Release Infoceutical, have been replaced by Energetic Star Infoceuticals, the newest class of remedies, which work as major "unblockers" of the body-field and energetically correlate to metabolic pathways in the body. Another class of Infoceuticals called Energetic Terrains also was developed. The Terrains deal with energetic environments in the body that can host pathogens, such as viruses and bacteria, or their energetic imprints.

Before we move to part 3 and the details of the NES system of healing, however, it is important to cover one last aspect of the theo-

---

*The Big Field, and the related Infoceutical, refers to natural Earth fields and is not to be confused wih the big body-field. The Big Field is discussed in detail in chapter 11.

retical development of NES—the physics that best explains Peter's data. We have alluded to this aspect of physics in this and previous chapters, but no real details have been provided. The next chapter explains that theory. You are free to skip it if you are not interested in the physics, but if you are wondering what those structures in space are that Peter keeps referring to, then you will want to read about Wolff and his space resonance theory. Wolff's theory provides a quantum window into understanding what may be going on in the human body-field, and for that matter, may explain how matter in general comes into being.

8

NES AND THE
FRONTIERS OF PHYSICS

PETER HAD SPENT DECADES amassing reliable experimental data, but he did not have a theory to explain it adequately. Various aspects of traditional and frontier physics—for example, Coopers Pairs, Feynman's path integrals, quantum entanglement, sync and complexity theory, and Harold Aspden's model of the electron's magnetic moment—have relevance to some of Peter's data, but no widely accepted physics theory could account for the entire body of his data.

Then, in 2005, Peter came across space resonance theory, a quantum electrodynamics (QED) theory proposed by US astrophysicist Milo Wolff, and it was as though the proverbial lightbulb went on. Wolff's theory provides a theoretical underpinning for the human body-field and, by extension, for biology in general. Space resonance theory (also called the wave structure of matter theory[1]) is itself frontier science because it is not widely known within the physics community and at first appears to be incompatible with the Standard Model of physics. However, as we discussed briefly in chapter 2, several recent experiments, such as those by Shahriar Afshar, lend credence to wave-dominant theories in general and to Wolff's model of the photon in particular.

What's so radical about space resonance theory? For starters, it suggests that there are only three fundamental particles—electrons, protons, and neutrons—but that they aren't particles, they are waves (although, as confusing as it is, Wolff, like all physicists, refers to them as particles as a matter of convenience and because that is the accepted parlance of physics). The theory states that they are the result of the interaction of two spherical standing waves, which Wolff calls the In wave and the Out wave. The photon, and all the other particles, are appearances created by the interaction of electrons as the quality—or resonance—of space changes during different kinds of In wave and Out wave interactions. We will look at Wolff's theory in detail, but let's first consider the challenges he faced in proposing any viable new theory at all. Quantum mechanics is the most well-verified theory in the history of physics, so overthrowing its main tenets would take persuasive evidence. It's worth our time to take a quick look at how science is not really as cut-and-dried as we have been led to believe. Within the scientific community, debate rages about what science means and how conflicting theories provide alternative explanations about how the natural world works.

SCIENCE AS COMPETING IDEAS

As quantum mechanics developed in the early- to mid-twentieth century, it became clear that it had to be joined with relativity theory if it was going to go the distance in describing nature. This was accomplished through QED, which grounds itself in Schrödinger's wave equation, which describes waves as having both quantum and relativistic properties. However, making that connection raised profound questions and involved some mathematical sleight of hand. As an illustration of the problem, let's look at the electron's spin.

Among QED's main difficulties was that it could not describe the electron's spin value. Spin is a curious property in quantum physics that describes a particle's intrinsic angular momentum. It is an inherent property of quantum objects, rather like mass or charge, and it can have a positive or a negative value. Quantum spin is counterintuitive, even bizarre. This is not spin as you might think about it in the physical world, such as a top spinning or Earth rotating on its axis. If an electron were to spin in the classical sense, like a rotating top, it would have to go around *twice* to get back to its starting point. In the classical sense of rotation, an electron's spin is 720 degrees, not 360 degrees. In the quantum sense, if you "rotate" an electron 360 degrees, you get the electron's opposite phase value.

What's more, although spin is often used as a defining characteristic of a *particle,* it actually refers to the quantum entity's *wave* nature. An electron with spin 1/2 is not the same particle as an electron with spin −1/2 , because their quantum waves differ. Wolff pointed out that calling electrons "particles" is a "historical blunder from the days before spin had been measured."[2] (Another point worth mentioning is that no two identical particles with the same spin can exist in the same state together. This is the Pauli exclusion principle, which has profound implications for chemistry. The periodic table of elements is built on this organizing principle, although no one knows why nature should be this way. However, the Pauli exclusion principle is violated in some cases, such as helium He^4.)

That the Schrödinger wave equation could not describe an electron's spin was a major problem in the then young science of quantum mechanics, one that was eventually solved by physicist Paul Dirac. The Dirac equation revealed not only the electron's spin but also its magnetic moment as well. (A particle's magnetic moment results from its spin within a magnetic field; ultimately the magnetic moments of groups of particles give rise to the magnetic field we feel in the real, physical world.) However, the Dirac equation had problems of its own; for one, it contained infinities. Infinity is a number to avoid in the mathematics of most physics theories, because no *measurable* value can have an infinite value. In physics, it is not useful for explaining reality to assume that an object or body has infinite energy or infinite mass. So physicists came up with a way to delete the infinities from their mathematics, using a process called renormalization.

How do infinities creep into quantum mechanics? Remember from our discussion in chapter 1 that a quantum particle is really not like a little billiard ball but is instead more like an inherently fuzzy probability cloud. Physicists reduce quantum entities to precise points, which they call particles, for various reasons, not the least of which are that they are easier to visualize than waves and the mathematics is more manageable. However, when they reduce a quantum object to a point-particle, that particle's self-energy becomes infinitely large, which is not only physically impossible but also makes the equations nonsensical and, hence, useless for describing the physical world. By using the mathematical technique of renormalization, physicists got rid of the infinities but still produced predictions that matched experimental results.

Although the mathematical technique worked beautifully, renormalization bothered mathematical purists. Dirac wrote, "This is not sensible mathematics. Sensible mathematics involves neglecting a quantity when it turns out to be small—not neglecting it because it is infinitely large and you do not want it! Of course, the proper inference is that the basic equations are not right. There must be some drastic changes introduced into them so that no infinities occur in the theory at all."[3] Richard Feynman, considered one of the fathers of QED theory, also was uncomfortable with renormalization, even though he helped develop it, calling it "hocus-pocus" and a "shell game." Other physicists weren't so bothered by the mathematics or their peers' objections to it, noting that the equations worked to make accurate predictions and that was all that mattered. Physicist Steven Weinberg, for instance, pointed out that "we very much need a guiding principle like renormalizability to help us pick the quantum field theory of the real world out of the infinite variety of conceivable quantum field theories."[4] To his credit, he recognized that although renormalization helped physicists pick a good theory, it didn't help them explain *why* that theory was the correct one to explain the real world.

Although most physicists jumped on the point-particle theory bandwagon, a few dissenters continued to look for alternatives, sticking more closely to field or wave theories. In the mid-1980s, two frontier theories emerged that solved the infinities problem in new ways: John G. Cramer's transactional interpretation (TI) and Wolff's space resonance theory. Cramer's theory does not do away with particles, although it posits a deep, intrinsic wave nature to reality that takes precedence over particles. He describes his theory as follows:

> The TI permits quantum mechanical wavefunctions to be interpreted as real waves physically present in space rather than as "mathematical representations of knowledge" as in the CI [Copenhagen Interpretation]. The TI is shown to provide insight into the complex character of the quantum mechanical state vector and the mechanism associated with its "collapse." The TI also leads in a natural way to justification of the Heisenberg uncertainty principle and the Born probability law, basic elements of the CI.[5]

Cramer's theory explains how "advanced" waves (waves moving backward in time) and "retarded" waves (waves moving forward in time) make a "handshake" in space that results in interactions we characterize as particles. They form a standing wave that appears to an observer as a particle. His theory resolves almost all of the paradoxes of quantum mechanics, many of which occur only when physicists insist that particles are real. These paradoxes include two of the most bizarre features of the Standard Model of quantum physics: wave-particle duality and nonlocality. (See discussion in chapter 2.)

Wolff's theory also explains away the same quantum paradoxes and is built around a spherical standing wave created by the interaction of what he calls In waves and Out waves. However, Wolff's theory goes further than Cramer's theory by positing that there are only three fundamental particles: the electron, proton, and neutron; all other particles are what physicist Erwin Shrödinger called Schaumkommen, or appearances.

A physicist who wants to do away with quantum particles is most certainly a heretic. Although the Standard Model has myriad problems, it also has been stunningly successful as a predictive theory. So beyond the problem of renormalization, why would anyone really want to get rid of most particles? Wolff, in his book *Exploring the Physics of the Unknown Universe,* lists the pros and cons of particles as follows:[6]

▶ Despite enormous effort at trying, no one has yet been able to detect a central structure for the electron. It does not appear to be particle-like in that it has no real structure.

▶ The mathematics of the Standard Model, and of other widely accepted quantum theories, cannot predict the electron's size, mass or charge. There are no meaningful calculations that quantify the electron, which means that you don't "need a particle concept because all the calculations are the same whether or not you believe in particles."

▶ Because mass can be converted to electromagnetic energy, which has no mass, there is no real "substantiality" to the concept of mass, and hence of particles.

Wolff finds only three plausible reasons for scientists' insistence on retaining a particle-based view of quantum reality:

▶ It is extremely useful in engineering calculations to approximate mass as being at a precise point, even if it really isn't.

▶ Particle theory has been taught in physics and engineering schools for decades and so is too useful a concept to throw out too quickly.

▶ Our sensory organs (particularly our eyes) and conventional technology (such as most microscopes) cannot distinguish wavelengths smaller than visible light. Smaller objects appear to be point-like. As a result, the concept of points, and by extension point-like quantum particles, is fixed in our senses, emotions, and traditions.

However, Wolff realizes that such quantum properties as spin, mass, and charge—which are associated in the Standard Model with particles—are real, so any quantum theory has to account for them. How do you do that without having particles? Let's look at Wolff's answer, although our overview of his theory by necessity must be brief and, hence, incomplete. We refer you to his book for a full explanation of his theory and its reconceptualization of some of mainstream physics' most ingrained and cherished assumptions.

MILO WOLFF'S
SPACE RESONANCE THEORY

Wolff's space resonance theory is built on the electron. However, because the Standard Model identifies the photon as the particle that carries force, or energy, between electrons, it is, by extension, also a crucial player in Wolff's theory, although he views it in radically different ways than do most physicists. In space resonance theory, coupled oscillators replace the photon as the energy carrier "particle" between electrons. As stated previously, oscillators are systems or entities that spontaneously begin to resonate, that is, to cycle together in a steady and repeating rhythm. Oscillators are said to be coupled when some mechanism allows two or more oscillators to influence each other and act as a single unit. As scientist Steve Strogatz wrote of sync, the science of coupled oscillators, "Planets tug on one another with gravity. Heart cells pass electrical currents back and forth. As these examples suggest, nature uses every available channel to allow its oscillators to talk to one another. And the result of those conversations is often synchrony, in which all the oscillators begin to move as one."[7] In Wolff's theory, spherical standing waves act as coupled oscillators, and they have a number of advantages over particles, such as being able to explain non-locality (Einstein's spooky action at a distance) without having to resort to faster-than-light-speed communication.

The assumptions of Wolff's theory can be summarized as follows:

▶ The de Broglie wavelength can be best explained by waves in space, not by wave-particle duality. The motion of coupled oscillators—at the dual centers of interacting electron In and Out waves—creates the de Broglie matter wave.

▶ Charge and mass are not fundamental to particles but depend instead on properties of space, which also are the basis for all of the physical laws of nature, matter, and the universe's structure.

▶ All matter is composed of space resonances, whose waves only rarely interact as they travel in space. When these waves do interact, however, the characteristics of space density that result at the point of the interaction of two or more of these waves are sufficient to explain all known particles.

▶ The motion of space resonances relative to each other produces all of the known laws of quantum mechanics and special relativity. Simply put, quantum mechanics, relativity, electrical charge, and conservation of energy arise from space properties, whereas other forces—gravity and inertia—emerge from perturbations of the electrical force (because of the Hubble expansion and the acceleration of matter).

According to Wolff, the "electron is composed of spherical waves which converge to the center and then become outward waves. The two waves form a standing wave whose peaks and nodes are like layers of an onion. The wave amplitude is a scalar number like a quantum wave, not an electromagnetic vector wave [a scalar wave is a mathematical wave of force, having quantity and magnitude without direction]. The Wave-Center is the apparent location of electron 'particles.'"[8, 9]

Among the most important, and revolutionary, aspects of Wolff's theory is that the solution to the quantum scalar wave equations involves three-dimensional, or spherical, scalar waves. What's more, these spherical waves are also scalar standing waves. A standing wave occurs when two waves of equal frequency are superimposed but traveling in the opposite directions.

We tend to think of waves as moving through a medium, but a standing wave remains stationary or constant as it moves through its medium. In other words, the crests, or amplitudes, of the wave always remain in the same place, even as energy is moving via the wave. We are most familiar with standing waves from our experience with string and wind instruments, such as a violin or clarinet. The waves that are set in motion along a violin's strings are standing waves, as are those within the cavities of wind instruments. Standing waves within a cavity occur when the waves bounce off the boundaries of the cavity. The frequency of the standing waves changes as the strings on the violin or the keys of the clarinet are pressed and so produce different notes.

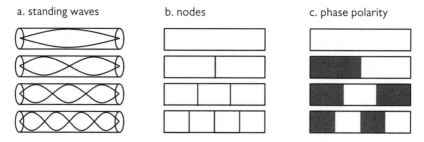

Figure 8.1. (a) Linear standing waves of various harmonics. (b) The patterns of nodes of the linear standing waves from figure 8.1a. (c) The phase polarities of the linear standing waves from figure 8.1a.

In Wolff's theory, there are two types of spherical standing waves, which have identical wavelengths: In waves and Out waves. All the quantum action takes place at the point of interaction when two or more of these waves meet, for energy transfer takes place at their intersection. As already explained, Wolff hypothesizes that all but three particles—electrons, protons, and neutrons—are appearances caused by this interaction and the resulting energy transfer. He says that "to 'find' a particle means to carry out an energy transfer since only a transfer can provide the data for measurement."[10] Wolff specifies three conditions for energy transfer. Without these

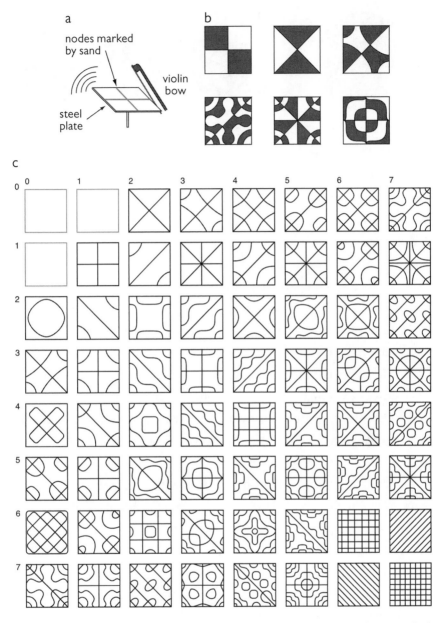

Figure 8.2. (a) When a violin bow is run along the edge of a steel plate on which sand is scattered, the plate vibrates, causing standing waves to form. (b) The standing waves cause the sand on the plate to form geometric patterns. Each pattern represents a different frequency of a standing wave oscillation, or resonance. (c) Graphical representation of Chladni figures, which are the geometric patterns formed by the varying resonances of standing waves.

a   b

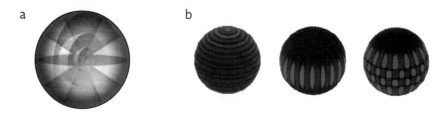

Figure 8.3. (a) Representation of a three-dimensional spherical standing wave. (b) Three patterns—of the nearly infinite variety that are possible—of spherical standing wave resonance.

following conditions present, waves travel independently in space and do not interact:[11]

▶ The wave-centers must contain a nonlinear region, at which the frequency changes (a transfer of energy occurs) between waves.

▶ The wave of each interacting resonance must overlap the wave-center of the others.

▶ Although the first two conditions explain the means for the energy exchange (change of frequency), a driving force is needed. This driving force determines in which direction the energy exchange goes.

In the Standard Model of quantum physics, the photon is the primary force-carrying particle. A startling implication of Wolff's theory is that the photon is not necessary to explain any of the forces, phenomena, or particle interactions in physics. (We will not deal with the photon's role as the particle of light, but suffice it to say that Wolff's theory provides explanations about light.) Wolff describes the photon not as a particle, but as an "energy exchange between particles that is a frequency change of the two resonances brought about by a modulation of the particle waves. The photon is not needed since there is nothing to be 'delivered' between particles."[12]

Wolff says that the conventional ideas about the electron arose historically in physics because of its role as a carrier of mass and charge.

Although he retains the electron as a fundamental quantum entity for other reasons, he rejects it as a carrier particle for mass and charge because these properties can be accounted for through wave interactions. What's more, he reminds us of a fact that conventional physicists chose to overlook, both because they idealized quantum interactions in their equations and for reasons of convenience: electrons can never appear alone. There always must be two or more in interaction, and any phenomena related to their interaction are always proportional to both charges. To put it another way that better highlights the bizarreness of the quantum realm: because there is no way to distinguish one electron from another in any interaction, you can think of all electrons that appear as being the same particle. As Wolff reminds us, it is curious that electrons ever came to be thought of as individual particles in the first place.

Wolff identifies the electron interaction as the simplest, most fundamental interaction that can take place between an In wave and an Out wave. When In waves and Out waves interact, the characteristics—what he calls the resonance—of space change. These changes determine the particle characteristics we can measure, with more complex kinds of space resonances producing characteristics that represent other kinds of particles.

In addition, because charge never appears alone, but only in relation to other particles' properties, such as mass, Wolff asks us to revise our understanding of what charge is and how it arises. He says, "In contradiction to popular opinion, we must conclude that charge is a joint property of both particles (space resonances) and of the space around them. It does not make sense to speak of charge as a property of *one* particle; instead, it is an energy exchange property between *two or more* particles. . . ."[13] Wolff's startling assessment means that properties such as charge and mass that are usually ascribed to individual particles actually result from the interaction of space resonances and their associated wave fields.[14]

It's easy to get caught in the details of Wolff's theory, for like any good theory, everything is connected to everything else, and it is difficult to summarize properly. Let's step back for a moment and look at the highlights of the complete theory and pull out those aspects of it that are particularly relevant to the NES theory of the human body-field. Wolff's theory of space resonances presupposes that space (which cannot be visualized as a physical substance, such as an ether) is the basic "entity" of the universe and is filled with spherical waves—what he calls In waves and Out waves. These waves can be thought of as convergent and divergent, that is, the two waves briefly combine at the center before reversing direction. Because they are of the same frequency, they form a standing wave. The amplitude of the standing wave is scalar, and it is finite at the wave center, which removes the infinities that plague much of current quantum mechanics point-particle electron model. If you could see the standing waves, they would look like the layers of an onion, for the In waves and Out waves are spherical waves. When they interact, they act as coupled oscillators. An energy exchange takes place only when the frequencies of the two oscillators match. A space resonance—a change in the properties of space—results from the interaction of these two waves. The resulting space resonance can take one of many different forms and so can display differing properties depending on how the In waves and Out waves interact, with the simplest resonance displaying the properties of an electron. The properties that we call different particles all arise from the changes in space, for space is the fundamental property of the universe. So it can be said that particles are located at the center of In wave and Out wave interactions, where the resulting space resonances produce the properties we have come to associate with the three fundamental quantum entities: electrons, protons, and neutrons. Finally, the laws of quantum mechanics and special relativity result from the motion of space resonances in relation to other space resonances. That's the gist of Wolff's theory, although he goes on to explain other assumptions and principles, such as the minimum amplitude principle. This principle is of primary importance, describing as it does that "the total amplitude of all particle waves in space always seek a minimum at every point. As a result, the centers of space resonances move, accompanied by frequency changes (energy exchanges), so as to approach the minimum value."[15]

On the basis of this model, Wolff is able to explain away many of the paradoxes of the Standard Model of quantum mechanics and account for all of the major forces (and laws) of physics, including gravity and inertia. The biggest mystery of space resonance theory itself, as Wolff freely admits, is the origin of the In wave, and as with any theory, there are many loose ends to tie up and mathematical proofs to be undertaken.

NES AND SPACE RESONANCE THEORY

So, what does space resonance theory have to do with NES? At the current time, it provides the most reasonable support for the physics underlying Peter's matching experiments. For decades, Peter wondered exactly what it was that he was measuring. An ampoule containing the energetic imprint of a tissue, element, or some other item matched with—or as Peter put it, talked to—certain items and energies but not with others. Why? What determined the match, the best possible answer in a range of possibilities? Space resonance theory provides a possible explanation. If indeed the fabric of space itself is the medium from which all properties of fundamental particles arise—if the point of interaction of an In wave and an Out wave actually changes the permittivity of space at that point, so that energy, and hence information, is transferred—then the matching experiments make sense. Peter has found a way to measure the conductivity of space where two waves meet and interact.

As Wolff explained, "An energy exchange only occurs when the frequencies of the two oscillators match each other. This can happen if the two atoms involved are the same kind of atom. It could also happen if different atoms have identical level differences."[16] These conditions are almost exactly those by which Peter's matches can be made!

These two criteria explain how things such as the body-field and physical body talk to each other, to use Peter's vernacular. Matches take place at many different levels. For example, the Energetic Integrators are the information highways of the body-field. When Peter calls them holographic structures in space, he is talking about them at the holistic, systems level. At this highest of structural levels, each Integrator can be thought of as a particular space resonance. However, each Integrator then links to the physical body based on other parameters, such as its frequency range and phase value, and at a still deeper subsystems level via the energetic properties of specific organs, cells, enzymes, hormones, and so on. They talk to each other because they share the same space resonances, and those shared resonances may explain how Peter discovered, for instance, that the liver meridian of traditional Chinese medicine (Energetic Integrator 8 in the NES model of the body-field) talks to the retina and iris, but not to other anatomical structures in the eye. You can think of these levels of resonances as a series of nested boxes, and as you move down into the next box, you find a different series of matches, each level being more and more specific and detailed. Energy exchange occurs at the point of interaction between two matches, and the result is a transfer of information. (Remember, you can only have information transfer when there is also an energy transfer.)

Wolff has calculated that the frequency of the de Broglie matter wave is in the realm of 10^{21} hertz, but there is no technology currently available that can detect energies in that range. So how can Peter know what he is measuring in his matching experiments and in the NES computer scan? It may be that he is measuring harmonics at half, quarter, and eighth wavelengths, with conductible losses of signal (if we think from an electrical engineering perspective) in the 15 decibel/harmonic range. Peter speculates that if the de Broglie wave is able to propagate itself, via Wolff's space resonance, and if there are indeed conductible signal losses, then harmonic resonance could be possible right down to a range as low as audible sound frequencies.

The Energetic Integrators may be representations of a mathematical structure within the entire electromagnetic frequency range and according to particular phase relationships. According to Wolff's theory, when an In wave and Out wave interact, there is a frequency change at that center point. (More accurately, heterodyning occurs at that point of interaction: two new frequencies are created.) However, Wolff wrote that "this change cannot happen to an atom spontaneously—there must be two atoms, one of which is decreasing frequency and the other increasing. The final combined arrangement of both atoms must be a net decrease of the total wave amplitude, to satisfy the MAP [minimum amplitude principle]."[17]

Peter and Harry had long known that frequency plays a role in the body-field, and Peter had amassed a lot of data from his matching experiments that indicated frequency plays a role in physical health, but he also had identified phase shifts as even more important. Phase shift refers to a change in a periodic signal, in this case a wave, in relation to a reference signal. To keep what can be a complex phenomenon simple, imagine two waves moving in relation to each other with peaks and troughs of the same strength. They are in phase according to amplitude. If one wave's amplitude changes, with its peaks and troughs losing strength, then it will fall out of phase with the other wave. (For a visual reference of phase shift in relation to time, see chapter 13, figure 13.4.) The Energetic Integrators appeared to each have a phase shift value, with the system reaching its limit at 180 degrees. However, Peter had no understanding of why this was the limit and what significance, if any, it might have. When he came across Wolff, who identified the phase shift of the In wave to the Out wave as being 180 degrees, the correspondence seemed beyond coincidence and its significance to NES became clearer. Wolff wrote, "At the center, the IN wave rotates 180 degrees converting it to an OUT wave. This fixed rotation creates the + or - quantum spin. It becomes an electron or positron, depending on the rotation direction."[18] Peter was intrigued to think that the range of Energetic Integrators, which represent the full body-wave, might have a correspondence to this phase shift from an In wave to an Out wave, for it is at this transitional point that an interference pattern is created and information conveyed. The Energetic Integrators are all about information regulation and transfer.

Peter explained that in NES, "We allow 15 degrees of phase for each of our Energetic Integrators, so we will get twelve of them in the 180 degrees of phase shift that occurs where the In wave turns into the Out wave at the center of the spherical standing wave, as per Wolff's space resonance theory. I checked this experimentally, and it works in practice; that is to say, there is a match between every Energetic Integrator structure and the 15 degrees of phase required. It appears that nature has arranged the body-field, in this respect, to work like a Swiss watch—very accurately. Accuracy, of course, is necessary for life to occur."

Peter's discovery that phase shift in some way has an impact on the state of the body-field, and by extension on health, moved NES even deeper into frontier territory. This discovery has important implications for formulating a truly comprehensive model of energetic pathology, as will be discussed in the Understanding the Energetic Integrators chapter in part 3. For now, it is important to realize, as Peter pointed out, that "all chemical reactions must result in a slight change of frequency of the atoms taking part in the exchange. If some chemical reactions advance the *phase* of the surrounding field, then the law of conservation of energy demands that other reactions will have a similar effect in retarding the phase. Phase and energy state are related ultimately. Put them together and chemistry, even biochemistry, is related to both frequency change and phase relationship. The new medicine must be involved in making sure that frequency and phase are both correct in the case of all of the body's chemical activities."

Other researchers are focusing on phase, especially former astronaut Edgar Mitchell and his collaborators, who are exploring the quantum holographic nature of consciousness and, indeed, of the universe. Mitchell refers heavily to the work of Dr. Peter Marcer, who proposes a theory of phase-conjugate-adaptive-resonance.[19] To briefly explain, he hypothesizes that all matter emits phase waves, as do all conscious beings. When the phase wave from a human being contacts the phase wave emitted from a physical object, the intersection of the two equal but opposite waves creates an interference pattern that imparts information. Information is carried via the phase relationships. He proposes that this phase-conjugate-adaptive-resonance functions at all levels of reality, from the quantum to the macroscopic and is at play in the biological functions of the body, from the level of DNA up through cells to metabolism. It even explains consciousness and perception. This research dovetails beautifully with Peter's, although Peter came to his ideas about phase independently of these researchers. While Peter embraces Wolff's theory, Mitchell and Marcer embrace the emitter-absorber model of Cramer and his transactional interpretation of quantum mechanics. However, the two theories have a lot in common, and while Mitchell and Marcer are applying quantum holography to consciousness and perception, Peter has applied it to the human body and body-field.

When Peter found Wolff's space resonance theory, he knew immediately that it had relevance not only to his own matching experiments and theory of the human body-field but also to all of bioenergetics. He felt that maybe, just maybe, Wolff's theory, with the addition of ideas about quantum holography such as Mitchell and Marcer's, might make the case for a truly quantum view of the human body, and of health. We will end this chapter with some of Peter's thoughts about both the possible impact of Wolff's theory and others' research on the coming revolution in medicine:

"How can the Wolff model change medicine?" Peter asked. "By leaving us with two worlds, *both of which are real*. The first world we already know a lot about: the laws of classical physics, the five senses, laboratory instruments, and time-related events. The second world is that of the quantum scalar wave interactions that are taking place all over the universe as a spontaneous activity of matter. This unseen but real quantum world affects what happens in the directly observed macroscopic world. In the scalar-wave world, matter has a 'knowledge' of the state of other pieces of matter. Without that, no chemical reactions could take place—ever! The interaction of In waves and Out waves can explain chemistry, and even action at a distance, for it provides a plausible way to explain how one molecule can 'know' if another is present, and even its state.

"There may be a prohibition on the distance over which certain energy configurations can extend their influence," Peter added, noting that much more research has to be done. "But the evidence suggests that frequency and phase represent the extent to which chemical reactions can influence the health of the entire organism, rather than just one part of a cell, or even less, a molecule. However, in therapy we need to not try to alter frequencies, because they are determined by the matter itself and where it is located on the periodic table. Instead, it should be possible to correct what we might call 'phase errors' between the In waves and the Out waves, which can lead to pathology, because it may be that the structure or shape of space is altered by all of these phase relationships. Every cell in the body, and in all of biology, has a characteristic phase shift value, and these are used as identifiers in NES technology, especially in relation to the Energetic Integrators.

"It may be that the structure of the immediately surrounding space changes[20] when there is a match between two test items," Peter explained, "and this phenomenon, whatever its explanation, has been the basis of natural medicine treatments for decades in Europe and North America. For forty years it has been accepted as though it were only an electrical effect. The fact is, it is not even primarily an electrical effect; it is a quantum field effect! Of that I am convinced! The body-field needs many types of energy to form and be maintained, and a weak electrostatic charge is among them. But the way information is transferred in the body is not primarily through electromagnetism, as so many people in bioenergetics think. We have to go beyond electromagnetics in alternative health and medicine and into QED fields, and phase shift, and more. As far as we know, NES is the only one doing this work now in relation to the physical body. We hope others will take up the challenge with us. All of these ideas are in their infancy, but they hold enormous potential for creating an entirely new model of biology and medicine."

PART THREE

The NES Model of the Human Body-Field

9

OVERVIEW OF THE
HUMAN BODY-FIELD

ALTHOUGH ASPECTS OF THE general configuration of the body-field—the external aura, chakras, meridians, and acupuncture points—have been described by others, Peter's work represents the first truly comprehensive systems-level mapping of the structure and mechanisms of the human body-field and their relation to biochemistry and physiology. Through Peter's work, we gain a better understanding of how the human body-field is the master control system for the physical body. Although there is an enormous amount of research that remains to be done, we can now, for the first time, begin to understand how the body-field's intricate, interconnected systems and subsystems—at the level of quantum electrodynamics (QED)—affect the state of the physical body. We can better understand how the body-field itself functions: what kinds of energies drive it; how information is created, distributed, and regulated in the body; and how the body-field is affected by external and internal influences, including Earth fields, diet, stress, toxins, pathogens, and other factors. We have a new basis for understanding how emotions and consciousness arise from or are affected by the movement of energy and information in the body-field. Also, we can directly correct body-field distortions through the use of the NES Infoceuticals.

The remainder of this book is devoted to the details of the NES model of how the human body-field works and how distortions at the bioenergetic level correlate to health. We trust that by the time you reach the final chapter you will be as awed as we are by the magnificent web of interconnections between the body-field and the physical body.

HOW YOUR BODY-FIELD FUNCTIONS

The human body-field is an intelligent, self-organizing, self-correcting, self-maintaining energetic and informational structure that functions at the level of QED and quantum holography. Your body-field and physical body are interdependent: one cannot exist without the other. Your physical body is dependent on chemistry, which drives the physiology of your body, allowing everything from DNA and cells to your nervous system and brain to perform the work that keeps you alive and healthy. Yet this same cellular activity gives rise, at least in part, to your body-field, which in turn directs and organizes the information that drives your biochemistry. It's a bit of a chicken-and-egg paradox, only in this case it is a quantum-level case of how the real and virtual are both necessary for all life processes. On the one hand, real chemical processes drive physiology, giving rise to the bioenergetic reality of the body-field, but on the other hand, the body-field is responsible for directing the information that maintains that biochemistry.

An analogy may make this concept easier to grasp. Let's say you have a ticket to the opera. You were issued a real paper ticket, but it is just a piece of paper unless it is printed with information that tells you what you are allowed to do with it. You can attend the opera, but you can't use this ticket to get into the rock concert. What's more, you can only get into the opera hall on a certain date, at a certain time, and will have to sit in a certain seat. So although you have to have the ticket, you won't know what you can and cannot do if there is no information printed on it. The ticket is meaningless without the information, but the information that gives the ticket its value cannot be easily transmitted without some form of physical scaffolding. So the real (paper ticket) and the virtual (information printed on the ticket) are interdependent. In a similar way, your body chemistry creates the very conditions of your health, but that chemistry is directed by bioenergetic processes (quantum processes, such as electron and photon exchanges or In and Out wave interactions). The real and the virtual work together.

From a bioenergetics perspective, all illness starts in the body-field, because all physiological processes that break down do so because of information distortions. Consider an allergic reaction. If you have hay fever, then inhaling certain pollen molecules sets off a chemical chain reaction in your body. You experience the effects of that reaction as a runny nose and watery, itchy eyes. There is nothing inherently wrong with your body chemistry. It is working perfectly, responding to protect your body from the allergen, which it considers to be a foreign substance. What is wrong is the *information* your body is processing. Your body somehow mistook harmless pollen molecules for harmful invaders, and your immune system mounted a defense. This is a case of mistaken identity—it is an incorrect match made by your body, at the level of information, that results in a real, physical reaction. You can have an allergy shot or take antihistamines to alleviate your symptoms, but they may not address the root cause of your problem. The cause is found in your body-field, where information is being blocked or distorted and so is affecting the way your body functions at a cellular level.

Everything that happens at a biochemical level in your body—amino acids arranging themselves only into allowable sequences, DNA unzipping itself to be copied, neurotransmitters cascading through your nervous system, electrochemical impulses firing muscle or heart cells—is mediated by information. Your body has to know what to do, when to do it, how much to do, and where the activity should take place, and it has to carry out millions of actions with breathtaking accuracy in milliseconds. So your body and body-field are interdependent, like two sides of a coin. Both aspects of your body—its biochemistry and its bioenergetics—mutually contribute to its homeostasis.

Illness often is referred to as the loss of homeostasis, because your body loses its ability to work properly, compromising your normal, vibrant state of health and well-being. The loss of homeostasis usually is a gradual process, not a catastrophic one, as your body-field's many information networks slowly deteriorate and that exquisitely organized web of interactions becomes increasingly chaotic. The symptoms of such a loss of physical equilibrium can be subtle or serious.

REQUIREMENTS FOR ESTABLISHING THE HUMAN BODY-FIELD

Peter's research suggests that at the minimum the following conditions are necessary to support, and perhaps even to create, the human body-field and to ensure its correct functioning:

▶ An electrostatic charge, which is created both by ionized particles in solution (such as in cells) and the action potential of the elements of the nervous system.

▶ Light, even in small amounts, of certain high-energy frequencies, both internal and external to the body. Biophysicist Fritz-Albert Popp has found that cells emit ultraweak light, so the body has an internal source of photonic energy. Peter said, "You don't need a lot of energy to make a human body-field, but you need energy of the right quality to make it work to carry information."

▶ Gravity and at least a weak source of magnetism, which is why Peter suggests that Earth energies such as those that contribute to geopathic stress and external magnetic fields such as the Schumann resonance may have subtle but profound effects on the body and body-field.

▶ *Magnetic confetti,* a term Peter borrowed from Reid, who believes that the electron has some sort of magnetic envelope or capsule. Information exchange takes place when an electron's magnetic capsule is broken open through an interaction with a photon. Magnetic fragments, which Reid called magnetic confetti, may be left over from the exchange. However, Peter believes that what Reid called the electron's capsule may actually be the electron's spherical standing wave, which has a charge and forms magnetic patterns in space, according to Wolff's space resonance theory.

All chemistry, including the chemical bonding processes that drive biochemistry, is based on the interaction of fundamental quantum particles, with the rules of physics determining how molecules can form and break bonds. The magnetic fragments are left over from the processes of molecular bonds breaking. In fact, magnetic confetti energies and bond energies may, in fact, be two terms for the same process in the body, for bond energies that are broken in metabolic processes are viewed by modern biologists as the main source of energy for the body.

Peter singles out the breaking of hydrogen bonds as a special case in biology and bioenergetics. He believes that "the source of magnetic confetti in the body is associated in a major way with gas exchange in the lungs, in particular in relation to Energetic Integrator 2, and oxygen exchange in the cells, in the circulatory process, which is described in NES in Energetic Integrator 10. My research shows an enormous increase in magnetic confetti wherever you get oxygen exchange, especially when carbon dioxide is exchanged for oxygen in the lungs. So the lungs and circulation are very special and important in terms of the body-field, but whenever there are chemical processes in the body, you get magnetic confetti, and there can be too many of these stray magnetic particles or not enough of them. You could say that according to NES theory, just as in biochemistry, we are all working off bond energy. A lot more research needs to be done, but magnetic confetti, especially as it relates to the hydrogen bonding process, is necessary to make and sustain a human body-field."

During a meeting with biophysicist Fritz-Albert Popp, at Popp's laboratory in Germany, Peter explained these conditions for the human body-field, and Popp asked Peter if he was sure he was talking about a quantum field in terms of the human body-field. Peter said, "It was a fair question. The only thing I could tell him, at this point in our research, is that it appears that if this is in fact a quantum structure, even according to the Wolff model, then it represents a *special case*, that is, it is a field specific to the biology of humans, or perhaps to warm-blooded creatures. It's going to take a long time to puzzle it all out, but I do think that, yes, we are talking quantum and that, yes, there is something special about how quantum relates to the biology of living creatures. All I can say with some measure of confidence is that these are the conditions, at a minimum, that my research indicates are required to form and support the human body-field."

THE BIG BODY-FIELD

We have talked about scale many times in this book, and in understanding the structure of the human body-field it comes into play again, for there is a "big body-field," that is the aggregate of all of the thousands, or perhaps millions, of smaller fields that arise in the body. Just as the physical body is made up of cells that aggregate into organs that form interconnected systems, which in turn all add up to what we think of as our body, the bioenergetic body is made from smaller components as well. Each cell creates its own minifield, as do all the cell's organelles (specialized components of a cell that serve functions similar to organs within the body). In fact, the fields from different types of organelles match with specific Energetic Integrators. There are even individual fields generated by the DNA contained in each cell nucleus. Each of the cell-level and below-cell-level fields aggregate to form the larger organ fields, and there are additional fields generated by the skeleton (bone is a living matrix), cerebral-spinal-fluid system, and the other large dynamic systems of the body. So, there are actually uncountable numbers of minifields within the body that together form the larger, structured big body-field (what we call the "human body-field" or simply the "body-field").

Through his experiments, Peter was able to simplify the organization of the system. For instance, he was able to collapse the ninety-six meridians down to a system of twelve Energetic Integrators. Many of the cellular minifields around organs could be grouped into sixteen Energetic Drivers. In this way, the map of the body-field emerged from the enormous complexity of these countless subfields through the process of aggregation.

HOW NES ANALYZES YOUR BODY-FIELD

The NES–Professional System is a computer program that provides a way to peek into the bioenergetic and informational recesses of your body-field to see what is going on. It's a snapshot that allows you to accurately assess the correlations between your body-field and your physical and emotional states at a particular moment in time. The scan itself is quick, easy, and noninvasive. You simply place your hand on the scanning device, which looks like a large computer mouse, and the software in the computer reads your body-field. How does it do that? You know from reading previous chapters about the quantum processes that are going on at the level of your body-field and you have read about Peter's matching experiments. You could say, then, that the scan is a QED matching test, and we are scanning for something that no one else is able to detect reliably—the waveforms of the body-field and the interference patterns that impart information. Both Wolff's space resonance theory and Marcer's ideas about phase-conjugate-adaptive-resonance relate to the NES scanning process.

Basically, the computer on which the NES analysis software is loaded sets up its own QED field (you have to have an electrostatic field to create the QED field and get information exchange, and the hardware of the computer creates a weak one that is sufficient to conjugate to the body-field). Your body-field and the QED field from the computer become entangled, and through a proprietary process, the scanning software is able to assess where matches are made between your body-field and the template of the body-field structures (based on Peter's research) that is encoded in the software. While the entanglement of the two QED fields allows the information to flow and thus be detected, the matching is of the structures in space whose qualities impart that information. Those qualities are themselves based on changes in the permittivity of space, according to Wolff's space resonance theory of physics. The NES system is, in effect, asking questions of your body-field and sensing information about the changes in space that are interpreted as responses from your body-field.

Unlike allopathic medicine, where tests seeks to determine baseline measures, such as your liver enzyme level, and then determine if there is a problem if your liver enzymes fall outside of what are considered normal parameters, the NES system is sensing the *quality* of response it gets back. It senses how strong or weak the match is and then prioritizes the responses it gets and returns them graphically for the practitioner to assess.

The NES system is not a biofeedback type of system, which, depending on the type of system, detects changes in the electrical characteristics of the skin or brain. The interaction that takes place during a NES scan between the computer and your body-field is a quantum process, perhaps similar to Marcer's theory of phase-conjugate-adaptive-resonance, and it happens almost instantly. Although each person has a somewhat unique biochemistry, our body-fields are all structurally the same. Remember, the Energetic Drivers, Integrators, and the like are really structures in space, and those structures are crucial to the proper functioning of everything that goes on within them. So it is not necessary, as it is in allopathic medicine, to get a reading of every item *within* a system, such as blood gases, cholesterol level, potassium level, and the like. Instead, we can look at the state of the larger energetic and informational structures themselves—your body-field's Drivers, Integrators, Stars, and others. (For a more detailed discussion of these components of the body-field, see specific chapters later in this part of the book.) By correcting distorted structures, everything within those structures is affected. So you could say that the NES scan is analyzing the *functional integrity* of your body-field. By "functional integrity," we mean that the objective of the scan is similar to identifying the weakest links in a chain, because your body-field is only as strong as its weakest aspects. A NES scan identifies those weaknesses, and you can use the NES Infoceuticals to correct them, if you so choose.

Ultimately, NES scans over time determine the body-field's correlations to the root causes of physical and emotional problems by working through the many layers of the holographic body-field to reveal the preferred sequence for healing. We do not address symptoms, which is what most allopathic diagnoses are based on. That's why we say we do not diagnose, treat, prevent, or cure disease. We are working at the holistic, systems level of your body-field and working with energy and information, not physical tissue or cellular processes directly.

The number of matches made in a single scan is about 145, and the information is correlated, sorted, and prioritized before being returned graphically in the analysis reports that show up on the computer screen. By sensing the quality of the matches between your actual body-field and the information about the body-field and its structures mathematically encoded in the NES software, the computer can detect where and to what degree your body-field is distorted. These distortions are prioritized according to Peter's research findings into the preferred sequence of healing, or in other words, by which distortions the body-field is indicating are best corrected first to support the body's own self-healing capabilities, which is what ultimately restores the body to homeostasis. One of Peter's most useful findings in terms of health is that there is a preferred sequence to healing. The sequence is that Big Field distortions are corrected first, followed by distortions in the Drivers, then Integrators, then Terrains, and finally Stars. Within each of these structural fields, there is also a preferred sequence for all the subsystems and subfields, and the Infoceuticals are sequentially numbered so that the order of correction is easy to follow, as will be explained shortly.

From a physics perspective, you could say that the moment you place your hand on the scanning device and the NES practitioner hits the SCAN button, the computer is probing the wavefunction of your body-field and turning what was virtual into something very real (i.e., measurable). The result is an informational snapshot of your body-field. To understand what this informational snapshot is all about, you have to know about certain other aspects of your body-field. For instance, your body-field is dynamic, which means it is always changing. Your body-field is a holographical structure that records everything that happens to you and everything to which you are exposed. As you can imagine, in any given second, millions of things are affecting you: your emotions and state of mind, other people around you, electromagnetic fields, light, heat or cold, toxins and pathogens, the food you have eaten and liquid you have drunk, and on and on. The NES analysis is a snapshot at one moment in time of the functional integrity of your body-field as it works to mediate all the influences on it and translate those influences into information the body can use.

In terms of prioritizing distortions, imagine everything in your body—every cellular process, tissue, organ, and more—as having a collection of little colored flags: red, orange, green, and yellow flags. When a body-field structure is distorted or information is blocked or degraded, there is a corresponding effect in your body, and the colors on the scan results (the "colored flags" in our analogy) indicate bioenergetic calls for help. It's like a cell, organ, or metabolic process is holding up a flag and waving it to get your attention, shouting, "Hey, I need your attention!" The cry for help at any of these subsystem levels is heard at the larger structural level of the body-field, at the level of the particular Driver, Integrator, or other body-field structure in which that lower-level problem is contained. The color of the flag indicates how badly help is needed. A red flag takes priority. It means, "Pay attention to me first. I need help *now!*" The other colors, in order of priority from highest to lowest, are orange, yellow, and green. If the test item needs no attention, the scan result shows as white.

NES practitioners are trained to prioritize the test results further, because there is more about knowing how to correct the body-field than seeing which color appears next to a test item on the results screens. Your practitioner will understand the implications of the *patterns* your scan reveals, including the preferred sequence of correction. Because everything of energetic and informational significance has its correlation to physical processes, NES practitioners must be licensed or certified health care professionals with an understanding of anatomy, physiology, and pathology.

Because your body-field is dynamic and a scan examines the subsystems of your field in relation to your entire body-field, there will always be something in your field that shows as needing correction. Even if we lived in an ideal world, with no exposure to toxins, pathogens, and the like, it is unlikely that a NES scan would ever be "zeroed out," that is, show that nothing needs attention. As long as you are alive your body-field is in constant interchange with the environment and subject to the influence of your own beliefs, thoughts, emotions, memories, and more, so distortions are inevitable. Although many people come to NES to address the bioenergetic aspects of specific physical or emotional problems, the fact is that NES is ideal for use as part of an ongoing wellness program because it can identify potential problems at the bioenergetic level *before* they manifest in the body.

It's difficult for people who are not familiar with bioenergetics to understand how, or even to believe that, the body-field can be decoded, but the process is not so different from many other tests you are familiar with and have probably had many times. Consider the following tests and technologies, all of which deal in some respect with real and virtual information, just as a NES scan does:

► *Electrocardiogram or electroencephalograph:* Your heart and brain emit many kinds of energies, including electrical energies. You can't see them, but they can be detected via certain types of machines. A technician places electrodes on your chest in the case of an electrocardiogram (ECG), which measures the heart's electrical rhythms, or your scalp for an electroencephalograph (EEG), which measures brain waves. The electrodes detect signals and processes them through the machinery to produce a visual output—the waveform "squiggles" that appear on a computer screen or a roll of recording paper. The doctor or technician can interpret those waveforms to learn about the functioning of your heart or brain. The NES software works in a similar way, although because it is not electrical, but quantum, in nature, electrodes are not necessary. The NES system reads the information in your body-field structures, translates it into graphics on the computer screen, and a trained NES practitioner can make sense of it.

In the case of the EEG, the information recorded can even reveal your *state of awareness* because different brain waveforms represent different qualities of consciousness, such as whether you are alert, relaxed, meditating, asleep, or even dreaming. In a similar manner, the NES system is reading the quality of the various aspects of your body-field (Drivers, Integrators, Stars, and so on). Just as the state of your awareness is always changing (think a different thought and your body responds instantly), so is your body-field. Just as consciousness is dynamic, but we can still measure brain states and learn something about the quality of your awareness, your body-field also is dynamic, and through a NES scan we can detect information that reveals something about its functional integrity.

▶ *Radio:* Think of the NES system as a radio receiver. Think of your body-field as the radio transmission station. A real wave is sent out from the station. Piggybacked on it is virtual information, which is the music, ad, weather report, traffic report, or talk show information encoded through modulation. The real wave, in effect, carries the virtual information, the music or discussion, that has meaning only when interpreted by the listener. In addition, you have to be able to tune into the real wave by tuning in the station to have access to the virtual information carried on that wave. If you have only AM tuning capability, you can't pick up any FM stations. Move the dial a little and you move from listening to 93.5 to 95.3. Each of these frequencies reveals different information. The NES–Professional System is the receiver that can pick up a range of signals (about 145 tests in each scan, so it's like listening to 145 stations at once) that your body-field is constantly broadcasting.

▶ *Computer:* Think of your body as the hardware that is running the software of your health. Software is a set of instructions that the hardware executes. That software is your body-field, which is telling your body how to function biochemically. If the software has glitches in it, the hardware won't run properly. You can think of NES as doing a status check on your software. Where it finds bad code, you can fix that code by using the Infoceuticals.

In fact, you can think of the NES scan as working rather like a word processor spell-checker for the body-field. A computer spell-checker, without your even knowing it, checks the document you are typing for errors by comparing every word against its internal dictionary. When it finds a word that appears to be misspelled, it flags that word. In a similar but more holistic and high-level way, a NES scan examines your body-field for distortions in the state of its many energetic and informational structures and substructures. But, in our spell-checker analogy, a NES scan goes beyond checking only spelling, for it examines the text at the sentence and paragraph level for meaning, determining if it is scrambled or otherwise degraded. The screen graphics show all the "mismatches" that the scan finds and the relative level of severity and then suggests Infoceuticals that can make the necessary corrections.

THE ROLE OF THE NES INFOCEUTICALS

Distortions in your body-field indicate where information transfer processes have broken down or where information regulation has gone awry. It takes information to correct information. So, to correct imbalances in your body-field, you need to provide your body-field with the information it needs to resume normal and efficient functioning. That's the job of the NES Infoceuticals, which are liquid remedies containing microminerals that are encoded with the QED information your body-field needs to "reset" itself. For example, the Infoceutical called Energetic Driver 1 deals with Source energy—the life-force energy your body uses to stay well or to restore wellness—whereas Energetic Driver 5 deals with the bioenergetic and informational correlations to circulation and processes connected to blood circulation.

Currently, there are sixty-two Infoceuticals, each one imprinted with precise information that affects a specific Driver, Integrator, Star, or other aspect of the body-field. The imprinting process is complex, involving a specially made machine that encodes information into the mixtures using high electrostatic fields, specific colors of photons, and more. The plant-derived minerals are not included for any nutritional value but only as carriers for the QED information. So while each Infoceutical is made of the same physical substance (water, microminerals, and a bit of alcohol as a preservative), each one is encoded with unique information that has a specific effect on the body-field.

You take Infoceuticals as a specific number of drops in a glass of water, always separately and at least ten minutes apart. (You should never mix different Infoceuticals together in the same glass of water unless instructed to do so. Mixing them actually creates something new, so the effect will be different from what your practitioner intended for you.) Your NES program might extend over many months and involve multiple scans, but for each scan you are given a NES protocol, which is a set of instructions on which Infoceuticals to take, in which order (order is important!), and how many drops of each. Over time, you might be asked to increase the number of drops, for example, starting with three drops of each Infoceutical, then working your way over a week or ten days to six, nine, or fifteen drops.

The number of drops is not arbitrary. Peter's research has shown that the Infoceuticals are, in effect, quantized. You might remember that the word *quantum,* from which the word *quantized* comes, refers to how entities in the quantum realm can occupy only certain discrete states and not others. For instance, electrons can be at only certain energy levels and are forbidden to be at other levels. If we imagine their energy levels as a flight of stairs, it's like electrons can sit on the first, third, and fifth stair, but can never be found on the second, fourth, or sixth one. If they need to go from the third stair to the fifth, they simply disappear from the third stair and show up on the fifth, never having traveled in between. That's just the way nature is at the quantum level! Something similar applies to the Infoceuticals. The restorative effects are quantized, that is, they occur at specific intervals of drops: three, six, nine, fifteen, and twenty-eight. It's fine if you measure out four drops instead of three, but you should know that there is no greater effect. The next leap in effect comes at six drops, not four or five. In the same way, seven or eight drops provide the same effect as six, and twenty-two or twenty-six drops provide the same level of correction as do fifteen drops. To not waste Infoceuticals, you are better off using only the number of drops your practitioner recommends.

THE NES SCAN
AND BODY-FIELD DYNAMICS

There must be a minimum of five days between body-field scans because the body-field, being quantum by nature, is affected—slightly perturbed—by the scanning process, and any rescan done too soon may not be accurate. Think of dropping a pebble in a pond. The pebble disturbs the water, sending out concentric ripples across the water's surface. It takes time for the water to return to equilibrium. Making a match with your body-field, which is what the scan does, disturbs your body-field, so you need to give it time to settle down again before rescanning.

Even though your body-field is dynamic, it is always recording everything to which it is exposed, from external factors, such as nutrition or exposure to pollutants, to internal ones, such as your thoughts, emotions, beliefs, and memories. In Wolff's space resonance theory, the spherical standing wave of the electron can be visualized as an onion because it has many spherical layers. That analogy works well for the body-field, too. Every moment, your holographic body-field is recording the state of your being, and over your life it builds up layer upon layer of information. Each NES scan probes deeper into the relative state of your body-field, peeling back these layers. The root cause of a physical problem may be correlated to a bioenergetic distortion deep in the layers, so it may take time to return the body-field to full functioning.

A scan, however, also is picking up the *patterns* that develop over time and that reveal themselves at the higher, systems level of your body-field, for instance, at the structural, informational field level of a particular Energetic Integrator. Again, we have to consider scale. Let's use another analogy to explain. Think of wind blowing through a field of grass. Individual blades of grass are being buffeted this way or that. One blade is bent, another straight. One is twisted around another. However, overall, as you stand back and look over the entire field, it looks fairly symmetrical, with wide swaths of grass moving gracefully together as the wind ripples across the field.

To look at it another way, the field of grass also is alive with other kinds of movement: bugs scurrying here and there, earthworms pushing dirt around, seeds germinating, and weeds growing. From that scale, the field is seething with activity, but from your normal viewing scale, it is just a plain old field of grass, with not much going on. In a similar way, scale is important when thinking about the body-field. Although the body-field is a dynamic system, always recording and being affected by what happens to you through its many subsystems, at a higher, systems level it has an integral pattern and structure that is fairly stable. In a similar way, your body-field is a stable pattern of information and energy, although it can be distorted by the microactivity at the subsystems level.

In the scanning process, distance matters. Contrary to many other bioenergetic researchers and complementary health care professionals, we believe at this time that the farther away the client is from the scanning equipment, the less reliable a body-field analysis is. The interaction of Out waves and In waves results in tiny phase shifts and frequency changes, which will affect how matching occurs in a computer. Our research has shown that the closer together the fields are that are going to be compared, the more accurate and reliable the scan results. In effect, the less "noise" there is to interfere with the scanning process, the better.

Wolff suggests that there may be a falling off, or attenuation, of the effects of space resonance caused by the interaction of In and Out waves with increased distance. It is generally believed by frontier researchers that in some nonlocal processes, such as remote viewing and intentional healing, distance does not matter because it is information and not energy that is exchanged in these long-distance connections, so any signal is not physical in nature. However, recent research has found that distance may matter, at least in terms of intentional healing. For instance, Dean Radin reports in his book *Entangled Minds* that the effect of intentional healing seems to drop off in proportion to distance, with effects diminishing steadily over increments of hundreds of miles.[1] More research is necessary before any conclusions can be reached about the effect of distance in nonlocal interactions and its relevance to bioenergetics, but as of the writing of this book, the NES system is designed so that the client being scanned should have contact with the input device to the computer. NES does not at this time endorse scanning at a distance with its system or testing via hair or saliva samples.

THE MAJOR SYSTEMS OF THE BODY-FIELD

We will devote a chapter to each of the components of the body-field later in this part, but here we will provide you a brief overview of each of the body-field's major energetic systems so you can get a preliminary sense of them. Over many decades of original research, and expanding on the knowledge of traditional Chinese medicine (TCM), Peter has come to identify three main systems of the human body-field: Energetic Drivers, Energetic Integrators, and Energetic Stars, as well as the Energetic Terrains and the body-field's relation to natural Earth and cosmic energies and fields that we call the Big Field influences.

Energetic Drivers

The Energetic Drivers are the powerhouses of the body-field. There are sixteen individual Driver fields, which together power the full body-field. Each major organ or organ system—the heart, nervous system, liver, thyroid, skin, and so on—produces its own energy and information Driver field, starting as the organ forms and begins to function during fetal development or soon after birth. If a Driver field weakens, then the organ system itself becomes compromised.

You can think of these sixteen Driver fields as imparting a kind of constitutional energy to each organ. When we think of people as being hearty or vigorous, full of enthusiasm and energy, we say they have a "good constitution." They rarely get sick, or if they do, they recover quickly. In the same way, we can think of each of our major organ systems as being hearty or not, according to how strong its bioenergetic field is. Just as the name implies, these fields power, or drive, our body and, hence, our state of well-being. If an organ field loses power, it is like a battery running down. Without the energy and information it needs to do its job, that organ begins to work less efficiently, but because its job in the body is crucial, the organ will put up a fight. It will work harder and harder to try to keep going—expending more and more of its dwindling energy supply faster and faster—and as a consequence of that struggle and stress, things will begin to go wrong. Finally, without the energy it needs, the organ will become seriously compromised and begin to malfunction or even to shut down. As that happens, other organs of the body and bioenergetic systems of the body-field will try to compensate, and then they, too, can begin to lose power. The loss of the integrity of your Driver fields can result in a cascade of problems in the body.

Interestingly, the health problems that correlate to a deficient Driver field can be associated with that particular organ or they can seem entirely unrelated. That's because bioenergetic physiology has more to do with TCM than Western allopathic medicine. An organ, such as the liver, can be connected via energetic circuits (in TCM, the meridians; in NES, the Energetic Integrators) to many other areas of the body. For example, in NES, as in TCM, the liver is correlated energetically with the heart, gallbladder, eyes, toes, jaw muscles and teeth, and many other seemingly unconnected parts of the body. So if your Liver Driver—the powering field of the liver—runs down, you might find yourself experiencing problems in your eyesight (perhaps retinal problems) or with your jaw muscles. Biogentically, it's because of the liver energy channel that people with gout often experience swelling of their big toe! The logic of many diseases defies explanation by allopathic medical standards but makes perfect sense by TCM, NES, and bioenergetic standards.

Driver fields become compromised for all kinds of reasons, from prolonged emotional stress, to exposure to toxins or pathogens, to genetic defects and chemical imbalances, to your body's misalignment with Earth fields.

Energetic Integrators

The Energetic Integrators direct and regulate information transfer in the body-field, and by extension among the DNA and cells of the body. There are twelve Energetic Integrators, each with a common structure that covers information relating to a range of physical aspects of the body, from elements (such as hydrogen, calcium, and potassium) through cells and tissues and on up through things as abstract as emotions.

Each Energetic Integrator covers a certain range of electromagnetic energy (frequency), and the twelve of them are in specific phase relationship to each other. We will discuss these aspects of the Energetic Integrators in detail in chapter 13, but for now it is important to note that the Integrators are the primary *information routes* in the body-field. The Integrators provide the information that allows cells to work properly, and they ensure that the right information gets to the right place in the body at the right time. Although each of the twelve Energetic Integrators covers specific kinds of information, as a whole they form a network that keeps the body-field functioning as a seamless web of information exchange.

Because the Energetic Integrators are communication networks in the body-field, a single Integrator links to many seemingly unrelated aspects of the body. It took Peter decades to carry out the matching experiments that revealed the complex links between each Integrator and specific cellular and physiological processes and also between the twelve Integrators in relation to each other. As an example of just how convoluted a single bioenergetic pathway can be, consider Energetic Integrator 9, which is called the Thyroid/Triple Burner Integrator. (In case you are wondering, the term *triple burner* is from TCM, in which it refers to the meridian linking the three major cavities of the body—the cranial, thoracic, and abdominal cavities, which generate what TCM calls "heat" in the body. In NES, this heat energy, via Energetic Integrator 9, is associated with Source energy.) You might think from the name that this Integrator deals mostly with thyroid issues (from a strictly bioenergetic perspective, of course), but from Peter's matching experiments, we know its links stretch far and wide in the body. It matches bioenergetically with the other major endocrine glands (specifically, the posterior and medial sections of the pituitary) and the adrenal medulla, but it also links to the mitral valve and right atrium of the heart (but not with other parts of the heart). It regulates information exchange to most of the mucosae (mucous membranes) of the body and to the lateral ventricles of the brain. It is associated bioenergetically with specific elements, such as iodine and selenium, and is intimately related to the energetic/informational aspects of the calcium-sodium relationship in the body. Thus, when function is restored to an Integrator by using Infoceuticals, everything within that communication channel is addressed.

Energetic Stars

The Energetic Stars are mini-information networks in the full body-field, in which multiple information channels converge to address a single issue. (Which is how they got their name, because you can think of all these channels converging as a sort of stick-figure drawing of a star.) The Energetic Stars differ from the Energetic Integrators because they represent specific metabolic pathways or multiple influences in the body-field that converge on one major function or mechanism, whereas the Integrators cover an amazing array of connections to dozens of specific aspects of physiology. What's more, the Stars are sequenced (numbered) according to the energetic and functional survival mechanisms of the body. So for instance, the Systemic Immunity Star comes before the Nerve Function Star, which takes precedence over the Enzyme and Muscle Star, and so on. The Star Infoceuticals are used when there are major energy blockages in the body-field that have not been taken care of by the other kinds of Infoceuticals and to support a radically weakened body-field when body-field processes have to be bolstered in significant core ways. Many of the Energetic Stars also are designed to correct distorted phase relationships in the body-field. (We will talk about phase relationships in more depth in chapter 13.)

Energetic Terrains

An Energetic Terrain is a not a structure of the body-field but is a type of body-field distortion that creates an environment in a body tissue that makes the tissue amenable to hosting microbes. Biologists recognize that certain types of microbes tend to infect or weaken certain types of tissues and not others—some microbes affect only your stomach, others only your eyes, still others only your muscles, and so on. Bioenergetics helps explain why: the field distortion in that type of tissue matches to the field signature of that family or type of microbe. Energetic Terrains are a bit difficult to describe succinctly, because the theory behind them presupposes that viruses, bacteria, and other pathogens have energetic fields every bit as real as the pathogens themselves. All living things, including viruses (even though they are not technically living) and bacteria, have fields to one extent or another. Peter's matching experiments have shown that certain kinds of body-field errors are energetically linked to the fields of disease-causing microbes. Microbiology recognizes categories of microorganisms, such as amoebas, fungi, yeasts, bacteria, and viruses, and in his testing Peter found that the Energetic Terrains matched to entire categories of microorganisms, rather than to specific, individual organisms. So the Terrain Infoceuticals cover these broad categories, and NES cannot be used diagnostically to identify a specific microbe.

In its Energetic Terrain theory, NES is dealing with the bioenergetic signature of a pathogen, not the physical pathogen. From a bioenergetic perspective, microbial or viral fields can remain in the body even when the actual pathogen is not present. For instance, you may have been exposed to a virus and experienced no symptoms. The actual virus itself may have been eradicated from your body, but the virus can leave behind an energetic imprint that can, at a later time and under certain conditions, cause bioenergetic problems for you. What's really tantalizing in terms of health and illness is that you may experience symptoms even if you were never exposed to the actual microbe, but only to its field. In other words, there is a second route of transmission for microbial infection, and it is entirely bioenergetic. Although this idea of what might be called a "virtual microbe" is a difficult stretch for many people, it makes bioenergetic sense and could explain why so many people experience the symptoms of microbial diseases but conventional lab tests fail to detect the actual microbes. It is the microbe's energy/information field that is causing the problem.

As explained, an Energetic Terrain is a bioenergetic field error or disturbance that affects specific organs or body tissues in such a way as to create an environment *attractive* to the energetic imprint of viruses, bacteria, and other microbes. The field error comes first, not the microbe, in the causative chain. The Energetic Terrain Infoceuticals provide the body-field with the information it needs to correct the Energetic Terrain, restoring the field of the organ or tissue so that the body can work properly to protect itself. By correcting the Energetic Terrain, your body-field, and hence body, in effect can "close the door" on microbes and pathogens, so they are less likely to gain hold in your body in the first place. This class of Infoceuticals also provides the restorative information to correct Terrain field errors for damage that might have occurred in the past.

PUTTING IT ALL TOGETHER

These different aspects of the body-field each have their own major function, their specific contributions to keeping us healthy and maintaining our well-being, but it can sometimes be difficult to see how they all form a seamless working whole. Here is a simple extended analogy that will help you to view the body-field as a dynamic, integrated, organized structure and to more easily remember what each aspect of the body-field does. Although we have not yet discussed the Big Field influences, the NES name for the natural Earth and cosmic energies that affect the body-field, we will include them in our analogy and so provide you with a preview of what they are.

Think of your body and body-field together as a car, as the vehicle that gets you through life.

  ▶ *Big Field:* Many of the newer cars have a global positioning system (GPS) device that works via satellite. The GPS allows you to know your position relative to the environment. It tells you where you are in relation to factors of Earth such as longitude and latitude or a location within a city. You can think of the NES scan results of the Big Field as telling you something about your body-field's state in relation to certain energy grids/fields of Earth (vertical, equatorial, and magnetic polar axes).

▶ *Energetic Drivers:* To drive your car, you have to fuel it. The Energetic Driver fields that arise from each organ provide power to that organ, and together they all power the big body-field. They are like each organ's gas tank. A NES scan tells you how filled each organ's gas tank is (energetically speaking, of course). If the scan shows a white bar, there is no distortion with the organ field that the body-field is flagging for correction at this time. A green bar means there is a slight distortion: you have a pretty good supply of fuel but not a full tank. A red bar, however, means you are close to empty and need to refill that organ's energetic gas tank. Usually the first symptom of illness or of a significant body-field distortion is fatigue, which is a signal that one or more of your body-field's gas tanks is running low. Taking a Driver Infoceutical is akin to filling one of your body-field's many gas tanks.

▶ *Energetic Integrators:* Health means being well enough to do what you want, when you want. It's about getting places and doing things. The Integrators are like route maps in your body-field, and you can think about how they work like you think about planning a trip in your car. You have to have information. If you want to go somewhere, you want to know the most direct and efficient way to get there and how long it will take you. You plot your journey by consulting a map. Integrators are like the route maps in your body-field that direct information to the right place at the right time, so your body works efficiently and correctly.

Let's say you are driving from Dallas to Boston. The most efficient route will be an interstate highway, which will get you there by the most direct route, so it takes the least amount of time and your car will use the least amount of fuel. However, if there is a problem on the interstate, you might get detoured onto a state road. There are already a lot of cars there (people who live in the area who are going short distances around their homes or work, so that is the shortest route for them). So, when you and others from the interstate are funneled onto the smaller state road, congestion occurs. There are also more stoplights and intersections, so the trip goes more slowly and you use more fuel. If something happens on the state road, all of you may be detoured onto a county road. The trip will now take even longer because the route will be more circuitous. You will use more fuel. Your car might even experience more wear and tear because the country road might not be as well maintained as the primary roads.

The body-field works in the same way. When your body-field Integrators are distorted, information gets shunted from fast and efficient routes to side routes. Your body needs to get that information, and your body-field must find *some* route by which to get it where it needs to go, so it will send it along secondary or ever tertiary routes, which will already have information traffic on them. By having to take a longer route, you will use a lot more fuel (your Energetic Drivers have to work harder to move the information). The more indirect the route, the poorer the quality of the information when it finally gets where it is going (more wear and tear, so to speak). Correcting Integrators keeps the information on the body-field highway it's supposed to be on to get the job in the physical body done quickly and efficiently, with the least use of fuel and the least chance of the information getting lost or corrupted.

▶ *Energetic Terrains:* When you are driving, you want to be at least minimally prepared to deal with any environment. You don't want to be driving through a hailstorm with the top of the convertible down. You don't want the windows down during a dust storm or snowstorm. You want your vehicle to protect you during your trip. You can think of an Energetic Terrain as exposing you to things in the environment you would rather be protected from. During your lifetime, you are exposed to all kinds of viruses, bacteria, and other microbes and pathogens (or the energetic imprint of them). You don't want your "top" down or "windows" open so that they can get in. If Terrains show up, it's like your body-field has its convertible top down during a rainstorm. By correcting a Terrain, you put the top up or close the window so the elements are kept out. By correcting Terrains, you ensure that no matter what shows up during your trip through life, you can deal with it.

▶ *Energetic Stars:* The Energetic Stars bioenergetically represent metabolic pathways. Functionally, the Energetic Stars act as powerful unblockers, for each Star matches to various information pathways that come together to effect a single, major aspect of the body-field. To continue our extended car analogy, using a Star is like calling in a master mechanic because the problem involves multiple causes. If your engine is not running smoothly, fixing only one problem might not improve its performance. You might need to change clogged filters, adjust the valves or cylinders, replace the timing belt, and service the battery. In terms of your body-field, you might find that an imbalance, say a problem with your Nervous System Driver, doesn't stay corrected through use of the corresponding Driver or related Integrator Infoceuticals. You might need the Nerve Star Infoceutical, which contains within it information for the Nerve Driver, Nerve Detox, Nerve Function, Regeneration, and other Infoceuticals.

In this chapter, we trust you have come to appreciate the logic of the body-field's structure and the beauty of its inherent order. You no doubt better understand how a NES scan reveals the condition of your body-field and how the Infoceuticals can help correct bioenergetic problems.

However, there is a lot more to know about how your body-field and physical body work together in harmony to keep you alive and healthy. You may know that there are all kinds of electromagnetic signals coursing through your body, for instance in your brain and in your heart, but did you know sound affects how your body works? You may know that your heart pumps blood, but did you know that it is a lot more than just a pump? It is actually a major imprinter and regulator of information in your body and body-field. NES and other research have revealed a whole new symphony of energies and bioenergetic processes at play in your body, and it is to these that we now turn our attention in chapter 10.

NES CASE OVERVIEW: RANDOLPH

This NES case overview, and the others that follow in this book, illustrate how energizing the body-field can help the physical body recover, even when the cause of the physical problems is unknown. Because NES works at the level of information and is not biochemical, it is compatible with pharmaceuticals, herbs, supplements, and other healing agents. Clients are counseled to continue their other treatments and to confer with their other health care professionals.

Randolph was eighty years old at the time he sought NES practitioner and naturopathic physician Jason Siczkowycz's assistance. Six months prior, he had been hospitalized with pneumonia, and since that time he had debilitating fatigue. He reported that he could barely function: simply showering and shaving in the morning would so exhaust him that he had to go back to bed. He visited Siczkowycz looking for an answer because his regular health care professionals were at a loss as to how to help him. His NES scan revealed that his Source energy was severely depleted. Siczkowycz instructed him on how to take the Source Driver Infoceutical, which he did for one month. When he returned for a follow-up visit, his Source Driver had fully corrected itself, and he was back to his vigorous self. In fact, a few weeks after that, Randolph called the NES US office just to say thanks. He said he had just about given up on life, telling his wife that his quality of life was so compromised that if he didn't find something soon to help him he felt he might as well be dead. He said that after using only the Source Driver Infoceutical, he felt like a "thirty-year-old again" and that NES had given him back his quality of life.

10

INFORMATION FLOW
IN YOUR BODY
AND BODY-FIELD

PETER WAS SIPPING COFFEE at a table in the main lecture room, waiting for the start of the first NES conference in Australia, when he noticed an elderly woman headed his way. He wondered, in amazement, how an elderly woman had become so avant-garde as to attend a NES conference. He was about to find out, for the woman came over and introduced herself. Peter cannot now remember her name, but he remembers their conversation.

"She told me she had driven seven hours just to meet me and to thank me," Peter recalled. "When I asked her what for, she told me about her husband. He was in his seventies, like her, but had been quite ill. Medical tests had revealed that his heart was badly enlarged, and he had been mostly confined to bed. I remember thinking that, at his age, none of this was a favorable sign because this kind of chronic frailty of the heart also puts a lot of pressure on the function of the lungs. The medical treatment then was to wait and see what happens, but she had taken him to see a NES practitioner, and the scan had indicated the most needed Infoceutical was Bone Driver. It sounded reasonable to me, because *Bone Driver* bioenergetically affects calcium metabolism, which will in turn affect all muscle tissues, and it combines three acupuncture meridians through which energy flows from the feet toward the head over the front of body, so it directs energy to the heart. She told me that after her husband had taken Bone Driver for only two days the swelling of his heart went down, to the point where he could get out of bed and function again, walking around and such. Everybody was amazed at his recovery, which his physicians had not expected. This woman had come a long way from her hometown, just to thank me and ask me more about what the Infoceuticals are and how they work. Her effort really meant a lot to me."

It was these kinds of fortuitous encounters that helped keep Peter focused even as he struggled, back in early 2000, to pin down a full theoretical framework for how the Infoceuticals work. This example shows how NES differs radically from conventional medicine. It does not deal directly with an impaired organ but instead focuses on the underlying energetic factors. Yes, this man's heart was enlarged, but the bioenergetic cause of the swelling likely had no direct connection to his heart tissue.

In this case, this elderly man's Bone Driver, not his Heart Driver, was waving the red flag, shouting, "Hey, fix me first!" Bone Driver, despite its name, does not deal solely with the bone. It also correlates to calcium metabolism (and calcium buildup in arteries), muscle contraction, virtual intercellular communication, nerve signal transmission, hormone release, blood coagulation, antibody production, and the red blood cells in relation to tissue and organ oxygenation. However, the real effect may have been even more theoretical in nature. Bone Driver combines all the Chinese acupuncture meridians that go from the feet to the head, so it directs energy upward toward the heart. This directed energy flow is well-known in traditional Chinese medical theory, and it could have been that this flow was what helped make the NES correction work so effectively.

In effect, NES and some of the other complementary medical systems, such as TCM, are working via the energetic and informational *feedback loops* that are not evident in the biochemical model of healing of most allopathic medicine. According to our research, these feedback loops are what drives the body's biochemistry. For people new to bioenergetics and biophysics, and even for those familiar with complementary medicine, it can take a huge conceptual leap to not think in terms of allopathic medicine, in which there is a one-to-one correspondence between a disease and an organ or physiological process. That is not usually true in bioenergetic healing. So let's take a moment to discuss the logic of bioenergetic healing, which can seem almost completely opposite to the logic of conventional medicine.

THE LOGIC OF BIOENERGETIC HEALING

In conventional biology, the body has a physical and a biochemical reality. When something goes wrong genetically or biochemically, it can result in illness or disease. The cure or treatment for the disease is nearly always tied to the particular offending organ and its biochemical processes. So, for example, there is no cure for Type I diabetes, but physicians can give the body the insulin it needs and that the cells in the pancreas are not making. Bioenergetics approaches the problem differently. It would ask, why are the cells not doing their job? What *information* are they lacking that is causing the breakdown in the biochemical processes they are designed to carry out? Can we supply the energy and information to restore or improve that process? The answers to those questions may have little to do with the physical processes of the pancreas at all. Instead, they would likely have to do with the energy and information used by the cells that make up that organ and all the other processes that affect those cells. That information stream may be quite complex and involve other organs and physiological processes that are far removed from the pancreas and its functions. In other words, bioenergetics looks for the web of interconnected root causes, whereas allopathic medicine, for the most part, looks at observable symptoms. Both approaches serve their purpose, but they are fundamentally different approaches to healing.

In some respects, NES goes even farther than most other complementary healing approaches and extends our previous understanding of bioenergetics, because Peter's research has identified a *structure* to the body-field. That structure affects how information moves between the body-field and physical body. For example, consider the spherical standing waves that form an electron (where the In wave and Out wave intersect). According to NES theory, when those wave phase relationships are out of sync in the body-field, then the body-field can tend to hide disease patterns. Where are they hiding? In the onion-like layers of the body-field. Especially in chronic diseases, the root cause of a problem may be in a deep layer of the body-field, and it may take time to work through the layers of the body-field to work through the related influences and to get to the root cause. Which is why the *sequence* of healing is so important. NES is the only theory that we know of that identifies the body-field's preferred sequence of correction. You can think of the sequence of a NES protocol as peeling back those layers.

The body-field layers are related to the development of the disease over time, so they may have taken decades to accumulate. In the NES sequence of correction, you are moving back through the layers according to the sequence of the body-field's structure. The NES protocol starts with the Big Field influences, then works through Source energy and the Drivers, asking in effect if the body-field is adequately powered. If not, then the organs might not have the energy they need to carry out their functions effectively. Information cannot be "pushed" properly in the body-field, and from layer to layer, if there is insufficient energy. So you first have to align the body-field via the Big Field and Polarity and then address the Energetic Drivers.

Next the protocol addresses the Energetic Integrators, the actual flow and regulation of information. A scan reveals if information is getting where it needs to go and arriving there precisely when it is needed. It asks if information is distorted or scrambled, if it is stuck in a layer or blocked from getting to another layer. By working with the Energetic Integrators over time, you work through layers of your body-field in terms of information.

The Energetic Terrains and Energetic Stars are addressed in later scans to follow the sequence of healing according to NES theory, but the Drivers and Integrators have the most relevance to body-field layers, as they are the two most crucial aspects for determining the energetic and informational state of the body-field.

So, although people expect to feel an immediate difference when they take a prescription drug or use allopathic medicine, their expectations have to be different when using complementary modalities such as NES. Relief might come quickly, but that does not mean that the root cause of the problem is taken care of. That process takes time. However, the ability to work through and correct the complex web of energetic and informational flows of the body-field, rather than just to lessen symptoms, is why NES and complementary modalities in general seem to have a better track record than allopathic medicine in helping people with chronic diseases.

Another major difference in healing approaches is the issue of "masking." To some extent, allopathic medicine recognizes the reality of masking, such as in pain referral, which is when a pain in one part of the body is really attributable to a problem in a different part of the body. For instance, pain radiating up your left arm might have more to do with the state of your heart than with anything going on in your arm. However, when we talk in bioenergetic terms about masking, we are talking about something much more subtle. In this case, masking means that the body is not *ready* or *able* to reveal, and thus to deal with, a specific distortion. This is rather like what happens in allopathic medicine when you have pain, but the doctors can find no cause for it. Your pain is real, but the mechanisms causing it are not evident. In bioenergetics, we see that kind of situation as quite normal, for there is rarely a clear one-on-one correspondence between a physical disease and a single or even a few bioenergetic distortions. At the level of information, the link between the body-field and a physical problem may be convoluted indeed! Distortions in the phase relationships in the In wave and Out wave may be at the heart of masking, but the simplest way to understand masking is that a problem may not show up in the scan analysis because it is out of sequence with what the body is ready and able to deal with.

Peter admits that there may be no lasting correction if the body-field is not corrected in the preferred order. You can sometimes address acute problems directly, but for lasting correction of the underlying problems, it is always best to follow the body-field's lead, that is, follow the scan results and protocol sequence, and honor what the body is flagging as being ready for correction. In this regard as in so many others, NES is quite different from other modalities. We do not attempt to overrule the body or the body-field, which each have their own kind of intelligence, but instead develop the patience to work with them. The only way to make a lasting correction is to allow the body-field, and by extension the body, to work with those problems that bioenergetically it is *capable of handling*. Otherwise, you simply trade one symptom for another and never reach the root cause of the problem. In allopathic medicine, masking may be why one person benefits from a drug or therapy while another does not, and why when one symptom or disease is taken care of, the person finds that soon they have an entirely different set of symptoms or health problems. There is no getting around masking, but you can learn to work with it.

Because the preferred sequence for correcting distortions in the body-field is not always intuitive or logical in an allopathic medical sense, you have to be prepared to release preconceived notions of what your scan should show. As an example, consider the case we mentioned at the start of this chapter of the elderly man with the enlarged heart. You might have expected that Heart Driver or Energetic Integrator 2 (which correlates with the Heart/Lung Meridian) would have been the most distorted items in his NES scan, but his NES scan showed that the priority for correction was Bone Driver. Bioenergetically, his heart was not asking to be dealt with; it wasn't the organ waving the red flag, saying, "Hey, pay attention to me first!" Instead, it turned out that his body-field flagged the Bone Driver as most in need of correction. Bone

Driver, you may remember, deals with many bioenergetic processes, including muscle physiology, antibody production, and oxygenation processes. Any of these bioenergetic processes could be part of the root cause of that man's heart swelling. You can think of this indirect correction process in terms of a construction analogy: it's best to build a strong foundation before you construct the house. After the body has supported itself in other ways, only then is it ready to deal with significant bioenergetic distortions in specific organs. In NES, we trust that the body's self-healing intelligence is at work, and we follow the structure of the body-field to make the correction the body is, in a very real sense, asking for (instead of imposing on it what we think it needs according to our own logic). We cannot stress enough how much rethinking you must do to truly grasp the mechanics of bioenergetic medicine. It is a radically different approach to health from allopathic medicine, in which treatment is almost always in a one-on-one correspondence to an affected organ.

There is one other aspect of the logic of bioenergetic healing that you should be aware of, and it is an aspect of NES bioenergetics that seems to turn logic on its head. Contrary to what you might expect, if you are ill by allopathic standards, your NES scan actually may show very few severe body-field distortions (red or orange items) in your first few scans. On the other hand, if you are relatively healthy, with few health complaints, your first few scans could show many red items. Both of those situations seem completely the opposite of what you would expect, right? Well, consider this analogy. Picture an old non-digital television—the kind whose picture, if the antenna wasn't strong enough, would become distorted with static, or what was called "snow." If the picture was already distorted but the distortion increased, you might hardly notice, because the increased snow wouldn't stand out sharply against the already static-filled screen, but if you had a crystal-clear picture and a little static occurred, you would notice it right away. It would really stand out.

A similar type of phenomenon may occur in your NES scan.

When there are a lot of severe distortions in your field, then nothing in particular may stand out as significant. In reality, many things are significant, but the body-field may not have the power or energy (via the Energetic Driver fields) to send out anything but a weak matching response. Remember, the scan seeks the best possible answers under the circumstances, and in some circumstances, such as in a person with a severely distorted field, the best possible answer is that the intelligence of the body-field is saying, in effect, "Don't mess with too much too soon." So it shows a relatively clean scan. But as the Infoceutical protocol is followed and the body is repowered via Driver Infoceuticals, the body-field has the energy to better respond and it reports on distortions that it is ready to have addressed. As those corrections take place, as a result of using the Infoceuticals, then down the road that person's scan could suddenly show up with lots of reds and oranges because the body-field is finally able to respond to the matching tests with the vigor and information that allow the distortions to stand out. They will be unmasked, so to speak and the body-field will be adequately powered and able to deal with them. In the same way, a relatively healthy person could show many red, or severe, items in a scan. There is very little static in his or her system, so even a slight distortion stands out sharply against the relatively clear screen that is the body-field.

This kind of masking is not common, but it can occur, so anyone using NES should understand what it means. Our main point in offering this information is that it is important to understand that you cannot compare your scan with anyone else's. It's about your field, and only your field.

One final point before we move on to examine other aspects of your body-field. We have already pointed out that no one will ever achieve a perfect NES scan. The fact is that we can never be isolated from our environment, so we are constantly exposed to all kinds of fields, toxins, pathogens, stressors, and the like. Our bodies will always be thrown out of balance by something. Plus, our emotions, beliefs, perceptions, memories, and more affect our biology, so as long as we are thinking, feeling, and emoting human beings, we will be experiencing the ups and downs of life and reacting to them, often to the detriment of our health.

An additional point is that the *functional* aspects of our illnesses tend to be more easily corrected than the physical symptoms. The nonphysical, nontangible aspects of ourselves, such as our emotions, thought processes, coping strategies, and decision-making abilities—tend to shift more quickly than do the denser, physical aspects of ourselves, such as our organs or joints. The bioenergetic patterns that lead to illness have to work down deep in the body-field before they can affect our flesh and bones, and therefore it tends to take longer to correct actual physical problems. So NES, and natural healing of any kind, usually improves how we function (how we relate to the world and our illness, our energy level, clarity of thought, evenness of emotions, and so on) before it improves our physical symptoms.

Although it might take time to correct a physical ailment, you don't have to use NES, or any other natural therapy, forever. You use it until you feel better, your symptoms abate, and your functioning as a full and vibrant human being returns. As with any health care modality, the choice is yours. Still, our system and most complementary health systems are best used as part of a long-term wellness program. Unlike your use of allopathic medicine, in which you usually wait until you are sick before seeing a doctor, with natural medicine you try to stay well, to prevent sickness from happening in the first place. It is proactive, rather than reactive, health care. Most of us take vitamins, exercise, and make other choices to maintain or increase our wellness. In the same way, periodic check-ups using NES or other energy- and information-based modalities can help you maintain the best bioenergetic health possible over the long term, helping to correct problems *before* they get to the level of the physical body. Each approach to health—allopathic and alternative—has its strengths and weaknesses. Remember, the body is like a coin with two sides: it has its biochemical aspect and its bioenergetic one, which are interdependent, and so both are necessary for the body's proper functioning. Ideally, we will attend to both aspects of our body to achieve our highest possible state of health.

Now that you have a more complete understanding of how the logic of bioenergetic healing differs from that of allopathic medicine, we can turn our attention to other important aspects of how these two healing traditions view health. In particular, we would like to acquaint you with two aspects of the body that conventional biology and allopathic medicine barely recognize, although both play major roles in keeping you healthy.

THE ENERGETIC REALITIES OF THE PHYSICAL BODY

In bioenergetic medicine, information holds the key to correcting a problem, but because the body-field and physical body are interdependent, the answers to staying healthy or regaining health do not lie in the body-field alone. The physical body has its own role to play in bioenergetics. In fact, there are many amazing ways that the design of the physical body enables it to work with bioenergy to power and regulate the physical and energetic bodies. We turn now to examine two of these areas: cavities and the heart.

The Bioenergetic Importance of Body and Organ Cavities

Modern science has shown how your physical body is awash in energy in many different forms, such as electrical pulses, vibrations and pressure waves, and sound energies of various frequencies. For instance, your brain produces different types of low-frequency electrical energy in the form of alpha, beta, delta, theta, and gamma waves. Traditional medicine can *describe* these energies, but it cannot *explain* them. Bioenergetics can—as frequencies, electromagnetic waves, pressure waves, and quantum fields that encode information that is crucial to initiate and manage neurological processes. What's more, bioenergetics recognizes that the shape of the organ and other purely structural aspects of it are crucial to how that organ works as a bioenergetic imprinter of information. This is an area of physiology that most biologists overlook or are not even aware of.

Although biologists and neurologists have little understanding about why or how the brain produces the many types of brain waves it does, the effects of these waves are fairly easy to study, for they are evident through states of consciousness. Your brain produces all types of waves at all times, but generally beta waves dominate waking consciousness, as you go about your day. Stop, close your eyes, and turn your thoughts inward in a relaxing and reflective way, and your brain switches to producing alpha waves. When you sleep, your dreaming brain is producing theta waves, but when it is in the deepest, dreamless aspects of sleep, it shifts to a delta-wave rhythm. In those rare moments of a natural ecstatic high or, at the other end of the spectrum, when you are seized by fear, your brain waves may switch to the gamma range. Brain waves are largely electromagnetic energies, but your brain produces other kinds of energies, such as slight pressure waves when it expands and contracts as cerebrospinal fluid flows through it.

All of your organs are vibrating, jiggling, twisting, or otherwise moving, even if many of these movements are micromovements. They produce many kinds of energies as a result of their motion, including pressure waves (sound energy), or what in physics are called phonons. Phonons are quantum particles of sound, a type of quantum vibration that moves through particular types of solids. As a photon is to light, a phonon is to sound. In the body, phonons move through solid matter, especially matter with rigid crystal lattice characteristics at the atomic level such as a cell or connective tissue. Although you can actually hear your stomach rumble or growl, you probably don't hear the myriad other sounds or feel the pressure waves made during peristalsis, during the nearly ceaseless contracting, twisting, pushing, and pulling that is going on in your intestinal tract, especially during digestive processes.

Perhaps the most familiar body sound is the "lub-dub" sound your heart makes as it beats. However, the contractions that produce that sound are also producing vibrations in your chest cavity and the phonons that, as we will soon explain, may be imprinting information into your blood. Physicians can tell many things about the condition of your heart from listening to it, but what they might not appreciate is that those sounds are useful for things other than diagnosis.[1] They may actually carry crucial biological information—vital body instructions—to cells throughout the body. If energy equals information, then the study of our organs must extend beyond cell biology and into biophysics.

The flows of cerebrospinal fluid, blood, and other body fluids are mostly nonlinear, which moves them into the realm of chaos theory, systems theory, and even quantum physics, areas that are not usually applied to biology. What's more, the body spaces within which these fluids move alter and augment the frequencies of the sounds, which has an important effect on any information content encoded by those sound waves. We don't often think about the shapes of our cells or organ systems and the anatomical structures that encase them, but according to NES theory, and a few other alternative health systems such as TCM, the body's cavities play an important role in health.

Different objects make distinctive sounds because of the way they vibrate, but the sound of the vibration depends on the shape of the object and the material from which it is made. Think of a musical instrument, such as a guitar or trombone. The configurations of the cavity (enclosed space) of the instrument help to determine its particular sound. The same connection between shape and sound holds true in the physical body. For instance, the cochlea of the ear is spiral-shaped for a reason—that shape heightens our sensitivity to low-frequency sounds.[2] The shape and orientation of red blood cells affects the sound energy in the blood they flow through, with certain shapes and orientations leading to a loss of sound energy and an effect on health.[3]

There is an entire subdiscipline in physics that is devoted to studying how energy behaves within cavities. The study of cavity physics has immense relevance to your health, for your body is full of cavities that collect and amplify energy that is stored within them. All of our major organs are encased, for instance, our skull encases our brain, the eye sockets our eyes, the rib cage our heart and lungs, and so on. Our cells and organs themselves are cavity-like in nature, most being sack-like or tubelike, for instance, the sinuses, the microtubules in the brain and kidneys, and the various organs themselves, such as the pineal and adrenal glands, ovaries, pancreas, and lungs. Obviously, the stiff or hard coating that surrounds or makes up the outer layer of vital tissues lends protection to these tissues and organs. However, nature's propensity for cavities may be more than a consequence of mechanical and structural physics; it may be a consequence of quantum physics as well, for cavities are excellent collectors of energy, and hence of information. These cavity-like organs and cells may act as organic capacitors, storing energy as charges in spaces. We know that there has to be a charge in a space for there to be a QED field and for information exchange to take place.

Conventional medicine and biology do not pay much attention to the physics of the body cavities, so they have mostly overlooked how cavities may play a role in health and in the dynamics of information flow throughout the body. However, in NES theory, as in TCM theories, cavities perform at least two crucial bioenergetic functions: they attract life-force energy and they store it. In NES, this life-force energy is called Source energy, which may in fact be zero-point energy. In other cultures, Source energy is called qi, *ki,* prana, and *yuan qi* (in TCM). When there is a depletion of Source energy in the body-field as a whole or in a particular cavity, then physical problems may result. We will discuss Source energy in more detail in the Drivers chapter (chapter 12), but here we want to examine how cavities enhance information exchange in the body.

As previously stated, NES, and other bioenergetics research, has shown that cells can form energetic connections with neighboring cells if they are arranged with adjacent flat surfaces that are within certain angular parameters. Almost all cavities in the body, including cavity-like organs and glands, are coated with epithelial cells, which are usually flat and overlapping or stacked in orientation, and are cuboidal or columnar in shape. NES theory proposes that these cells act as energy connections and information conduits between cells, forming a distributed information network in the body (epithelial cells cover just about every cavity in the body). The epithelial cells, because of their shape, attract Source energy into the cavities and facilitate information exchange between cells that make up the cavities and organs. Peter's research shows that the angular orientation of the epithelial cells must be within 5 degrees from parallel to each other in their layer, or else the connection between cells is lost. So the shapes of the cells that line the outer surfaces of cavities, organs, and glands and their orientation to each other play a crucial role both in energy storage and information exchange in the body.

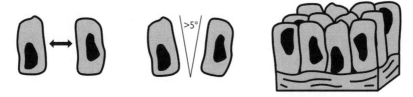

Figure 10.1. The orientation and alignment of cells, especially epithelial cells, affect their ability to communicate at a bioenergetic level. NES research shows that a deviation of more than 5 degrees from parallel appears to break field communication between cells and other structures. Epithelial cells envelop organs, presenting flat surfaces to neighboring cells and creating the conditions that help organs—as cavities—attract and store Source energy.

In NES therapy, because practitioners don't deal with a damaged organ or gland directly but instead work with the information of the body-field, this might mean working with the larger body cavity in which the organ or gland is located. So, for example, if there is a problem with kidney function, one option for addressing the problem is to support the abdominal cavity, which stores the life-force energy for that area of the body. Every cavity, even those that are glands or organs, can store Source energy, but the three major cavities of the body—the cranial, thoracic, and abdominal—store huge quantities of it. Sometimes simply by "powering" the main cavity itself, everything within that cavity is corrected.

Practitioners also can work to correct Source energy deficiencies by using certain Energetic Integrator Infoceuticals. So, in addition to the Source Driver Infoceutical, particular Energetic Integrator Infoceuticals, such as Energetic Integrators 9 (Thyroid/Triple Burner), 2 (Heart/Lung Meridian), 6 (Kidney/Kidney Meridian), and 11 (Bone Marrow/Stomach Meridian) and the Energetic Star 4 Infoceutical (Triple Cavity) could prove helpful for specific types of cavity energy-depletion problems, although the NES scan would indicate what is most needed at that time.

NES research has shown that certain elements, about twenty of them, collect especially easily, physically and via their fields, in the cavities; and their information is particularly important (in a supportive or detrimental way, depending on the element) to the bioenergetic functioning of the cavities of cells and organs:

Aluminum	Molybdenum
Boron	Nitrogen
Cadmium	Oxygen
Calcium	Phosphorous
Carbon	Potassium
Chromium	Rhodium
Cobalt	Ruthenium
Hydrogen	Scandium
Magnesium	Silicon
Manganese	Vanadium

Although the Energetic Integrators link energetically to these and other elements, Peter's matching experiments showed that the cavity–Source energy system linked only to these specific elements. Source energy in the lungs and kidneys in particular, but in other cavities and tubules as well, may be what allows cavities to interact with the matter waves of only these elements. Source energy may be conjugate with these elements and thus easily make energetic matches to them. If this is true, and further experiments need to be conducted, then it may be that the human body-field interacts especially strongly with certain parts of the zero-point field and not with others, which would have enormous ramifications for health.

At a more practical level, these experiments suggest that one of the best ways to restore Source energy is to breathe! Breathing has been at the forefront of many esoteric health systems across the globe and throughout the centuries, especially the yogic traditions. NES cavity theory suggests why this may be true, especially breathing sea air, for the sea spray would release many micronutrients and other beneficial elements into the air. It also suggests, contrary to popular opinion, that vitamin or mineral supplements may *not* be effective sources of these elements, for ingesting them bypasses the important cavities (lungs especially) that are bioenergetically important in how the body uses them.

In TCM, yuan qi, or the life-source energy, collects primarily in the brain, lungs, and kidneys—all of which are made of millions of microtubules. TCM identifies the heart as the master organ—the "emperor" of the body and the "ruler" of the five major organ networks. Peter's research has extended that idea in important ways by explaining the links between the heart–midbrain system and modern biochemistry, proposing a biophysical explanation for the heart's special status: the heart, in concert with the midbrain, is the primary conduction system for Source energy. *It is the master imprinter of information in the body.*

The Heart as Imprinter

The conventional view of the heart is as a pump, that through its strong muscular contractions it drives the blood flow of the body. You might be surprised to know that some researchers take issue with this view. They feel that from a purely mechanical point of view, the heart is neither designed solely as a pump nor is it a very efficient pump.[4] What NES research has shown is that on the virtual level, the heart is a lot more than simply a pump.

In embryological development, the heart is among the first organs to form and the first to work. It starts to beat at about twenty-one days, when the embryo is only about 5 millimeters in size and the heart itself has formed only two rudimentary chambers. The embryo gets most of its nourishment and oxygen via diffusion from the mother and the yolk sac. At this early stage, it has formed a neural tube, but the brain is just beginning to form and the lungs won't form until the sixth week of development. So what is the heart doing if it is not needed as a primary pump for blood? From a bioenergetic perspective, it is beginning its work of imprinting information that is crucial for the fetus's continued development. In other words, the fetus is forming not just according to genetic, chemical, and anatomical templates, but through a quantum informational template as well. The heart produces myriad sounds (phonons) and various kinds of waves, from pressure (sound and vibrational) waves to electromagnetic waves, that help direct fetal development. In fact, other major systems of the body, such as the connective tissue matrix and the nervous system, imprint information, but the heart is a primary imprinter of information bodywide.

Of course, once the fetal brain develops, it works in concert with the heart to direct development. It is interesting to note that Peter's matching experiments have shown that the heart has the same energy type as the midbrain. The midbrain, according to conventional biology, is known to process certain kinds of sensory input and to control parts of the autonomous nervous system. For instance, it controls movement. However, research by Walter Rudolf Hess, Nobel Prize winner and among the greatest of modern physiologists, has detailed previously unknown or little understood functions for the midbrain, such as how it influences blood circulation and respiration. What's more, the new science of neurocardiology has shown that the heart and brain share an undeniable link at the cellular level because the heart actually contains neural cells of exactly the same type as are in the brain. So Peter's matching experiments are being validated by conventional, allopathic research. In NES, the heart and brain also are linked energetically via many different Energetic Integrator channels, as we will soon discuss. Our point here is that it is erroneous to think that the heart's only function is to pump blood. It may be that it is a kind of second brain in the body, as people in so many cultures, especially the Chinese, have suggested.

How might the heart work as an imprinter of information? Every time your heart beats, it creates strong pressure waves and phonons within its chambers. Your heart produces dozens, if not hundreds, of different frequencies, each of which is capable of carrying a different type of information, although research into this area is still in its infancy, so not much is known about this encoding process. The phonons may imprint information onto the lipids in your blood, which then are carried throughout the body. It is interesting to note that some statins and cholesterol-lowering medications have the curious side effect of disrupting short-term and long-term memory.[5] These side effects are often dismissed because there is no known mechanism in conventional biology to explain them. However, they make perfect sense in NES theory because the information imprinted into fats in the bloodstream may act as a kind of body-wide memory storage and retrieval system. In addition, phonons stream through your blood plasma, carrying additional information from the central nervous system to the hemoglobin, which also carries oxygen throughout the body. It is interesting that red blood cells, which carry hemoglobin, have no DNA of their own, so they are neutral carriers of information.

We know from recent conventional research that the pattern of your heartbeats can be a predictor of the overall state of your health.[6] Whereas once it was thought that a healthy heart kept a regular, consistent beat pattern, medical professionals now understand that just the opposite is true: the more variable your heartbeat frequencies, the healthier you tend to be. In fact, the lack of beat-time variability has now become one of the indicators for how ill someone is. However, researchers do not yet fully understand how the types of heartbeats and the rate variability of those beats correlate with health, despite the abundance of biochemical and bioelectrical heart data. From a bioenergetics point of view, heartbeat variability makes sense, for each type of beat encodes particular types of information into the blood (or tissue such as connective tissue) for transmission to the trillions of cells throughout the body. The fewer types of beats the heart is able to make, the more degraded this information function of the heart becomes.

In addition to the pathway by which hemoglobin is imprinted, there are three other possible avenues of information transmission. Some of the phonons may travel out of the heart chambers and spread through the blood in connective tissue as pressure waves. The heart also may produce small numbers of free electrons, which are electrically conducted via the blood and skip between ionized molecules. Finally, the heart may produce and transmit ultraweak light (or photons, if you think of light as being composed of particles) that also carries information. The functions of the phonons, electrons, and photons at play in this information system overlap, providing redundancy, which is crucial for critical biological processes.

The phonon represents the slowest, yet most reliable, method of information transmission. We know from studies of sonoluminescence (a process by which sound transmitted through water produces light) that phonons don't need or use much energy and that they are not adversely affected by electromagnetic fields. Because of their generally slow velocity in the body, phonons may act as a sort of buffer for the body, via the heart, from the many signals that inundate it, so that for short periods of time they can help the body adapt to sudden changes. If the body is shocked or unexpectedly stressed, a sudden increase in pressure inside the heart may emit a burst of phonons, which may help raise the blood pressure, as part of the fight-or-flight survival mechanism. The higher the blood pressure, though, the faster phonons travel, so they can, if they need to, race to all parts of the body to transmit crucial information to the cells.

Can pressure waves, frequencies, and phonons really accomplish what we are suggesting they can? Recent research from conventional researchers provides support. It has always been thought that molecules of chemical messengers such as peptides have to dock on cell receptors to activate or deactivate a cell, basically giving it the information to know what to do and when. However, psychopharmacologist Candace Pert and others have recently discovered that sound can activate the receptors on cells. In other words, sound can act on a cell in exactly the same way a biochemical molecule does! Pert refers to music in her work, but her point can be applied to any type of coherent sound. She wrote,

> Music, which is a patterned vibration, can bypass the ligand and directly resonate those [cell] receptors, interacting like a peptide or drug—or an emotion. The vibrational frequency of the notes turns on the receptors, setting in motion all kinds of cellular activities. That's how music can heal, interacting directly with your molecules of emotion to charge you with energy, get your juices flowing, and make you feel good.
>
> These molecules are not only vibrating to cause bodywide changes, but they are "hearing" each other through the psychosomatic [mind-body] network of cellular communication. You can see that we don't just hear with our ears, but we "hear" with every receptor on every cell in our bodymind. We're literally alive with the sound of music![7]

This is an amazing discovery that has provocative implications for bioenergetic health and bolsters the NES research showing that the patterns of phonons generated by the body's organs and physiological processes can be considered the quantum music of the body. As our various organs emit phonons, they are flooding our system with information that is every bit as real as the peptides that activate cells. The phonons that cascade through our body can change our very biochemistry, and the research into how heartbeat variability equates with health is only one of the areas of academic study that is providing convincing evidence for the reality of these underlying quantum processes.

Magnetism also plays a role in information transfer in the body, although this role is not well understood, even within the NES model. Modern science has shown that the blood has magnetic properties; for instance, oxygenated blood is polar magnetic, that is, it displays both a north and south pole axis, whereas deoxygenated blood is paramagnetic (has no poles). It may be that this difference in blood magnetism acts as a driving force for blood circulation. We also know that blood tends to spiral through our blood vessels, rather than flow in a linear way. (Quantum physics underlies many nonlinear dynamic processes.) Both the opposing magnetic forces and the nonlinear spiraling dynamics of blood flow may contribute to blood circulation, in a sense causing the blood to partially "pump" itself, so that the heart does not have to function as the sole pump.

Information distribution in the body, according to the NES model, occurs by all three routes: electromagnetism, phonons of various frequencies, and electrons. These are the "real" information transfer mechanisms, but the information itself is part of the body-field dynamics, the realm of the "virtual." Think back to the opera ticket: you have to have an actual paper ticket on which is printed the virtual information that gives the ticket its meaning and usefulness. What is unique in the NES model, although it arises from TCM, is the realization that our blood transfers information from our central nervous system to all the cells in the body via the heart, which serves as the main imprinter of this information into the blood. There is a virtual feedback loop between the heart and central nervous system, with the central nervous system sending information to the heart, where it is imprinted into the blood and carried throughout the body, and then back from the heart to the central nervous system.

It is interesting to note that this theory of the heart as information imprinter can explain why some patients who received heart transplants report that they take on the feelings, habits, and likes and dislikes of the person whose heart was implanted into them. For example, in one of the most publicized reports, a woman, Claire Sylvia, received a heart-lung transplant, and afterward she suddenly began craving chicken nuggets and beer, two things she had never particularly cared for.[8] She later discovered that her heart donor was a teenage male who had died in a motorcycle accident. He loved chicken nuggets and beer. Other transplant recipients have reported major behavioral changes, only to discover later that they had begun speaking and behaving like their donors. Allopathic doctors for the most part write off such reports, but bioenergetics provides a perfectly logical explanation: although the heart may be in a different person's body, it still imprints vestiges of information that are particular to the body, mind, and spirit of the person who was its donor.

However, let's return to the more physiological effects of the heart as imprinter. NES research suggests that if this heart-brain flow is blocked in either direction (heart to brain or vice versa), there are consequences for the body. For example, if information sent from the heart to the brain is not being processed properly by the brain, then the flow in the feedback loop slows and energy levels within the brain rise, which correlates to an increase in migraine headaches. As the heart tries repeatedly to get this information to the brain but can't, the information/energy overload in the brain spills over and affects the sensory nerves in the brain, which may account for a migraine headache–sufferer's heightened sensitivity to light and sound. Conversely, if the midbrain is sending information to the heart, but the heart is not processing it correctly or efficiently, then energy builds up there and can correlate to heart problems. It also may cause systemic problems bodywide, for the heart is not taking in the information and imprinting it into the blood for the rest of the cells in the body to use. The body may begin to lose its ability to regulate itself at a systems level, that is, it begins to lose equilibrium (homeostasis). The information being blocked or degraded can be of a specific type, depending on the problem with the heart, so the results might be felt only in a specific type of cell that is not receiving the information it needs. When an information route in the body is blocked or distorted, the body will try to find another less direct or efficient route to get the information to the necessary cells. However, if heart function is compromised, rerouting often is not an option because the heart itself is the primary imprinter of the information to the rest of the body. Symptoms of an information blockage in the heart can rapidly worsen as the cells lose access to crucial, life-sustaining information. The heart is so crucial a bioenergetic organ that NES has three primary Infoceuticals that directly correlate to correcting the heart field at a holistic bioenergetic level and many others that indirectly address specific parts of the heart field.

There are other ways that information is encoded for use by the body, such as through frequency and perhaps even phase relationships. These bioenergetic mechanisms are tightly correlated to the Energetic Integrators in particular, so we will cover them in chapter 13. In each of the next six chapters, we will introduce you to a specific aspect of the body-field. The interconnections are amazing, and we will be able to provide only a glimpse into the intricate web of information and energy that you are. We will begin with the Big Field and move through the Energetic Drivers, Energetic Integrators, Energetic Terrains, and Energetic Stars, in that order.

NES Case Overview: Helen

For nine months, Helen had suffered from severe abdominal pain, with no cause discovered by her primary health care providers. On a scale of one to ten, with ten being most severe, she rated her chronic pain as an eight. When she visited NES practitioner and naturopathic physician Jason Siczkowycz, her scan showed her Source energy was severely depleted and her Stomach Driver was severely weakened, so she took these two Infoceuticals daily for six weeks. When she returned to Siczkowycz's office for another scan, she reported that her abdominal pain was gone. The new scan showed her Source Driver and Stomach Driver as fully functional.

11

BIG FIELD INFLUENCES

IN THE SUMMER OF 2005, a woman named Ann e-mailed the NES US office to ask about the Infoceuticals. She explained that she had taken her daughter to a NES practitioner and while there had been scanned herself. Her NES scan showed that her body-field was misaligned with aspects of the Big Field. In NES, we sometimes talk about the Big Field as an aspect of body-field structure for simplicity's sake, but it is actually a relationship of alignment between your body-field and natural Earth and cosmic energies and fields. When this interconnection is distorted (or another item called Polarity, which we will discuss at the end of this chapter), it must be corrected before other areas can be dealt with because it tends to make subsequent body-field readings less accurate. Ann was given the Big Field Aligner Infoceutical, and after only a few days of using it she felt a marked difference. "What has been happening to me is absolutely amazing," she wrote. Ann did not have a clear idea of how the Infoceutical worked, but the NES employee who answered her e-mail took the time to send her a comprehensive explanation. She then wrote back to report in more detail about the changes she was experiencing. Between her two e-mails she reported:

> I'm experiencing improved memory, bursts of creativity [she's an artist who had not been productive for some time]. . . . My creativity is unbelievable, and I have several projects going now. I am not

procrastinating when it comes to household bills and instead I have become this organizing fanatic. I have never been organized and I believed I, like my sisters, had inherited the family gene [for being disorganized]! I've bought countless books trying to learn to become organized, but they never helped. I also have better stress management, better sleep, memory, and moods. I could go on and on.

The Big Field Aligner Infoceutical does just what its name implies—it aligns your body-field with the Big Field of Earth. Its effect is to stabilize and better organize your body-field, so it tends to "ground" you, to make you feel more stable within your physical body. People whose body-field is seriously misaligned with any of the three axes of Earth's Big Field can tend to become unfocused and unorganized, what others might call "spacey." Although the Big Field Aligner Infoceutical affects different people in different ways, Ann presented a classic case of how aligning yourself with Earth's Big Field correlates to improved focus and lessens erratic emotions and behaviors, allowing your talents (in her case, her creativity) to flourish.

So just what is the Big Field test in a NES scan? It is an analysis of the basic way in which your body-field is placed, or oriented, in relation to the three principal axes of a larger natural Earth field that NES calls the Big Field. The three aspects of the Big Field are the vertical, equatorial, and magnetic polar axes. Our orientation to these axes correlates to aspects of our emotional state, as energy moves through the heart area of the body. As you may remember, the heart is a major "emotional" and sensory organ in the body, according to both NES and TCM. However, before we describe these axes in more detail, let's briefly examine what kinds of fields arise from or permeate Earth and how they might affect us.

EARTH FORCES AND FIELDS

The ancient Chinese, and the people of many other ancient wisdom traditions, taught that the human body is an energetic reflection of natural fields. Their idea of "as above, so below" yokes our bodies to the energies of both the heavens and Earth. The subtext of much of their natural medicine approach was to help the sick person achieve harmony between heaven and Earth, to align with the natural fields and to avoid the geopathic stress fields that adversely affect the energies of the human body. Geopathic stress relates specifically to the health effects of vibrations and fields that emanate from Earth's interior and flow across its surface. The energies detrimental to health arise especially from caves and subterranean caverns or from certain types of underground streams and aquifers, fault lines, and particular kinds of mineral and coal deposits.

Modern scientists, except perhaps for those involved with protecting the health of astronauts and those who work underground, such as miners, barely acknowledge that natural energy fields have any real impact on the state of our health. Although physicists and cosmologists know a great deal about the many kinds of forces and fields that permeate the universe—cosmic radiation, electromagnetic fields, nuclear energies at the center of stars such as our sun, geothermal energies within the earth, and the like—they still don't know how to measure, by conventionally accepted methods, the geopathic stress fields as they affect the body. In the conventional biological paradigm, the causes of disease are almost always limited to biological and genetic processes and environmental factors such as toxins and infectious agents.

In terms of public health, with the exception of the negative health effects of ultraviolet radiation from the sun and radon gas from the earth, there is little scientific agreement about the health effects of energy fields, natural or man-made. Debate rages about the effects of the loss of the ozone layer and the output from high-power electrical transmission lines on health. Despite reams of studies, we are left with contradictory guidelines about the safety of cell phones, microwave ovens, computers, and other electronics that emit low-level electromagnetic or magnetic fields. We know even less about how the huge fields of energy that encompass Earth affect us. For example, we are only now beginning to explore how the electromagnetic fields that fill the ionosphere impact us. Let's explore the potential implications of these energy fields by looking at one phenomenon, called the Schumann resonance, which was named for its primary discoverer, German atmospheric physicist W. O. Schumann, who confirmed its existence in the mid-1950s.[1] The Schumann resonance is of special interest to us because it deals with two phenomena of physics that are at the heart of the NES model of bioenergetics: resonant cavities and standing waves.

The ionosphere is a layer of the atmosphere that is located at the edge of the larger magnetosphere about 34 miles above Earth and is filled with ionized radiation from the sun. It is rife with electrical activity and is of major importance to the conduction of radio waves. What Schumann proved was that the space between the earth's surface and the ionosphere forms a resonant cavity. Lightning, which strikes somewhere on or above the earth tens of thousands of times a day, pumps energy into the ionosphere (more specifically, into the cavity formed between the ionosphere and the earth), and this energy causes quasistanding waves of extremely low frequency, a phenomena called the Schumann resonance. The Schumann resonance frequency ranges from about 5 to 50 hertz, with an average frequency of between 7 and 10 hertz. That average just happens to match the alpha range of human brain waves, so there is wide speculation, and growing evidence, that the Schumann resonance affects the human brain. The heart also is tuned closely to this range of frequencies.

The late New Zealand scientist Neil Cherry was among the most well-known of researchers who studied both the Schumann resonance and extremely low frequency (ELF) waves in relation to human health.[2] He noted that they almost certainly play a role in the human circadian rhythm, which includes the wake-sleep cycle. Other research shows levels of melatonin—a hormone associated with sleep—significantly drop in response to ELF waves in the range of 16.7 to 50 hertz. For a more comprehensive overview of the research in the field, we refer you to Dr. Robert O. Becker's book *The Body Electric,* which discusses the myriad ways that electromagnetic signals, especially very low frequency and extremely low frequency electromagnetic waves, affect physiology, from cell division to wound healing. Most of the focus of this kind of frontier research is on man-made electromagnetic pollution, so very little is known about how natural geomagnetic and atmospheric fields may adversely affect human health.

Interestingly, we can turn to Europe to explore the detrimental health effects of geopathic stress. The reality of such fields is much more accepted, and thus more widely studied, there than it is in the United States. Part of the reason for this wider acceptance is that dowsing—the ancient art of using rods, pendulums, or other implements to detect the subtle shifts in underground energies, particularly those associated with caverns, mineral deposits, and certain types of watercourses—enjoys widespread practice throughout Europe even today. Dowsers, using various methods, but today usually employing wooden or metal rods as "antennas" to pick up energies, can detect where the best place might be to drill a water well or to prospect for oil or minerals. The energies dowsers are able to detect are not measurable by conventional standards, such as in terms of frequency or amplitude, so scientists, for the most part, dismiss them and their techniques, although modern businesses, especially those of the mining and petroleum industries, have used dowsers for decades. Dowsers and NES practitioners face the same challenges in terms of finding acceptance by conventional scientists. Dowsers may in fact be performing a kind of resonant conjugate matching, as is Peter in his matching experiments.

Dowsers, like the practitioners of feng shui and other Eastern health traditions, tend to warn against living near certain kinds of Earth features, such as deep caverns, or situating your house, or bed in particular, over certain types of underground watercourses. They also believe that Earth itself is crisscrossed with natural channels of energy in the form of meridians of concentrated geomagnetic energy, some types of which are called ley lines. It is claimed that many of Earth's "power places" and sacred sites are situated at the intersection of multiple ley lines. However, prolonged exposure to these sources of geopathic stress and other concentrated Earth energies can be detrimental.

Officials in Vilsbiburg, Germany, take geopathic stress seriously. When they detected an unusually high cancer rate in their town, they set about trying to track possible causes. Finding no obvious mechanism for the cancer rate, such as environmental hazards in air or water, they decided to commission a medical study that compared the health records of residents to dowsing charts that pinpointed geopathic stress hotspots in the area. They discovered that there was a strong correlation between sources of geopathic stress and the incidence of cancer.[3] Other studies elsewhere in Germany and in Austria have shown a similar correlation. In fact, geopathic stress as an indicator of or a possible causative factor in cancer and other diseases is now taken so seriously in parts of Germany that officials have begun to keep health records for individual homeowners, presumably those whose houses have been identified as situated over or near areas of high geopathic stress.

Now that we have reviewed the links others have made between Earth fields and health, let's look at what NES research and theory have revealed about this correlation.

NES AND EARTH FIELDS

In NES, the body-field scan is designed to take readings about the relationship of your body-field to many kinds of field energies, including those associated with the earth. The primary natural Earth field—called the Big Field—is composed of three axes, which are each considered separately in the NES scan. These are the vertical, equatorial, and magnetic polar axes. According to NES theory, for optimal health your body-field, as a quantum structure in space, must be aligned properly with these Earth fields. The three axes form planes that intersect your body very close to the center line of your body, slightly to the left, where the heart is located. Peter's research shows that a misalignment can distort the communication networks in your full body-field, in large part because the heart cannot imprint information properly. The closeness of the intersection of the planes to the heart could also explain why the Big Field Aligner Infoceutical, which corrects distortions in these three fields, impacts emotions and even memory, which are bioenergetically connected to the heart. In addition, we know from the work of cell biologist Bruce Lipton and others that cells are tuned to the environment with the cell membrane serving as a kind of receiving and transmitting medium for environmental signals. NES research confirms and extends these findings: cells are not only tuned to the external environment but also to the energies of the three axes of the Big Field as well. When the body is misaligned with one or more of these axes, information imprinting at the cellular level can go askew, so cells themselves become a source of body-field errors.

You may remember that in one of Peter's experiments with Dr. Bevan Reid, the connection between the fields of two matching items was broken when the plates they were tested on were moved from the perpendicular by more than 5 degrees. Something similar may be going on in relation to the orientation of your body-field and the Big Field. As your body-field moves out of alignment with one or more of the axes of the Big Field, the communication routes in the body that are correlated with that field (or fields) become blocked, interrupted, or distorted. Overall, the misalignment can make you feel that you are not securely "in" your body. The effect of not being energetically grounded can take myriad forms but generally correlates to flightiness, disorganization, scattered thoughts, lack of focus, impatience, erratic emotions, and even insomnia. In fact, an unaccountably disrupted sleep pattern correlates bioenergetically to misalignment between your body-field and Earth's Big Field.

More specific to biology and anatomy, Peter's matching experiments showed that the Big Field is linked to immune system function via yellow bone marrow. There are two kinds of bone marrow, red and yellow. Yellow marrow develops in the long bones of the body, especially the arm and leg bones. Although we have mostly red marrow when we are young, yellow marrow increases as we age, filling our bone cavities with fatty tissue. Most red blood cells, platelets, and certain types of white cells are made only in the red marrow, but under emergency conditions, such as during extreme blood loss, yellow marrow can turn into red marrow. As we age, we are more susceptible to infections and cancers partly because we have less red marrow, and hence fewer immune cells, and more yellow marrow. However, when we have an infection, yellow marrow can be converted to red marrow to increase the number of immune cells available to combat the infection. Yellow marrow is an energy-storage tissue because it is composed mainly of fats. During extreme conditions, such as a period of starvation, the body can use yellow marrow as a source of energy and fuel. Why there is an energetic connection—a conjugate relationship or match—between the Big Field and yellow marrow is one of the myriad questions about bioenergetics that remains to be answered.

In addition to the bioenergetic health ramifications of the Big Field, there is also a technical reason for making it a priority for correction. As mentioned briefly earlier, if your body-field is not properly aligned with one or more of the three primary Earth field axes, then readings for all the substructures of your body-field may be skewed. NES theory identifies an optimal sequence to healing, an order of correction that is based on the bioenergetic dynamics of the body-field as revealed over Peter's decades of exploration. Those dynamics require that, under almost all circumstances and especially at the beginning of your use of NES, you must align your body-field with the Big Field before you go deeper into the body-field layers to correct Integrators or Terrains. It's possible to correct those aspects of the body-field when your body-field is misaligned to the Big Field, but it might take longer and the correction might not hold over time. The single NES Infoceutical called Big Field Aligner works to correct an imbalance or distortion in any of the three axes of the Big Field.

Let's take a brief look now at the specifics of the three axes of the Big Field.

The Vertical Axis

The vertical axis is intimately related to gravity and its numerous effects on the body. Gravity is a field of attraction. Of all the forces of nature, the gravitational force is the weakest and yet is the one we are most familiar with because it is the one we can most easily sense. When you step on a scale to see how much you weigh, what the scale is measuring is how strongly Earth's gravitational field is pulling on you. When a ball bounces, it comes back down to Earth instead of flying off into space because of the pull of Earth's gravity. We can't escape gravity, although the farther from Earth's surface we get, the less we feel its pull on our bodies.

The National Aeronautics and Space Administration (NASA) in the United States has done an enormous amount of research into how gravity affects the body, because lack of gravity, which astronauts experience during space flight, can have adverse effects on health. For example, without the constant pull of gravity, astronauts lose bone mass.

The vertical axis also is associated with geopathic stress. Although NES cannot make a direct one-to-one correspondence between cause and effect in this case, Peter has found that there is a strong bioenergetic correlation between the vertical axis of the Big Field and the human nervous system. Among the most common symptoms of a Big Field distortion is a disrupted sleep pattern. As previously stated, there is evidence that the human circadian rhythm—our internal biological sense of time, or "body clock"—is linked subtly with the Schumann resonance, so it is not a huge leap to think that Earth's Big Field also is an influence on our body-clock. NES research also shows that the Nervous System Driver is energetically linked with brain waves, specifically alpha waves, delta waves, and the low-frequency waves prevalent during relaxation and the sleep cycle. So, in many cases of clients who complain of erratic sleep cycles, their NES scan shows that both their Big Field (and specifically the vertical axis of the Big Field) and the Nervous System Driver are out of balance.

The Equatorial Axis

The equatorial axis is associated with Earth's rotation. In terms of bio-energetic health, it is related to how the body responds to electrons and ionic charges, such as those associated with oxygen and hydrogen, so it is intimately connected to cell function and, thus, to normal physiological functioning. This axis correlates energetically to detoxification processes in the body via free radical and antioxidant formation. Free radicals are molecules that are missing an electron, so they scavenge in the body, "stealing" electrons from other molecules, which can eventually damage cells. Free radical damage is often equated with the aging process because the negative effects of aging are associated with loss of cell function. Antioxidants are molecules that counteract the effects of free radicals because they give their own electrons to free radicals and so prevent them from taking electrons from the atoms in cells. Because the equatorial axis appears to link energetically to these molecules, it may be an important bioenergetic link to the aging process. Some metabolic diseases and certain types of arthritis also correlate bioenergetically with a misaligned equatorial axis, as do problems of the large bowel, colon, and liver.

The Magnetic Polar Axis

Earth is cocooned in magnetic fields, which emerge both from the interior of Earth and from cosmic phenomenon throughout the universe. The movement of electrically conductive molten iron in Earth's outer core generates its polar magnetic field, which is so large that it extends far beyond Earth's surface and into space. Magnetic fields in space, called the Van Allen belts, are made up of an inner belt of protons that are left over from cosmic ray collisions and an outer belt of ions and electrons that are trapped by Earth's magnetic fields. The belts make up a magnetic field that is oriented perpendicular to the gravitational field of the earth, and they help protect us from many of the harmful effects of cosmic radiation and other cosmic fields.

There are many biological processes that are magnetic in nature.

For example, we earlier discussed how an fMRI machine works by affecting tiny biomagnets in protons in the hydrogen nuclei of water molecules in your body. Your brain has magnetic aspects to it, as does your blood. In fact, hemoglobin is rich in iron, an element that is strongly affected by magnetism.

This axis also is intimately connected with circadian rhythms, and by extension with the wake-sleep cycle. Research has shown that most living organisms, from coral polyps to human beings, are affected by the pull of magnetism from the moon and by Earth's own magnetic field. Our internal body clock is set and can be reset, not only by light, but also by magnetic fields.

In bioenergetics, however, cause and effect can be less clear-cut. NES research has shown that when your body-field is misaligned with the magnetic polar axis, you may experience problems that don't appear to be causally linked to magnetism. For instance, you may experience thermal regulation problems—a breakdown in the way your body creates and distributes heat.

Although both static and fluctuating magnetic fields external to the body have been implicated in health problems, including cancer, conventional science has reserved judgment because epidemiological studies in humans are inconclusive and the physics seems dubious. Magnetic fields, such as those from high-tension power lines or natural fields around Earth, are thought to be too weak to break the chemical bonds of molecules in the body or even to heat those molecules. However, recently biochemists have uncovered evidence that magnetic fields are not as innocuous as first thought. As reported in *New Scientist* in 2002, biochemists have found that proteins in our bodies "can act like magnets themselves, and that steady external magnetic fields of fridge-magnet strength can force them to bend in line. If the same happens in the membrane of living cells, magnetic fields could have a host of knock-on effects such as slowing down ion transfer and disrupting cell signaling."[4] Although the jury remains out on the overall health effects of magnetic fields, NES research has shown that for ideal bioenergetic health, it is best if your body-field is in alignment with Earth's Big Field, including the magnetic polar axis.

THE POLARITY FIELD

In NES, the term *polarity* refers to a negatively charged electrostatic field that permeates the physical body, forming in part from the overall biological and energetic activity of the body and playing a vital role in the formation and functioning of the human body-field.[5] Peter's research suggests that the body-field, and the physical body, prefers a slightly negatively charged field and that when electrostatic fields are too positively charged, exposure to them could correlate to increased chance of pathology. His research also suggests that the main link between the electromagnetic Polarity field and the physical body is via the stem cells in the red marrow of the bones. Biologically, this link could be quite important in health because marrow stem cells are precursors of many types of immune cells.

Polarity is especially upset by travel, especially airplane travel, and it must be corrected through use of the Polarity Infoceutical early in any NES protocol because the body-field resists changes in other areas until its Polarity field is corrected. Because the Big Field often also shows distortions when Polarity is distorted, the Polarity Infoceutical also contains Big Field Aligner Infoceutical within it. So, if Big Field and Polarity both show as distorted in a NES scan, only the Polarity Infoceutical need be taken.

There are many lines of investigation begging to be followed about the links between natural Earth and cosmic fields and our health, and it will take specialists from many disciplines to sort out those links. NES research has only teased out the barest connections and plans to continue its research into this most important, but overlooked, aspect of bioenergetic health.

NES Case Overview: Rosa

Rosa came to NES practitioner and naturopathic physician Jason Siczkowycz because for nearly five years she had suffered from severe bouts of nausea and vomiting. Her medical doctors had conducted a battery of tests over the years, but the tests were all negative and a cause for her problem was never identified. Rosa had taken various prescription medicines, but none helped much. When she visited Siczkowycz, her first NES scan showed that her Big Field alignment was distorted and her Kidney Driver was severely distorted. She was given the Big Field Aligner and Kidney Driver Infoceuticals and followed the NES protocol for two months. When she returned for another scan, the Big Field alignment was no longer distorted, but her Kidney Driver still showed as severely distorted. So, she continued taking the Kidney Driver Infoceutical, only she upped the number of drops she took daily from nine to fifteen. After another two months, when she returned for a scan, she happily reported that the nausea and episodes of vomiting had diminished by 80 to 90 percent, for the first time in five years.

12

THE ENERGETIC DRIVERS

THE ENERGETIC DRIVERS ARE FIELDS that generate power for the body-field and the physical body. They arise from the major organs of the body. According to NES theory, both the functioning of the organs and their shape contribute to the creation of these Driver fields. Energy is needed for the body-field to form at all, and the cavities of the body appear to be excellent collectors of zero-point energy.

Almost all the major, and even the minor, organs of the body form cavities. That is, they are roughly oval or tubular, hollowed or spongy structures. We know that cavities can attract energy and store it and that they can act as tuned resonators for that energy, setting up electrostatic fields and facilitating the information exchange that takes place in QED fields. Whereas the physical body and its metabolism are fueled via various processes such as the carbohydrate and sugar cycle, the citric acid cycle (Krebs cycle), and so on, the bioenergetic body is fueled by various processes involving energy and information exchange within and around the cavities. For example, organs acting as resonant cavities can produce, tune, and amplify sound (phonon) waves. The yogis of Eastern traditions, from wandering Hindu ascetics to formally trained Tibetan monks, use sound and vibration to effect real physical changes. The yogic breathing practice of *pranayama* and the Tibetan chanting and breathing practice of *tummo* both can produce heat in the body. By raising the vibrational state of their bodies, these adepts

233

can produce so much body heat that they can dry wet blankets draped around their shoulders even if they are sitting outside in the cold and snow.

Western science cannot explain such anomalies very well. The thermoregulation of the body is very much tied to the conversion of food calories to heat. Breathing and chanting should accomplish little more than raising blood pressure, and so generate only the minimal heat (and the sweating by which the body releases excess heat) that comes with minor physical exertion. However, bioenergetics can explain how such practices work because the causal mechanisms are found at the level of the energetic body and body-field. The healing effects of music also are widely touted in the alternative health community, as are laughter and humor, deep breathing, chanting and toning (directed vocalization of sounds or mantras, such as *Aum* or *Om mani padme hum*), and many other techniques that involve sound and vibration. One way to explain these healing effects is through the movement of sound at the quantum level through the orbs—as traditional Chinese medicine would call the organs or resonant cavities—of the body.

It is no great leap of logic, then, to think that the cavities of the body—the organs, microtubules, and the like—might create their own fields. According to the NES model of the human body-field, they do. These fields are called Energetic Drivers—the "gas tanks" of the body-field. For most people, the first inkling that they might be getting ill is that they feel tired. They speak of feeling "run down." This is because one or more of their Driver fields are compromised.

It was not until after Peter had developed his theory of the Energetic Drivers that he realized his theory meshed with biology. Throughout his research, he had been drawing heavily from his knowledge of traditional Chinese medicine, which designates the orbs of the body—its major organs—as both generators of the energy that powers the physical body and reservoirs where that energy is stored for later use. However, he didn't blindly accept the wisdom of the traditional Chinese system. He preferred to perform his own matching experiments to determine how the body-field works. Over his decades of testing, he was able to determine not only how many Energetic Drivers there are in the body but also their preferred order. In other words, he was able to establish that there is a sequence to the bioenergetic arrangement of the Drivers and that this sequence matched well with embryological development and generally with the importance of the organ or organ system in relation to its survival importance for the body. These correspondences confirmed yet again how Peter's map of the body-field correlated bioenergetics with biology.

The Energetic Driver Infoceuticals are numbered—from one to sixteen—according to this sequence of survival importance to the body. You always take the Infoceuticals in order, taking the lowest numbered

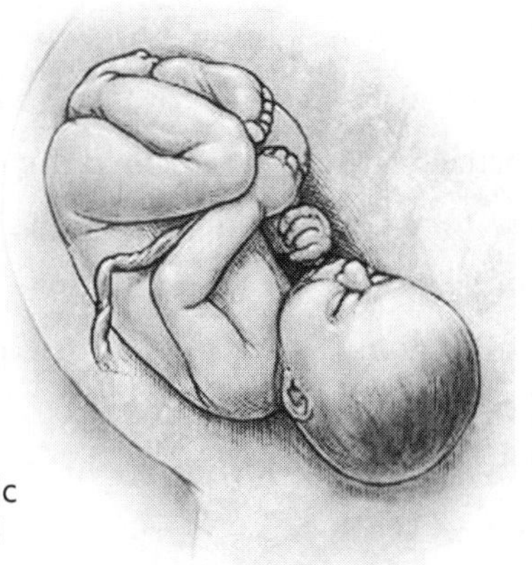

• **Source Driver** is the major biofield that is correlated to Source energy, which is a motive force for growth and homeostasis.

• The **Imprinter Driver** field supports information transfer from the heart to the entire body.

• The **Cell Driver** field correlates to cellular metabolism, especially as relates to cell organelles.

• The **Nerve Driver** field mediates ionic waves and electrical charges that travel through neurons.

• The **Circulation Driver** field helps power blood circulation.

• The **Heart Driver** field is produced by the physical action of the heart, especially electrical conduction and pressure waves.

• After birth, when the baby begins to breathe on its own, the **Lung Driver** field is activated.

• As the baby develops after birth, other Energetic Driver fields—such as those for the stomach, muscles, and skin—are activated.

Figure 12.1. The sixteen Energetic Driver fields arise from organs more or less following fetal development, with some not becoming fully functional until after birth.

one first and following the numbered sequence. For example, suppose that your NES scan showed Energetic Driver 13 as the most distorted Driver, followed by Energetic Drivers 3, 1, and 14. Your practitioner recommends that you take only three Energetic Driver Infoceuticals during the protocol, choosing the most distorted: 13, 3, and 1. Even though Energetic Driver 13 is the most imbalanced Driver field, you take the Infoceuticals in order, from the lowest number to the highest. So you would take Energetic Driver 1 Infoceutical first, followed by the Driver 3 Infoceutical, and then the Driver 13 Infoceutical, all taken at least ten minutes apart. Following this sequence—the order of the survival importance of the fields in the larger body-field—supports and speeds the healing process.

The Energetic Drivers, like the Energetic Integrators, are fields that bioenergetically correlate to a wide array of seemingly unconnected aspects of the physical body. For instance, you might assume that the Heart Driver would cover the whole of the heart field, with an adjunct correlation on heart-related systems, such as lungs, blood, and the circulatory system, but NES bioenergetics shows that is not the case. So the Infoceuticals are designed to bioenergetically affect only the aspects of physiology that a specific Driver field links to. The Heart Driver field matches only with specific tissues and structures of the heart: it "talks" only to the outside of the heart and to the electrical conduction system within the heart, such as the bundle of His, which is a group of cardiac nerves that sends electrical signals to regulate the heartbeat. The Imprinter Driver field, in contrast, correlates to the heart's bioenergetic function as an imprinter of information into the body, so it is linked with structures inside the heart organ.

We will now provide a brief overview of the sixteen Energetic Drivers. Each Driver field talks to the items listed in its overview, powering the system for a specific organ and bioenergetically correlating to the anatomical structures and metabolic and physiological processes listed. Although the explanations that follow contain biology terms with which you may not be familiar, we have included this level of detail so that you can understand how the NES system of bioenergetic health is furthering our understanding of the biophysics of the body.

ENERGETIC DRIVER I: SOURCE DRIVER

Source energy, as already explained, can be thought of as a kind of life-force energy, perhaps representing energy from the quantum zero-point field. From a body-field perspective, this Source energy forms a Driver field in the body, being attracted by and stored in the body cavities and microtubules. In NES theory, Source Driver is bioenergetically the "Driver of Drivers" because it powers all of the other Driver fields. When correcting the Drivers of the body-field, it always takes priority, so any distortion in the Source Driver is corrected first, before any other Driver field imbalances are addressed.

In TCM, yuan qi is considered to be the ocean of life-energy, and the NES model retains echoes of that tradition. Yuan qi is derived from the energetics of respiration (breathing) and the functioning of the kidney-adrenal complex. In the NES model of the body-field, however, Source Driver correlates to a wider array of bioenergetic, anatomical, and physiological structures and processes. For example, Source Driver matches to the reticuloendothelial system, a part of your immune system that produces cells that tend to aggregate in your lymph nodes, spleen, and reticular connective tissue. Generally, these are cells, such as monocytes and macrophages, that defend against invader organisms and microbes. In particular, Source Driver links particularly strongly to megakaryoctyes, a type of large cell made in the red bone marrow that produces blood platelets.

According to bioenergetics theory, before any illness can take hold in the body or before a gene is "turned on" to express itself as the cause of a genetic error or predisposition to a genetic disease, there usually is a problem with Source energy. If your Source energy is strong, your body does what it is designed to do, which is work properly and keep you healthy. So just the fact that you are expressing symptoms of illness provides a clue that your Source energy may be low.

You may have heard of medical experiments in which volunteers are exposed deliberately to a pathogen, such as flu virus. Some of the people exposed get the flu, whereas others don't. In conventional medicine, one explanation for this result is that those people who did not get sick have strong immune systems. From a bioenergetic perspective, however, we would say that those peoples' Source energy is strong. (There could be other bioenergetic explanations as well, such as that their bodies did not harbor the Energetic Terrain in which that virus could take hold in the body, and we will talk about this in chapter 15.) Such tests show us that simple exposure to a pathogen or microbe is not enough to make us ill. Our body has to be unable to deal with the invader organism to which it is exposed, and that process starts at the level of the body-field.

Our stores of Source energy tend to become depleted by prolonged stress, being indoors too much, chronic shallow breathing, poor nutrition, and exposure to toxins, among other factors. This depletion increases the probability that our bodies may not be able to maintain homeostasis, so symptoms of that loss may develop. If you do become ill, then as your illness moves from being acute to chronic, your Source energy becomes further weakened, and your body has less and less of a reserve of energy to deal with the illness. So, it is important in healing that your Source Driver field be restored or supported before the actual bioenergetic correlations to any illnesses are addressed. By correcting how your organs attract and store Source energy, your body is strengthened and can begin to better deal with the illness through its own natural healing responses.

ENERGETIC DRIVER 2: IMPRINTER DRIVER

This Driver field plays a crucial role in information transfer between your nervous system and cells, via your bloodstream. As previously explained, bioenergetically your heart is not only a pump, it also is an organ that imprints information into your bloodstream—by using pressure waves, phonons, photons, and electromagnetic signals—so that information can be distributed quickly throughout your body via blood circulation. This is the field that correlates to the heart's information regulation and transfer role.

The Imprinter Driver links energetically with the endoplasmic reticulum, an organelle found in all eukaryotic cells, that is involved with the process of protein folding. Specifically, Imprinter Driver bioenergetically links to both the rough and smooth endoplasmic reticulum. The rough endoplasmic reticulum is involved in how your cells use proteins, whereas the smooth endoplasmic reticulum is involved in such metabolic processes as synthesizing lipids and converting carbohydrates or cholesterol. The smooth endoplasmic reticulum also connects strongly with calcium uptake and regulation and with your body's use of substances such as glycogen and steroids.

Your emotions are not separate from your physical body, so correcting the fields connected to your physical body also may help address the bioenergetic aspects of psychological problems and so may enhance your emotional health. Peter's research has shown how the heart links to the brain and nervous system, and the work of other people and organizations such as HeartMath supports his findings.[1] Their research shows that the heart can be thought of as a second brain and an independent generator of emotions. Research in the relatively new field of neurocardiology lends credence to this rather radical new view of the heart, for heart tissue has been shown to be comprised of 65 to 75 percent neuronal cells—exactly the same types of cells that are in your brain. This research has revealed that the heart has its own internal nervous system that synthesizes and releases catecholamines and artrial naturetic factor, which are neurochemicals. Some neurocardiology researchers claim the heart can communicate via these neurochemicals with the brain, immune system, pineal gland, thalamus, and pituitary gland, concluding that the heart has the capability to function as a center of emotion, learning, and memory.

Because the Imprinter Driver field is linked to body-wide communication via the signals transmitted from your heart through your blood circulation, it is connected to an overall feeling of well-being on an emotional level as well as a physical level. The Energetic Driver 2 Infoceutical, therefore, is sometimes called a "Feel-Good" Infoceutical and the "Charisma Infoceutical."

ENERGETIC DRIVER 3: CELL DRIVER

The Cell Driver field is connected to cellular respiration and excretion and to the enzymatic powerhouses of your cells, the mitrochondria. It also links to adenosine triphosphate (ATP) because mitochondria produce ATP, which is believed by conventional biologists to be among the most potent of biological energy sources for your cells. However, Peter's matching experiments showed that mitochondria also match to Source energy, so they may play a role in energizing the body that conventional biology has yet to reveal. His matching tests also showed that Cell Driver "talks" to mast cells, which are crucial in the process of blood coagulation, and to immunoglobulin E, a molecule active in allergic reactions.

More generally, the Cell Driver field bioenergetically optimizes cellular activities including creation of heat, absorption of oxygen and nutrients, excretion of cellular waste products, and cell replication. All of these processes are dependent on information—on the cell knowing what to do, when to do it, and in the case of cellular production processes, how much of an enzyme, hormone, or other molecule it should make. Cell Driver also correlates to liver function because your liver is the powerhouse of cellular energy metabolism and waste disposal. In addition to what is noted above, the Cell Driver field is bioenergetically linked to:

▶ Centrioles, which process biochemical information in cells
▶ Golgi bodies, which are cellular structures that at a biological

level process substances made by cells and at a bioenergetic level may process photons and their information

▶ Centricenar cells, which are located in the pancreas

▶ Lymphobloasts and lymphocytes, which are cells of the immune system

▶ Myocardial tissue, which is heart tissue rich in mitochondria

▶ Spleen cells

▶ Von Kupffer cells in the liver, which recycle worn-out red blood cells

Proper cell function is, of course, fundamental to your overall good health. It can be compromised for any number of reasons, from poor nutrition to invasion by viruses to exposure to environmental toxins. Peter's matching experiments have shown that cell function, at a bioenergetic level, may be distorted particularly easily by the following pollutants: dioxins, phencyclidines (PCPs), xlyenes, electromagnetic radiation, and heavy metals. The Cell Driver Infoceutical bioenergetically helps to restore cell function. It generally tends to have an energizing effect on your body, so it is best not to take it around bedtime.

ENERGETIC DRIVER 4: NERVE DRIVER

The nervous system is particularly complex from a biophysical perspective. Bioenergetic studies have revealed that during prenatal development, the fetal nervous system produces low-frequency sounds, which are likely imprinting information that is crucial to the continued development of the growing fetus. As fetal development nears completion and soon after the baby's birth, its nervous system becomes heavily dependent on electrical-chemical signals, such as those that produce the different types of brain waves (alpha, beta, theta, and delta). This Driver field showed particularly strong bioenergetic correlation to low-frequency brain waves.

The various energy fields of the nervous system are variable, that is, they tend to fluctuate throughout the day and night, with especially low levels of activity occurring during sleep. For example, the sleep brain wave—the delta wave—has a particularly low amplitude. However, the lifestyle realities of the modern world—with electric lights that turn night into day and our penchant for staying continually stimulated via TV, computers, and other media—mean that your natural rhythms are continually disrupted and your mind-body overstimulated. More often than not, your circadian rhythms are affected in ways that can carry serious health consequences. When your nervous system is on perpetual overdrive, you may experience a range of effects, including insomnia, personality disorders such as anxiety and attention deficit disorder, and a general immune suppression that decreases your ability to fight off colds, flu, or more serious pathogens, microbes, and toxins.

The Nerve Driver Infoceutical bioenergetically addresses these nervous system issues, helping to restore system integrity. It is energetically linked to the dendrites, nerve cells, nerve axons, and the perineurium, which is a sheath of connective tissue that surrounds bundles of nerve fibers. In terms of cell maturation, this field links strongly with neuroblasts, which are embryonic nerve cells. Surprisingly, Peter's matching experiments did not show a strong correlation between the Nerve Driver field and structures in the brain, such as synapses. That may be because the NES system is working at the informational level of the body-field, not at the electrochemical level.

The Nerve Driver field appears to be bioenergetically sensitive to specific pollutants, chemicals, and other substances, such as butanol, a hydrocarbon solvent; chlorpyrifos, a common organophosphate pesticide; and heptane, a neurotoxic solvent. It has a correlation bioenergetically to vaccinations for diphtheria, rabies, and tetanus.

From a bioenergetic perspective, it is not too dramatic to say that the nervous system lies at the root of most illness, for our nervous systems tend to be overloaded and assaulted to the point that this most vital of information networks gets scrambled or partially breaks down.

Information that influences your core physical and emotional health is affected when the Nerve Driver field is compromised, so the effects of a Nerve Driver weakness tend to be systemic and can affect your overall sense of well-being.

Because the nerves are mostly sheathed by protective cells and tissues, it is a particularly difficult system to energetically detoxify. The Nerve Driver Infoceutical represents a starting point, but achieving the best bioenergetic correction may require the use of an appropriate Integrator Infoceutical. The Energetic Integrators, you may recall, are specific bioenergetic information regulation pathways in your body-field, and many of them connect to your nervous system: Energetic Integrators 1 (Neurosensory/Colon Meridian), 3 (Mucosae/Small Intestine Meridian), 4 (Neurotransmitters/Heart Meridian), 8 (Microbes/Liver Meridian), and 10 (Circulation/ Pericardium Meridian). So these particular Integrators work in tandem with Energetic Driver 3 to bioenergetically support your nervous system field.

ENERGETIC DRIVER 5: CIRCULATION DRIVER

As the name implies, this Driver field deals at the bioenergetic level with blood circulation. It comes before the Heart Driver but after the Imprinter Driver in the NES sequence because in NES the heart is not primarily a pump but is an imprinter of information. The arteries themselves may play a crucial role in blood circulation, for your blood may be self-propelling to some degree because of its spiral flow through your arteries. A motive force for that propulsion may be magnetism, arising from the iron content of hemoglobin.

Even though the heart begins to beat in a developing fetus before blood is being pumped, after the baby is born and living as an autonomous biological entity in its own right, the circulatory system becomes paramount for efficient and accurate information transfer. So, if both Energetic Driver 5, the Circulation Driver, and Energetic Driver 6, the Heart Driver, were to come up as *equally distorted* (both the same color, say red, indicating a severe distortion) in a NES scan, generally you would correct the Circulation Driver first because it comes first in the protocol healing sequence.

The Circulation Driver field bioenergetically connects to plasma-blasts, which are precursors to blood plasma cells. The action of this field promotes overall blood health, especially through its bioenergetic effect on red blood cells and because it is intimately correlated with the cellular-level processes of oxygen transfer, excretion of cell waste products, cell nutrition, and hormone production.

ENERGETIC DRIVER 6: HEART DRIVER

Whereas the Imprinter Driver is connected to the inside of your heart organ and to its information imprinting processes, the Heart Driver field links bioenergetically to the exterior structures of your heart and to cardiac function in general, especially your heart's electrochemical conduction system. Your heart, obviously, does not function in isolation, but its connections are much more diverse than conventional cardiology admits. According to TCM and NES research, it is intimately associated with the lungs, nervous system, and stomach at the level of energy and information. Because the heart is the major organ of the thoracic cavity and the stomach is a major organ of the abdominal cavity, there is a strong bioenergetic link, and errors in the stomach's overall field may cause secondary errors to appear in your heart's field.

The Heart Driver field is generated by the chemical and electrical activity of the heart and the process of blood oxygenation in the lungs. However, the action of the Heart Driver field also influences most other systems in your body, because it sits at a point of integration for the three planes of your big body-field and it correlates with the three axes of Earth's Big Field (the vertical, equatorial, and magnetic polar axes). It has a particularly strong link to your midbrain, and thus to sensory and perceptual processes such as visual and auditory acuity. At the cellular level, it bioenergetically matches with immune system platelets, lymphocytes, and monocytes. The Heart Driver field also correlates to linguistic skills, so using the Heart Driver Infoceutical, if it is called for in a NES scan, may generally correlate bioenergetically to enhanced language and other intellectual skills such as decision-making. It also correlates to increased mental integration overall, and it appears to bioenergetically enhance even more intangible aspects of your mind such as your sense of self-identity and mental clarity.

NES research shows that the Heart Driver field can be compromised easily by viral infections in the heart organ, and it is especially susceptible because of its bioenergetic link to the stomach field, which is the point of entry into your body for many toxins and pathogens. It can also be weakened by stress, emotional or physical shocks, and particular pollutants, especially 4-phenylcyclohexene (from carpet backing and carpet off-gassing), dioxane (an industrial solvent), and the measles-mumps-rubella vaccination.

ENERGETIC DRIVER 7: LUNG DRIVER

The Lung Driver field, as the name implies, is concerned with the pulmonary system. However, this bioenergetic field is generated not only by the actual oxygenation function of your lungs but also by the vibrations, phonons, and pressure waves that result from the expansion and contraction actions of your lungs. The lungs also produce sound via the larynx, which itself generates specific kinds of energy flows in your body.

The Lung Driver Infoceutical was designed to enhance all of the energy flows from the lung field and to bioenergetically reactivate various isotopes of oxygen that are crucial to a healthy metabolism, such as those produced through the exchange of gases in the bronchioles—the small cavities within your lungs. Because many pathogens and toxins are introduced into your body via your lungs and they tend to thrive in oxygen-deficient conditions, the Lung Driver Infoceutical bioenergetically aids your body by ensuring that your lung field is working efficiently and oxygenation is adequate.

There also is a bioenergetic link between the Lung Driver field and mental acuity. Metalloid toxins that may accumulate in your lungs may, on a bioenergetic level, affect the frontal lobes of your brain, so a weakened Lung Driver field may impact the proper functioning of that area of your brain. The Lung Driver field correlates strongly to higher mental functions in children and to nonordinary states of consciousness in adults. The latter finding is, of course, not new, as healers from cultures throughout the ages and across the globe, and especially those from the Far East and Himalayan regions, have developed breathing and toning techniques to aid healing and encourage mental and spiritual growth.

Specific toxins that may on a bioenergetic level particularly compromise the Lung Driver field include butanols and asbestos. The vaccinations for influenza, polio, yellow fever, and tuberculosis (BCG vaccine) may also bioenergetically weaken this field. The Lung Driver Infoceutical can help restore correct functioning to your lung field, especially through its energetic link to erythroblasts, which are the cells in the red marrow that synthesize hemoglobin.

ENERGETIC DRIVER 8: STOMACH DRIVER

The major organs of your digestive tract, including your stomach, intestines, and bowels, generate the Stomach Driver field. However, the main bioenergetic mechanism by which this field is generated is the electron transfers caused by the myriad activities that take place in this region of your body. According to NES theory, the constant metabolizing and processing of fats, minerals, proteins, and carbohydrates in the stomach and bowel linings actually generates an energy field of what is known as magnetic confetti, those tiny bits of magnetic energy left over from the forming and breaking of bonds and other such biochemical processes. However, the huge toxic load that can accumulate in these organs because of foods contaminated by chemicals from pesticides and fertilizers may severely compromise the bioenergetics of your stomach field. A further insult to your system may result from overconsumption of heavily processed and synthetic, lab-engineered foods.

In TCM, and as confirmed by NES research, your stomach field is bioenergetically linked to your lungs, heart, and muscles. The connection to muscles is especially strong because diet and nutrition in general affect muscle function. Blood sugar and amino acid levels, which are tied to nutrition quality, provide signals for muscle proteins. Muscles provide a reserve for protein, carbohydrate, and mineral metabolism in the body. The heart is made from muscle fibers, so in diabetics, for example, poor blood sugar regulation can affect heart muscles. (However, as explained later, the Muscle Driver field itself does not match or "talk" to the heart.) Glycogen, a factor in blood sugar metabolism, acts on liver and kidney tissue as well. So the muscles, which we tend to think of only in terms of locomotion, are intimately linked to metabolism.

In terms of specific cell correlations, your Stomach Driver links bioenergetically to granulocytes, which are white blood cells that defend against foreign invader organisms, such as viral particles and bacteria. Bioenergetically, the Stomach Driver field links to your brain, especially to the prefrontal lobes, and to mental functioning via the physical connection to blood sugar. The stomach meridian in TCM and the stomach Energetic Integrator route in NES branch to cross the prefrontal lobes, so the Stomach Driver field has an energetic link to higher brain function, especially as related to intellect and learning. There may even be a bioenergetic link to the physical symptoms allopathic medicine associate with Alzheimer disease. However, as with most things bioenergetic, many systems come together to form complex informational networks, and the brain is an integration point for most of these networks. So, as an example, while the Stomach Driver links to the prefrontal lobes, Kidney Driver links bioenergetically to brain tissue as a whole, and Heart Driver links bioenergetically to the midbrain. Therefore, trying to bioenergetically correct the fields that may correlate to an illness such as Alzheimer disease takes a multilayered approach, which is why in NES we let the body-field reveal what it is most important to correct and what it is ready to address, rather than trying to treat symptoms or diagnose illness.

As we have already indicated, your stomach is an organ that can become heavily contaminated because it is a major point of intersection between the world outside of you and the one inside. Homeopaths have long said that cadmium salts accumulate in the stomach, and from a bioenergetic perspective, NES matching tests confirm this. Even if physical cadmium is not found there, if it is present in other areas of the body, its energetic influence seems especially to affect the Stomach Driver field. NES research also finds that lead has a special bioenergetic affinity for the large bowel, and it can be a strong blocker of your Stomach Driver field. Other things that have a particularly adverse bioenergetic effect on this field are fungicides, electromagnetic radiation, heavy metals (especially arsenic, lead, antimony, and cadmium), and the hepatitis A and B vaccines.

The Kidney Driver field (Energetic Driver 12) is tightly correlated to the Stomach Driver field, so if it turns out to be a challenge to correct the Stomach Driver field, you can sometimes "go around to the back door" and work with the Kidney Driver field. Correcting the Kidney Driver field or even the Pancreas Driver field may sometimes "kick start" the Stomach Driver.

ENERGETIC DRIVER 9: MUSCLE DRIVER

This Driver field is generated by the extension and contraction movement of your striated, or skeletal, muscles and by the chemical activity involved in muscle movement. However, as previously mentioned, it is not connected to heart muscle, which is a different type of tissue. The Muscle Driver field bioenergetically maintains efficient muscular function, including metabolic waste excretion that takes place via your muscles, muscle growth and repair, and regulation of how your muscles use calcium and magnesium. Because muscles may become the repositories of pollutants, such as lead, if your body cannot excrete or otherwise deal with such pollutants, this Driver field generally aids bioenergetically in the detoxifying process. At the cellular level, the Muscle Driver is linked specifically to monocytes, which among other functions act as scavengers to clear dead cells from your body, especially around the site of infections.

Bioenergetically, muscles can retain the imprint of physical and emotional shocks, having a kind of muscle memory of childhood trauma and other psychological wounds and of severe physical assaults, such as car accidents.[2] The deep myofascial connective tissue and muscle network of your body can hold these imprints over the course of a lifetime, and many types of deep-tissue massage techniques, such as Rolfing and myofascial release, can help you to release the emotions that are stored in your physical muscles. The Muscle Driver field also holds these imprints, and the Muscle Driver Infoceutical can help your body-field bioenergetically process them and so help release them from the physical muscle tissue.

As we have said before, the bioenergetic approach of treating disease differs greatly from the allopathic one, so when addressing specific muscle diseases, the process is not based on symptomology or even biochemistry. Instead, correction is addressed according to what the body-field reveals as being most compromised, which might be counterintuitive to conventional physiology and anatomy. For example, osteoarthritis, a disease that is rampant in modern society, is said to be caused at least in part by a calcium sheath that builds up around the tendons, especially at the joints. The bioenergetic approach, however, is not to address the muscles and joints directly, but instead to address the information networks that affect these body areas. So, in the case of arthritis, you might have to address the efficiency of the liver by taking Energetic Integrator 8 Infoceutical and bioenergetically improve oxygenation efficiency in the body by taking Energetic Integrator 2 Infoceutical. Those are possibilities, and only a NES scan can indicate whether they are called for in a particular case, as other Integrator and/or Driver fields might have to be strengthened or corrected first.

ENERGETIC DRIVER 10: SKIN DRIVER

The Skin Driver field is generated by the movement of subatomic particles and molecules through the layers of your physical skin, especially via respiration. Your skin is the largest organ of your physical body, so if the Skin Driver field is bioenergetically compromised, it can have serious ramifications on your physical well-being. This field can be weakened by many things but is especially compromised by environmental toxins such as fungicides, insecticides, and agricultural chemicals.

As your largest organ, your skin performs myriad functions, among them maintaining fluid balance in your body, helping with thermoregulation, maintaining mineral balance, protecting you from ionizing radiation, and aiding in detoxification. Of course, it is also your body's first line of defense, providing a protective barrier between your body and the outside world. It repels toxins, microbes and viruses, ultraviolet light and other forms of radiation, chemical and physical threats, and the like. As an organ, your skin is active metabolically; for instance it is instrumental in vitamin D absorption. It is also a major sensory organ, linking you to the environment, and so bioenergetically it has a strong connection to Earth's Big Field.

Your skin also responds almost instantaneously to conscious and unconscious emotions, changing color (blushing) and texture (goose bumps) according to your thoughts, feelings, and perceptions, so it is part of the nervous system information network. It also is linked to the action of your muscles, connective tissue, and the fascia that lies just below it. Because of its immense range of regulatory functions, such as those involved with blood and body heat, this field also is energetically linked to the Lung Driver field, so using the Skin Driver Infoceutical may have a residual beneficiary effect on the Lung Driver field. This connection between skin and lungs is also acknowledged in TCM.

Finally, because the skin is made of epithelial cells, it is strongly linked with the mucosae, especially of the bowels, lungs, and other large organs. In fact, Peter says that calling this field the Skin Driver is a bit of a misnomer because its major bioenergetic effects are not on skin per se but on mucosae in general.

The Skin Driver Infoceutical is designed to bioenergetically support immunity, toxin excretion, metabolic regulation, oxygenation, and other processes that underlie the symptoms of a skin condition, which may in fact be more related to mucosae than to your skin. Inflammations tend to show up as skin problems, but their causes go much deeper. So, for example, the Skin Driver Infoceutical might help bioenergetically address an allergy-related skin condition because it is dealing with the information the body needs to deal with the bioenergetic root cause of the allergy, not because it is lessening the irritation at a particular site on the skin directly. The same is true when a skin condition results from an underlying autoimmune disease. NES would deal with the body-field breakdowns that correlate to a compromised immune system, and by clearing that underlying cause, your skin may clear up, too.

The skin and mucosae in general are bioenergetically networked via all of the Energetic Integrators, either directly or indirectly. The Integrators are similar to acupuncture meridians, forming interconnected channels of information throughout the body and linking organs and processes that are anatomically or metabolically unrelated by allopathic standards. For this reason, the Skin Driver Infoceutical often is paired in a NES protocol with one or more Energetic Integrators. For example, from a bioenergetic perspective, a skin condition affecting mainly your face might be addressed with the use of the Skin Driver Infoceutical along with Energetic Integrator 1 Infoceutical in the same protocol. A problem with the skin on the trunk of your body might call for Energetic Integrator 2 Infoceutical, and a condition affecting mainly your hands might pair best with the Energetic Integrator 8 Infoceutical. The bioenergetic bottom line with skin conditions, however, is that the root cause is rarely the skin itself, so a NES scan may not even show the Skin Driver field as distorted if you suffer from a skin condition. Instead, it will identify contributing bioenergetic causes of your problem, which may seem entirely unrelated.

ENERGETIC DRIVER 11: LIVER DRIVER

The Liver Driver field is generated by the chemical and cellular activity of your liver, and it directly correlates bioenergetically to liver cells and their functions. The liver is the largest organ, after the skin, and it is the site of some of the most crucial biochemical processes in your body. It is a major site of metabolic functions, including those affecting protein, fat, minerals, and vitamins. It processes the internal wastes your body produces during the normal course of metabolism; produces or aids in the manufacture of bile, hormones, and enzymes; and stores and processes fats and carbohydrates. It is a major detoxification organ in your body. However, it can become overtaxed because of the enormous load of chemicals from the highly processed food we tend to ingest, pesticides and other toxins to which we are constantly exposed, and the many other assaults of modern living. The consequences of a bioenergetically compromised liver may be enormous, for your liver is involved in filtration processes that directly impact your immune system. What's more, it plays a primary role in blood clotting, regulating your body's acid-alkaline balance (pH level), and blood sugar regulation, among other critical physiological and metabolic functions.

At the cellular level, the Liver Driver field is linked bioenergetically to reticulocytes, which are cells that help regenerate blood, and to pro-thrombin, which is a precursor to a blood-clotting agent. It also links to pancreatic cells, such as beta cells, because bioenergetically the pancreas is considered a companion organ to the liver. The Liver Driver Infoceutical bioenergetically affects lymphatic cells in general.

The NES approach to bioenergetically rebalancing a compromised Liver Driver field is to proceed with great care because this field is so crucial to the body's homeostasis and is such a potent detoxifier. For this reason, a NES practitioner will almost never use the Liver Driver

Infoceutical on a client's first use of NES. As a general rule, the Liver Driver field is supported by the Pancreas Driver, Cell Driver, or Bone Driver fields, but the NES scan will reveal the specific fields that are best dealt with first, before the Liver Driver field is addressed.

The Liver Driver field also is closely linked to geopathic stress, so if the Big Field is distorted, Liver Driver is likely to be as well. Correcting the Big Field may clear Liver Driver distortions. The latest NES research also reveals a bioenergetic correlation between a compromised Liver Driver field—specifically correlated to liver cell function—and overexposure to electromagnetic radiation, which we call "e-smog."

ENERGETIC DRIVER 12: KIDNEY DRIVER

The Kidney Driver field is generated by the chemical and cellular activity of your kidneys. In TCM, the kidneys store *jing*, which is a constitutional energy that is one of three major life-force energies (along with yuan qi and *shen*). It is indicative of your essence, especially your physical essence, and is responsible for strong growth and development. It is akin to the Source energy in NES, for the kidneys are composed of millions of tiny microtubules that attract and store Source energy. However, many of the bioenergetic functions of your kidneys as described in TCM, such as their links to your brain and emotions, are located in the information network covered by the kidney pathway for Energetic Integrator 6 (Kidney/Kidney Meridian) in NES, rather than in the Kidney Driver field.

Interestingly, the essence of a cell is the cell nucleus, and bioenergetically Kidney Driver is so tightly correlated to the nuclei of cells that Peter says you can think of Kidney Driver as a kind of cell nucleus driver. The Kidney Driver field also resembles, on a bioenergetic level, the energy field of brain cells. So when Kidney Driver comes up on a NES scan, the root of the distortion may not be in the kidney organs at all.

This Driver does, of course, bioenergetically link to the kidneys themselves, especially to their filtering functions. Your kidneys are primary organs for filtering waste from your blood, producing urine, monitoring and maintaining electrolyte and fluid balances, assisting in the regulation of blood pressure, and aiding blood cell production. They are bioenergetically linked to lymphocytes and monocytes, both of which provide defense against invader organisms. The Kidney Driver Infoceutical helps ensure that this field is properly powered so that your physical kidneys and all bioenergetically related systems and cells work optimally.

ENERGETIC DRIVER 13: IMMUNITY DRIVER

Your immune system is partly a search-and-destroy system, keeping you safe from a constant assault of external threats, such as pathogens and toxins, and from cellular and internal metabolic breakdowns, such as the growth of defective cells. Bioenergetically, the Immunity Driver field is strongly correlated to red blood cells—especially to blastic cells created in the bone marrow, such as plasmablasts and leukoblasts—rather than immunity provided by white cells or viral antibodies, which is covered by the Spleen-Omentum Driver. It is also bioenergetically connected to your spleen, which has a strong immunity function. Powering the Immune Driver field can help increase the production of plasmablasts, leukoblasts, and other immune system cells, although it can take time—from a few days to as much as a month—because there is a development process cells must go through before they are active in the immune system.

The Immunity Driver Infoceutical pairs well with the Lung Driver Infoceutical, especially to bioenergetically address respiratory infections and to generally enhance your immune system to ameliorate the field effects of toxins. The Cell Driver and Energetic Integrator 12 Infoceuticals also pair well with the Immunity Driver Infoceutical. In fact, the Cell Driver and Immunity Driver Infoceuticals can powerfully support each other.

From a bioenergetic perspective, immune problems often can be traced back to field distortions in the bone marrow, especially because there is usually a toxic heavy-metal load in the bones and muscles. So the Immunity Driver Infoceutical also pairs well with the Stomach Driver Infoceutical because the Stomach Driver field is a kind of gate-keeper for preventing contamination in your body. Its action as an energy channel crosses the long bones of your legs, where mercury, cadmium, and lead can accumulate.

ENERGETIC DRIVER 14: SPLEEN-OMENTUM DRIVER

The Spleen-Omentum Driver field is bioenergetically linked to both the red and white pulp of the spleen as well as to the omentum, a type of mesenteric sheet that lines the abdomen. It also links to all parts of the thymus. In fact, originally this Driver field was called Thymus Driver, but in early 2007 Peter's research revealed its strong correlations to the spleen and omentum, so this Driver Infoceutical was reformulated, the Driver field renamed, and its bioenergetic correlations expanded on.

The spleen organ has three functions: elimination of older red blood cells, blood regulation, and most important, the production of lymphocytes and plasma cells, which make antibodies. The omentum also has an immune function, although it is targeted more specifically to the peritoneal cavity and is most active if there are problems such as peritonitis. The omentum supplies leucocytes to the abdominal cavity, and it is so dynamic a tissue that it will even form collagen to engulf and seal off contaminated areas of that cavity when necessary.

In TCM, there is an energy and information link between the spleen and the lungs, but NES research extends the spleen's links to include the thymus, an immune system organ that is located in the midchest region. From a bioenergetic perspective, long-term immunity against viral threats depends on the thymus, which also appears to have an important bioenergetic role in addressing allergies. It is also of enormous interest that the Spleen-Omentum Driver has a robust bioenergetic link to the following varieties of bacteria that may infect both the peritoneal cavity and the lungs: *Bordetella pertussis* (cause of whooping cough), *Haemophilus influenzae* (cause of chest infections), *Klebsiella* (some types may cause pneumonia), and *Moraxella catarrhalis* (cause of upper-respiratory infection). Normally, Klebsiella bacteria are harmless in the gut and abdominal cavity, although they become dangerous in the chest cavity, where they can destroy lung tissue.

The Spleen-Omentum Driver Infoceutical, therefore, may be useful for bioenergetically addressing a range of immune defense functions, especially when the problems are affecting the abdominal cavity and lungs. This Infoceutical also pairs well with Energetic Integrator 8 Infoceutical (Microbes/Liver Meridian) because of that Integrator's bioenergetic link to low-frequency electromagnetic radiation. Such e-smog may bioenergetically compromise the immune system if you are overexposed to it. In the case of e-smog, the Liver Driver and Energetic Star 1 (Lymphatic Immunity and General Radiation) Infoceuticals may also be beneficial, but the NES scan is the final indicator of what in the body-field needs to be corrected.

The Spleen-Omentum Driver is important because of its many bioenergetic links, especially to the thymus. Whereas Immunity Driver is focused bioenergetically on overall cellular immunity, especially as it relates to cells produced in the bone marrow, the Spleen-Omentum Driver, through its link to the thymus, correlates bioenergetically to antibodies and white blood cells generally. It is linked more with long-term immunity. In allopathic medicine, the thymus was not a very well understood organ until fairly recently, with major breakthroughs in understanding occurring as late as the mid-1960s. For decades the thymus was thought to be a rudimentary or vestigial organ that played no major role in the body and could even be harmful to it. The thymus tends to atrophy, or shrink, as you grow older, so researchers thought that its function was important only early in life, as the immune system forms and matures. Now, however, there is increased research into the thymus as a gland that may play an important contributory role in regulating your long-term immune system, especially via thymosin, thymopoelin, and serum thymic factors.

Bioenergetically, the Spleen-Omentum Driver, through the energetic and informational pathway of the thymus, links closely with specific types of immune cells, including T-lymphocytes, T-helper cells, T-suppressor cells, and natural killer cells. It also supports your body's bioenergetic resistance to molds, parasites, and allergic responses and plays a bioenergetic role generally in helping to prevent autoimmune disorders.

ENERGETIC DRIVER 15: PANCREAS DRIVER

The Pancreas Driver field is generated by the action of pancreatic cells. It bioenergetically connects to the vagus nerve and, at the cellular level, to lymphocytes in the spleen. It further correlates to the production of digestive enzymes for carbohydrates, proteins, and fats, and, in relation to endocrine function, is concerned with the islets of Langerhans, which are involved in the production of glycogen and insulin. The Pancreas Driver field also correlates to blood sugar regulation in general.

The pancreas is closely linked bioenergetically with your liver and also connects strongly with Energetic Integrators 4 (Neurotransmitters/Heart Meridian) and 12 (Shock/Spleen Meridian), in which the vagus nerve also plays a crucial bioenergetic role.

ENERGETIC DRIVER 16: BONE DRIVER

Generated by the compression of osteons, the Bone Driver field exerts its bioenergetic influence on calcium metabolism in all its forms, such as in the formation of bones and in muscular contraction, and on hormone release, blood coagulation, and intercellular communication on an energetic, not a chemical, level. The Bone Driver Infoceutical, therefore, is designed to help address any field errors that occur in calcium-related diseases, such as calcium deposits in your arteries or organs (such as gallstones). Calcium metabolism is involved in tens of thousands of body processes and so may be involved bioenergetically in a staggering range of health problems in ways that allopathic medicine has yet to identify.

The Bone Driver Infoceutical contains information related to the kidneys, liver, and pancreas because all of these information channels are interconnected. In TCM, the major acupuncture point *sanyin-jiao,* which is located on the inner leg above the ankle, is a meeting point for the channels for the kidneys, liver, and spleen. (The spleen and pancreas are not clearly distinguished from one another in TCM.) The Bone Driver Infoceutical in NES is based on this knowledge as well as on Peter's thousands of matching experiments. (The Energetic Integrators linked to these same three organs also affect bone, primarily via calcium use in the body.) So, the Bone Driver Infoceutical may be useful in correcting bioenergetic processes that may contribute to allopathic diagnoses of osteoarthritis, calcified tendons and organs, and even brain anomalies that express themselves in conditions such as Alzheimer disease.

In addition, the Bone Driver field appears to be strongly connected bioenergetically to red blood cells and to the antibody system generally. The Bone Driver field is particularly sensitive to, and thus is easily weakened by, heavy metals, especially lead, mercury, and aluminum.

NES Case Overview: Heidi

In 1998, Heidi had been diagnosed with Crohn disease, an inflammatory bowel disease, with the most persistent symptoms being loose stools and chronic diarrhea, with blood occasionally present in her stool. She was treated for years by her primary physician, who prescribed various drugs, most recently Asacol, but by 2006 she was still suffering symptoms, especially diarrhea. Although she continued to see her allopathic physician, she decided to also see a naturopathic physician who also is a NES practitioner. The NES scan showed Skin Driver as the most distorted aspect of Heidi's body-field, so that was the Infoceutical she was given. Skin Driver links energetically to epithelial cells and to mucosae, especially of the bowels and lungs, so it was not surprising that it showed a severe distortion in her scan. Heidi took the Skin Driver Infoceutical as instructed for three weeks and then returned for a follow-up scan, during which she reported that her bowel movements had returned to normal, for the first time in nearly eight years. The new scan showed Skin Driver as balanced. Two months later she returned for another scan, which showed that Skin Driver remained undistorted. During that visit, Heidi reported that her physician had reduced the amount of Asacol she was taking and that she was symptom-free, with totally normal bowel movements.

13

UNDERSTANDING
THE ENERGETIC
INTEGRATORS

THE ENERGETIC INTEGRATORS are the "information highways" of the body-field. To do them justice as an integral part of the NES model of the body-field, we feel obligated to provide some theoretical background and technical explanation about the Energetic Integrator system before we detail how each Integrator bioenergetically links to the physical anatomy of the body, which we will cover in chapter 14. This chapter, then, provides an overview of the Energetic Integrator system from the view of both physics and psychology. The physics discussion describes the wave dynamics of the Energetic Integrators, showing how NES moves bioenergetic theory beyond accounting only for the frequencies of the body-field to including a consideration of phase shift. For those readers with less interest in the technical explanations, we suggest that you just dip into sections of this part of the chapter here and there to get a general overview.

In addition, since bioenergetics is not just about the body, but the mind-body, we have concluded this chapter with a brief discussion of how NES body-field theory provides a radical overturning of commonly held views about consciousness. Our theory has major implications for the practice of psychology in general and for medicine in terms of how emotions may affect health.

--------◆--------

Although we've described the Energetic Integrators as channels or routes of information in the body-field, similar to but more extensive than the meridians of TCM, it's more accurate to describe them as *structured fields* for the transfer and regulation of information. However, when discussing the bioenergetic, and certainly the quantum, realm, you have to get beyond thinking in spatial terms. This realm is not spatial in a classical, geometric sense, so it is illusory to think of the Energetic Integrators as actual physical channels in the body-field or body. Terms such as channels, rivers, or routes of information are metaphors that describe bioenergetic fields of information. It's more accurate, but still metaphorical to some extent, to think of them instead as an inter-locked network of information "resonances," where like matches with like to make discrete subnetworks within the larger network we call the human body-field. The body-field has an energetic structure formed by the aggregate of the fields at the next lower level of structure—Big Field (connections to Earth fields) and Energetic Drivers, Integrators, and Stars—and each of these fields is composed of subfields itself.

Academic and independent researchers—in particular biologist Rupert Sheldrake—have proposed theories about how life is dependent on large organizing fields. Sheldrake proposes that morphogenetic fields are the organizing informational and energetic templates for life, with each species having its own template field. Then there is a larger field that links all life in an interconnected web. However, as far as we can discern, Peter is the only person who proposes a theory for the deeper structures of the human body-field that explains its interdependence with the biology and biochemistry of the physical body in detail and with precision. Only NES provides a purely bioenergetic model of anatomy and physiology, and a corresponding bioenergetic model of pathology, that integrate biology and physics. Peter goes much farther than even

Sheldrake, identifying energetic and informational fields for structures at all levels of the body, from the microscopic level of proteins and cells to the larger organ structures to the overall human body-field.

That said, we should point out that the body-field cannot be seen, as in an aura, which we will discuss briefly at the end of this chapter. The body-field is also not a static system that can be easily visualized or fully described. The reality of the quantum realm precludes us from ever having a firm grasp of the totality of the body-field because it is a *dynamic* web of interrelated flows of energy and information. It changes constantly, at quantum speeds, as it responds to everything in the internal and external environments that affect it.

In reality, the human body-field may be a *special case* of quantum field interactions that are taking place in the realm of biology, a special case that arises only in the realm of organic, living systems. The body-field appears to be a structure formed from the dynamics of uncountable numbers of electrons—which in the Wolff model are dual oscillators—that interact and whose influences aggregate to form a "structure in space" (the body-field) that serves as a master control system for all physiological processes.

Within each Integrator are links to elements, cells, organs, organ systems, and higher level, nontangible aspects of ourselves, such as our emotions, as illustrated in figure 13.1.

FREQUENCY AND PHASE

If there are twelve Energetic Integrators, then an obvious question is, what distinguishes one Integrator from another? Although the same classes of information (elements/compounds, proteins, cells, organs, emotions, etc.) are found in each Energetic Integrator, each Integrator links to specific items within each class. For example, in terms of elements, copper matches only to Integrator 6 and nickel only to Integrators 7 and 10. Each Integrator also links to different specific aspects of our physiology. However, an important part of the answer about what dis-

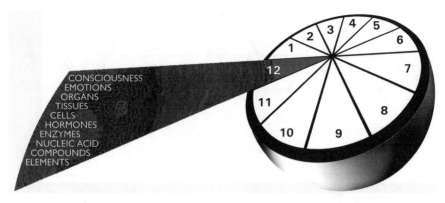

Figure 13.1. The twelve Energetic Integrators are structures in space arranged around the spherical scalar standing wave. Each Energetic Integrator correlates to specific information in the body from the subcellular level up to emotions and consciousness.

tinguishes Energetic Integrators also lies in frequency and phase shift, which describe how waves move. In case you are unfamiliar with wave dynamics, here are some basic, if elementary, facts about waves that will be helpful to know as you continue with this chapter. The illustrations that follow are mostly of linear matter waves. Spherical wave dynamics and matters of phase in the quantum realm are much more complex.

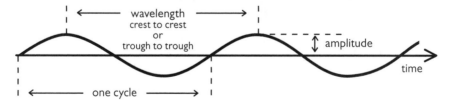

Figure 13.2. For a linear matter wave, a wavelength *is a measure of any two corresponding parts of a wave, such as the distance between two wave crests. The length of the wave determines its type—a radio wave, light wave, infrared wave, or other type of wave. For waves of visible light, the wavelength determines the color of the light. One full wave crest and trough is considered a* cycle. Amplitude *is concerned with a wave's size or strength, which is determined by the height of the crests.*

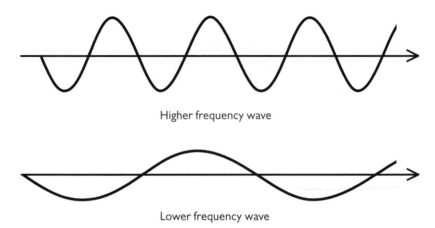

Higher frequency wave

Lower frequency wave

Figure 13.3. A wave's frequency *is measured in cycles per second, notated as hertz. The shorter the wavelength cycle, the higher the wave's frequency. (For a standing wave, which oscillates in place, the cycle is the number of oscillations per second or unit of time.)*

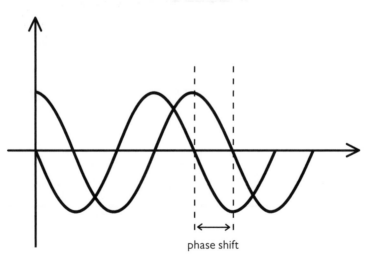

phase shift

Figure 13.4. A wave's phase *relates to how a feature of a wave's cycle is displaced from a reference point. In terms of two or more waves, phase can be thought of as how the waves line up or match in relation to each other. The two waves can be said to be in phase with respect to their amplitudes (the size of their peaks and troughs is the same), but displaced (shifted out of phase) in relation to time (represented by the horizontal axis, where one wave is moving ahead of the other).*

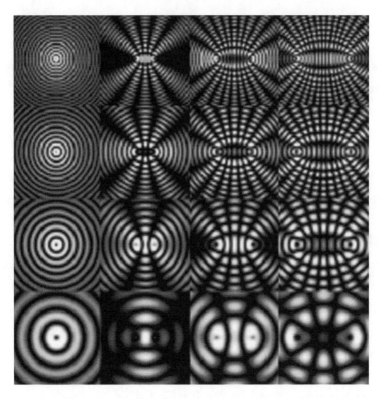

Figure 13.5. Waves create interference patterns. Matter waves that are in phase are said to have constructive interference, that is, they add together and their energy increases. In contrast, waves that are out of phase have destructive interference, wherein they cancel each other out. Interference patterns convey information, for the shape of the medium in which the two or more waves are moving together changes as a result of their interaction. In this series of illustrations, two circular scalar waves interact. Over time, the waves move apart from their centers, but areas of destructive interference remain stable.

In the NES model of the body-field, phase shift appears to be at least as important, if not more important, than frequency in terms of the state of our health—because frequency tends to be stable whereas phase can shift. Peter's research suggests that measuring both Integrator frequency and phase shift is necessary for interpreting body-field dynamics. His research into the phase shift aspects of the body-field is still very much in its infancy. We present what we think we know in the interest of potentially stimulating further research by others and to demonstrate to readers how our understanding of the information routes of the body-field goes well beyond the concept of meridians in TCM, and to highlight the intricacy of the bioenergetic influences that may be important for restoring and maintaining health.

In the Energetic Integrator system, each organ has a primary frequency range. The heart, as an example, produces many frequencies but primarily is a low-frequency organ. It correlates to Energetic Integrator 2, which covers a frequency range of 10 to 100 hertz. However, in NES theory, frequency alone is not sufficient to explain body-field energetics. Phase shift also is important. According to both our model and Wolff's space resonance theory, *energy exchange* in the universe takes place via the matching of space resonances (or what researchers who subscribe to the Standard Model of physics would see as particle interactions). However, *information exchange* is dependent on the interference patterns created by the interaction of the space resonances associated with waveforms of the three major particles—electrons, protons, and neutrons—via phase shifts. As previously explained by space resonance theory, the three major particles are dual oscillators, and as their waves interact they create interference patterns at the central part of the particle, where the In wave changes to the Out wave. As the In wave changes to the Out wave, there is a phase shift of 180 degrees, a figure that agrees perfectly with Peter's experiments: through his matching experiments he found that the twelve Energetic Integrators each cover a 15-degree range of what appears to be phase shift, thus covering a range of 180 degrees total for all twelve. Peter had gathered that data years ago but was not sure what it meant until he came across the Wolff model of the electron. It seemed beyond coincidence that the total range of the Integrator system's phase shift would match the phase shift of 180 degrees as the In wave turns into the Out wave. That is the point, according to space resonance theory, where energy exchange takes place and, hence, where information can be imparted. How the electron's phase shift relates to physical health is a heady question that remains very much open to question, but at this early stage of his research, Peter feels that phase shift may play a significant role in the proper functioning of the Energetic Integrator system, the crucial information routes of the body-field.

Peter proposes that "the information the body needs is carried in the heart of the electron, neutron, or proton, although in biology it may be the electron that is most important. The electron has within it a very dense area of space—the link between the In wave and the Out wave. We can make a link between the varying densities of this space with each of the Energetic Integrators. Each Integrator falls within a specific frequency range, but each also relates to specific ranges of phase shift. In NES, we found there was 15 degrees of phase shift for each of our Energetic Integrators, so all twelve of them fall within the 180-degree range of phase shift allowed by the Wolff theory of quantum. This does not prove anything, of course, but it does tell us that we can fit well within the Wolff model of physics. We know, too, that phase can be altered when there are abrupt changes in electromagnetic waves, and this may relate to what we call shock in NES and in natural health care in general. A shock or trauma to the system—physical, emotional, or bioenergetic—may have adverse effects on health, especially in the development of cancer."

Peter further explained that "every cell in the body, and in all of biology, has a characteristic phase shift value, and these are used as identifiers in NES technology. Pathology may result when the Energetic Integrator becomes distorted, covering more or less than its characteristic 15 degrees of phase shift value on the spherical standing wave. If an Energetic Integrator becomes compressed or, alternatively, expands, then contiguous Integrator structures are affected and these distortions will have consequences for how information is routed from the body-field to the body."

The Energetic Integrators make up an exquisitely organized system in which minute changes can result in major effects in the body-field and, ultimately, in the body. Although the body-field is sensitive to change, it is also a robust, self-correcting system. As Peter has already said, the Energetic Integrator system works like a Swiss watch—very accurately— which is a condition necessary to health and to life itself. He said, "If we allow our Integrators, our 'information packages,' to represent a range of phase shift—to indicate where the information belongs in the NES Energetic Integrator system, which, in effect, correlates to its position on the spherical standing wave—and include a vector, so as to recognize the three-dimensionality of space, and also include the sum of the In wave and Out wave, then we have a data set that could form nice mathematics. We also have a *pattern* that could be recognized by the body-field."

The chart below shows how the Energetic Integrators arrange themselves from very-low-frequency sound up to a frequency just below that of visible light, and the corresponding phase shift range for each Energetic Integrator.

NES ENERGETIC INTEGRATOR FREQUENCY AND PHASE CHART

Energetic Integrator	Frequency Range (hertz)	Phase (degrees)
Energetic Integrator 1	0–10 Hz	15°
Energetic Integrator 2	10–100 Hz	30°
Energetic Integrator 3	100–1,000 Hz	45°
Energetic Integrator 4	1,000–10,000 Hz	60°
Energetic Integrator 5	10,000–100,000 Hz	75°
Energetic Integrator 6	100,000–1,000,000 Hz	90°
Energetic Integrator 7	1,000,000–10,000,000 Hz	105°
Energetic Integrator 8	10,000,000–100,000,000 Hz	120°
Energetic Integrator 9	100,000,000–1,000,000,000 Hz	135°
Energetic Integrator 10	1,000,000,000–10,000,000,000 Hz	150°
Energetic Integrator 11	10,000,000,000–100,000,000,000 Hz	165°
Energetic Integrator 12	100,000,000,000–1,000,000,000,000 Hz	180°

Biochemists recognize the processes of energy exchange but for the most part miss the phase-dependent *information exchange* processes that may be affecting the state of the body. Frequency and phase may represent the extent to which chemical reactions can influence the health of the entire body, rather than just one part of a cell, or even less, a molecule. As Peter points out, "Conventional medicine and biochemistry are right on the verge of looking into what controls the biofield surrounding the chemical reaction. They are on the verge of taking a revolutionary step—into quantum field energetics. What seems to be most important in bioenergetics is frequency, phase, and space resonance, or what we call 'structure.' If you think about it for a moment, you will see that when you have frequency and phase, you must also have a structure. This structure is really what our information is. We are correcting these distorted information structures in space. It's hard to wrap your mind around, I know. But that is what our tests are indicating is going on, and we are only following where Nature is leading us."

THE BIG BODY-WAVE VERSUS THE BIG BODY-FIELD

We've talked about the big body-field as the aggregate of the body-field's energetic subsystems—the Drivers, Integrators, and Stars. To fully understand the Energetic Integrators, you also have to have an understanding of the big body-*wave* and distinguish it from the big body-*field*. The big body-wave can be thought of as the systems-level *waveform* for the entire body-field, in contrast with the countless waves from all the smaller subsystems such as those that arise from the individual organs or different types of cells.

The big body-wave is the *carrier* for the Energetic Integrator system. The big body-wave "begins" at Energetic Integrator 1 and "ends" at Energetic Integrator 12. The "signal," for want of a better word to describe how information is carried via the big body-wave, feeds back from Energetic Integrator 12 into Energetic Integrator 1, so the wave constantly loops or cycles. However, if information is distorted anywhere along that waveform, in any of the twelve Integrators, then the distorted information gets fed back into the start of the wave, at Energetic Integrator 1, and that distortion may become chronic. Over time, the distortions can so deform the information carried via the big body-wave that activities and processes in the physical body become affected, resulting in what we call the symptoms of disease. It's rather like a game of telephone, in which one person whispers a message—let's say, "You are an energy being"—into the ear of another person, who whispers it to still another person, and so on through a line of dozens of people. When the message is whispered back to the first person, it can bear little or no resemblance to the original message. "You are an energy being" has become "Your car has an engine ping." The longer the chain of people, the higher the probability the message will become distorted.

In an analogous way, the longer a small distortion in your body-field cycles unchecked through the network of twelve Integrators—through the big body-wave—the higher the likelihood that the distortion will become larger and work its way down through the layers of the field to affect the physical body. The body is very adaptable and flexible, so it can deal with small distortions, but as a message becomes more and more distorted, the body is less able to understand and use that information. Ultimately, the message becomes so scrambled that the body cannot compensate, so physiology breaks down. The symptoms of disease may result. This is one of the reasons that so many complementary health care professionals stress the value of preventive health, and it is why NES is so useful as a part of a wellness program. When the distortion becomes so gross that it affects the physical body, it may take a long time to correct that problem. It's wiser to correct energy and information distortions *before* they affect the physical body.

The big body-wave cycle through the twelve Energetic Integrators happens many times a second. You can think of the end of the wave— at Energetic Integrator 12, where the wave reforms—as an "adaptation point." It is a transitional moment in the sequence of the big body-wave cycle, the last chance to check the information in the waveform before it is sent back to the start of the wave at Integrator 1.

Information can be inserted into the wave at any Energetic Integrator point in the big body-wave for any number of reasons—physical shock or trauma, emotional shock or trauma, toxins, microbes, parasites, bacteria and fungi, ionizing radiation, X-rays, microwaves, poor nutrition, geopathic stress, and the like. The opposite also is true. If *corrective* information is inserted into the wave at an Integrator anywhere along it, then that information also can change the wave, reforming it in a way that is more in tune with the body's natural state. Corrective information also can take any number of forms—emotional or perceptual epiphany or insight, positive change in your belief system, physical cleansing or detox, improved nutrition, or bioenergetic correction from massage, acupuncture, herbs and supplements, homeopathic remedy, or NES Infoceutical. (Of these corrective substances, only the NES remedy *directly* corrects any distorted phase shift relationship affecting the Energetic Integrators; all the others, such as herbs or homeopathic remedies, produce indirect corrections to the body-field.) The adaptation point, then, is crucial to homeostasis, for it either supports or hampers the body from regulating itself.

It is at Energetic Integrator 12 that the disruption or correction of the body-field wave has its consequences, because the adaptation point gives the physical body its ability to change, to respond to everything to which is it exposed. Every cell of the body contributes, through its DNA fields, to the changing nature of the big body-wave. However, if the waveform is badly distorted at Energetic Integrator 12, at the end of the wave cycle, the consequences are especially serious, for the waveform cannot start up again properly, or perhaps at all. If the adaptation process ceases to function properly, the result is what in NES we call field collapse. Of course, the ultimate field collapse is physical death.

Although the Energetic Drivers, Terrains, and Stars are extremely important in terms of the functioning of the body-field, the Energetic Integrators are at the heart of the system. Yet in the NES sequence of correcting the body-field, the Energetic Integrators are not addressed until Source energy, the Big Field and Polarity alignments, and the Energetic Drivers are relatively balanced because it takes energy (Source energy and the Drivers) to push information (the Integrators), and the states of the Drivers and Integrators cannot be determined accurately until the big body-field is correctly aligned as to its electrostatic Polarity and with Earth's Big Field (vertical, equatorial, and magnetic polar axes).

THE NES VIEW OF THE VISIBLE AURA

The human body-field is both an energetic and informational structure, and there are many traditions that have devised systems for interpreting its information visually or intuitively, with ancient concepts such as the meridians, chakras, and the aura. We will take a moment to discuss the aura because it often is evoked as the visible part of the human energy body from which information may be gleaned. Some readers may confuse it with the NES body-field, so we want to be clear about how they relate to each other. In the NES model, the external aura can be thought of as a sort of corona of the dynamic body-field, but not as an integral part of its information network.

The aura is largely electromagnetic in nature but composed of visible light (it can be seen by the human eye or detected through certain photographic methods, such as kirlian photography; its visibility also is why it is often referred to as the "light body" in metaphysical parlance). Visible light covers only a tiny range of the electromagnetic spectrum, which is vast, with energies (frequencies) such as radio and infrared waves extending below the range of visible light, and others, such as ultraviolet, X-ray, and gamma rays, extending far beyond it. Because it covers so small a portion of this range of frequencies, the aura is severely restricted in the amount of information it can encode. In contrast, the human body-field, according to NES, includes much more of this spectrum of energies, especially via the Energetic Integrators, which include frequency ranges in hertz from near 0 to 10^{12}, as shown in the chart earlier in this chapter. We are not denying that those perceptive people who can see the aura and its colors can extract information, including health information, from it, but we are suggesting that the information will always be partial at best.

To use an analogy to make this distinction clear, think of how a mechanic can extract information about how your car's engine is performing by analyzing only the emissions from the tailpipe. He'll know a lot about the engine, but not everything. In the same way, information is encoded in the visible aura, but it is scant compared with what is contained in the vast network of the body-field. Peter quips that the visible aura is the "off-gassing" of the body-field. So, in actuality, it may be that people who can "read auras" may in fact be mostly *intuiting* information from the larger body-field rather than extracting information from the visible aura.

THE ENERGETIC INTEGRATORS, CONSCIOUSNESS, AND EMOTIONS

We've talked a lot about how the NES model of the body-field correlates with the physical body, but we are more than blood and bone. What about emotions and consciousness? These, too, are "contained" within the Energetic Integrators, and we will now provide a quick tour of what Peter's research has revealed about how the Energetic Integrators correlate to emotions and consciousness.

Every aspect of our being is covered to one degree or another by the information network we call the Energetic Integrators, with more biologically complex aspects of the body falling at the higher end of the frequency and phase shift ranges of the Integrators. Each of the twelve Integrators contains information about every aspect of the body—including elements, cells, tissues, organs, emotions, and aspects of consciousness. At the very "top" of each Integrator, after emotions and consciousness, is what we call *self-organizing breakdown,* which is a NES term for the adaptation point of the wave—the crux of homeostasis, where the information the body needs either contributes to health or to the breakdown of health and well-being.

Mind-body medicine has shown us how emotional tape loops—habitually replaying emotions or behaving according to mostly unconscious emotional patterns—can affect the body-field just as physical habits can. It also has shown how stress, beliefs, attitudes, and other emotional states can directly affect our health and well-being. For instance, meditation and relaxation practices can beneficially affect our physical state, lowering our blood pressure, alleviating pain, and more. Researchers such as Candace Pert, author of *The Molecules of Emotion,* and others have shown that the neuropeptides—the molecules of emotion, which were once thought to be manufactured and circulated only in the brain (hence the term *neuro*peptide)—actually are found everywhere in our body. Researchers are beginning to understand what wisdom traditions have told us for thousands of years—that emotion is actually distributed body-wide.

NES has produced a general Infoceutical, called Emotional Stress Release, to address the effects of stress on our body-field. This Infoceutical is correlated to the medulla oblongata, the hindbrain, the seat of the autonomic nervous system (which controls such functions as breathing and heart function). There is also a Star Infoceutical, Energetic Star 8–Chill, that addresses deeper, long-term, stress-related issues. It is bioenergetically correlated to the cerebral cortex, which can become overloaded with sensory data and so contribute to our forming perceptual/emotional tape loops. In contrast with these general stress-relief Infoceuticals, the Energetic Integrator Infoceuticals address specific emotions.

How did Peter know which emotions are bioenergetically correlated with which Energetic Integrator? Originally, he built on the information already available from TCM through his matching experiments to discover, when possible, how the Energetic Integrators correlate to parts of the brain and extrapolated how those parts of the brain are known to affect emotions. Later, he was able to amass information from his own and his clients' use of the Infoceuticals. As an example, Peter discovered that Energetic Integrator 1 is linked energetically with our ability to be organized, hopeful, and considerate of ourselves and others. However, it is important to note that if there is a distortion in an Integrator, that does not mean we are incapable of feeling an emotion or feel an overabundance of it. It means, instead, that we have less of an ability to *manage* that emotion or to be able to deal with situations in which that emotion or condition comes into play. So for instance, in our example of Integrator 1, if the distortion was with organization, it could mean that this person might feel unsettled by a messy environment or feel overly stressed if things or events in his or her life are not predictable and orderly, or it could mean that he or she is having to deal with others who have problems with organization and so is impacted, too. In other words, a distortion of an Energetic Integrator in terms of emotion relates to how well the person tolerates those types of emotions in himself or others and does not mean that he or she has too much or too little of that particular emotion. It is also important to note that some of the terms used by NES to describe emotions are imprecise because emotions are decidedly nuanced. The specific emotions correlated to each Integrator are covered in the next chapter.

How do the Energetic Integrators correlate to consciousness? Peter has reached some fascinating, if tentative, conclusions about how consciousness fits into the body-field. However, because there is so much more to discover about the body-field and only so much time to carry out the research, he has chosen to focus most of his energy on studying the body-field's correlations to physical health. Thus, he has only scratched the surface of how the NES model of the body-field can impact psychology and contribute to consciousness research in general. That said, what he has found is immensely provocative!

Peter wouldn't be the first researcher to say that consciousness, when it becomes incoherent and disordered, contributes to the formation of disease or that when it is coherent and ordered it contributes to health. The science of physics, however, does not have anything to say about such speculations. Consciousness cannot be "found" in the brain, although various states of consciousness and memory can be correlated to brain activity and, according to conventional imaging techniques, even to specific areas of the brain. The general philosophy of consciousness has been labeled metaphysics by allopathic researchers, so they tend not to include it in their realm of inquiry. Conventional medicine practitioners make few definitive statements about the relation between consciousness and disease, and when they do, they tend to do so only within specific and narrow parameters, statements that we can summarize very generally as:

▶ There are diseases caused by biochemical errors in the body, which includes the brain, and these can sometimes be corrected by altering biochemistry, that is, by using pharmaceuticals.

▶ There are diseases of the brain that involve some degenerative damage to brain structures, which can affect the mind. These can sometimes be addressed mechanically, that is, by surgery.

▶ The mind is an emergent property of the brain and is but tenuously linked to health. For diseases of the mind—generally called psychosomatic diseases—treatments are limited mostly to reconditioning, behavioral modification, and other psychotherapeutic methods. For healing effects that are said to be mind-mediated only, the placebo effect is provided as an explanation.

▶ So far as consciousness goes, we have two discrete categories—awake/aware and asleep/unaware—and a third called the subconscious/unconscious, which tends to play a slight to nonexistent role in conventional medicine. Generally, the subconscious is considered to be linked to "unknowing" and consciousness to "knowing." In other words, consciousness is linked with the sensorium, that is, the sensory apparatus of the brain.

Peter postulates that every one of these statements is incorrect! He said, "Once you accept the idea—the evidence!—of a complex set of energy fields flowing through the body, together with the idea—and the evidence!—of the ability of the body to self-generate these fields, there is a true revolution in the way we understand how we work and indeed who we are."

Peter thought that the twelve Energetic Integrators might play a role in consciousness. He explained his line of reasoning and the results of his years of matching tests, stating "The Integrators turned out to have *inner structure* and a preferred sequence, an order that the body 'likes' because it helps it to achieve or maintain homeostasis. When I tested each tissue of the body, it matched with one or another of the Integrators only. So, of course, it was of interest to see where the parts of the brain wanted to go in the Integrator system.

"It is of enormous interest to the development of bioenergetics that the Integrators all showed similar arrangements of items within them. First of all, the lowest frequency area contains certain elements, and moving up the frequency ranges, they contain compounds, followed by simple things in biology like amino acids, followed by proteins, tissues, organs, and so on. As complexity increases, so does the frequency of the compartment. These things match in space *in a certain order.*

"Higher up in the frequency domain," he continued, "I finally was able to place the emotions. This was not entirely new at all since the Chinese had linked a prevailing characteristic emotion with every main group of meridians, and this is taught widely around the world and occurs in the basic ancient texts on the subject. However, I found that something as tenuous as a personality characteristic, such as charisma, which can be thought of as a characteristic of a person rather than an emotion, also appeared in the high frequency region near the end of the Integrator!

"What came after emotions? Consciousness! There appeared to be a place, or twelve places really since it happens in each Integrator, where there is a system for consciousness to be expressed, and even measured. Whoa! This stuff surprised even me. I had to wrap my mind around it for a while before I could continue to explore it.

"What really boggled my mind was what appeared to be taking place *between* the Integrators, or rather at the point where one Integrator became another. The Integrators appeared in my experiments to act like separate but contiguous compartments, and I found an esoteric mathematics by which the energy from one compartment transformed into the energy of another compartment, from one constant to another constant, in fact. What I found is that this is where consciousness fits into the system, *in the transformation areas*. Just as the big body-wave has an adaptation point at Energetic Integrator 12, and to some extent also at its beginning, at Integrator 1, so do the Integrators. It's like the transition point from one Integrator to the next is a miniadaptation point, and these are especially important in terms of consciousness."

As Peter gathered data and tried to make sense of it, he became aware that what he was discovering about the Energetic Integrators, emotions, and consciousness could have profound ramifications in psychology. His research suggests that when energy and information cannot flow properly or at all from one Energetic Integrator to another, a sort of psychic blockage occurs. This blockage might be what psychologists call resistance and even repression. It is not uncommon in psychotherapy for patients to resist the efforts of their therapists, to resist seeing their problems in perspective, or to not be able to access feelings or even memories about events in their lives. This kind of resistance, of course, does not happen only in therapy. We are all prone to it. Memory is dynamic and malleable. We don't like to have our beliefs challenged, and we resist radical shifts in our worldview. As Peter says, when our beliefs about ourselves or our views about the world are challenged, "the inner brakes go on." In the NES system, the brakes are represented by the divisions, the transition or adaptation points, between each of the twelve Integrators. If energy and information does not flow through the Energetic Integrator network, through the entire big body-wave, then the wave breaks down and does not restart properly.

"So the idea of resistance," said Peter, "takes on a new meaning. You can think of the process this way: the *energy* goes through the

Integrators but the *information* is left behind at some point. Where it is stuck, at which Integrator, can indicate a lot about what the problem is, as each Integrator matches to specific emotions and aspects of consciousness. The body-field is a dynamic system, so when something within it becomes static, there are consequences!"

The NES Infoceuticals are designed to support normal emotional functioning—to help energy and information flow properly again. The initial effects of the Infoceuticals usually are on the *functional* aspect of clients' problems or their disease, that is, on their emotions and perceptions: how they feel about and perceive their state of health or lack of it, how well they can cope, how well they function generally in their lives. These types of functional changes often occur before the physical body changes.

Peter said, "You might now be able to imagine the implications of this bioenergetic system as it relates to consciousness. The awareness of the communication taking place between the Integrators in our body-field may actually *be* what we call consciousness! When this awareness of the communication is inhibited for any reason, we get something that has been called, perhaps incorrectly, the subconscious, but the subconscious may simply be the way we explain information that is *not available right away*. It is stuck between Integrators, and so not flowing through the big body-wave. Perhaps you and your therapist can retrieve it at great expense, since data is not lost, just hidden.

"Consciousness is then linked inevitably with memory," Peter continued, "and one can influence the other. One can inhibit the other. In this regard, it means that the information in the field is not freely available. So memory is not just a field, it is certain parts of the general field that store information. Information is stored in every cell of the body, including the brain. So you were not entirely wrong when you thought that the brain 'does' memory, but now we have to entertain the idea that the whole body retains memory, as so many recent scientists, such as Candace Pert, have been telling us."

Peter reminds us, however, that consciousness is different from memory. The Integrator fields can be thought of as having thresholds between them—those adaptation points—and sometimes the doorway is wide open, sometimes partially open, and sometimes closed. Perhaps the doorway, the adaptation point, is a protective mechanism to stop us from knowing too much too soon. This fits with many long-term observations by psychologists. It also might explain what we mean when we talk about attaining higher levels of consciousness, or enlightenment. That could be a state with all the doors wide open, with all information and energy available to us consciously, in full awareness. However, as Peter said, "For most of us, some doors are open and some partially closed, and a few shut tight, maybe even locked!"

The beauty of the NES model is that the scan can show us the status of the Integrators and the NES Infoceuticals can correct the problems without our having to know explicitly what is going on in each of the Integrators. We don't have to have a physical diagnosis, as in naming our problem as lupus, asthma, pancreatic cancer, or whatever, or a psychological diagnosis, as in naming our problem as anxiety or panic disorder. We don't even have to blame ourselves for what we perceive as our inadequacies, such as being trapped in our childhood trauma or unable to resolve grief. From the NES perspective, our root problem is stuck, or static, information in one Integrator or another. Of course, it might serve us as human beings to strive for awareness of our problems, but in terms of our physical health, naming and knowing are not necessary prerequisites to healing.

One other point about the Energetic Integrators and emotions and consciousness that will be of interest to readers is that the heart, not just the brain, is also a seat of emotion. Peter's matching tests revealed that emotion, and by extension memory, is inevitably linked back to the heart, its tissue, and the nerves surrounding it. Peter explained, "I give traditional Chinese medicine credit for exploring this, but I have also gone farther in explaining the processes. Modern science tells us that the brain is the seat of our mind and hence of our emotions, but esoteric systems have always said the link was through the heart. What is the connection? You might be surprised!

"An experiment I once did involved a matching experiment between an Infoceutical preparation called Field Stabilizer—which has since been reworked into an Energetic Star Infoceutical—and all the tissues of the brain that were available for the test, as well as other tissues of the body. Field Stabilizer is about correcting the big body-wave, the overall field. So it includes just about everything, including the twelve Integrators and emotions. The results were as usual quite astounding. There were *no* matches between the Field Stabilizer and the parts of the brain or to any of the various organelles of most cells. *The only match found was to the cells and structures of the heart.* For example, it strongly matched to myocardial tissue, which is the tissue that plays the most important role in imprinting memory into a certain type of fat cell.

"You have fat cells all over your body, so the implication is that the heart as imprinter affects the whole body via the blood. *So, you have both memory and consciousness over all of your body,*" Peter stated. "Your body is a holograph of memory, and when a bit of that memory 'goes missing,' it is simply no longer available to awareness because it is not moving through the Integrators. Information cannot be destroyed but it can be compartmentalized, static rather than dynamic, so that it is not *available* information. This is complicated by the fact that we have both conscious awareness and subconscious awareness, but bioenergetically it may be that those are just labels for how information is moving, or not, through the Integrator system. For us to remain sane, for our survival, it serves us to compartmentalize some kinds of information from our lives, to keep it static rather than dynamic until we can deal with it, but the bioenergetic fact is that this information—memory—is *always* available to be accessed, and the NES system can help people access it when they are ready. NES theory and experiment show us that you cannot treat the body and psychology/consciousness separately. So, this is some of what I have found out about how the Energetic Integrators—as a collective field system for moving information through the big body-wave—are at the foundation of both our physical and emotional selves."

NES Case Overview: Paula

Paula had a family history of heart disease. In fact, both of her parents and all of her many siblings had been diagnosed with heart-related problems. Two brothers died of heart problems in 2004.

Paula was under a doctor's care to monitor her own heart health. She had previously suffered two small strokes, although she had fully recovered. Exacerbating her family medical history was Paula's use of tobacco and her environmental exposure to pesticides and fertilizers because she worked intermittently in commercial farming in rural Australia. She was on a regular regime of pharmaceuticals, including medications to thin her blood and help control high blood pressure and an elevated cholesterol level.

In 2002, Paula failed a stress test. An angiogram revealed that the main artery to her heart was 80 percent blocked. When she sought out a NES practitioner, Debra Carter, in late 2004, she had been on a list for bypass surgery for nearly two years, but her blood platelets had been chronically low, too low for her to be a good candidate for the operation.

Paula's first NES scan showed Muscle Driver, Cell Driver, and Bone Driver as the most distorted aspects of her body-field, and these were the three Infoceuticals she was put on. Carter also advised Paula to quit smoking, take a B-complex vitamin, and take red cayenne pepper capsules to strengthen her nervous system and possibly stimulate her circulation.

Several weeks later, Paula returned for a second NES scan, which revealed a host of body-field distortions, including Polarity, Nervous System Driver, Stomach Driver, Muscle Driver, Kidney Driver, Bone Driver, and Energetic Integrator 10 (Circulation/Pericardium Meridian). Although a NES protocol customarily does not include more than four or five Infoceuticals, Carter had Paula take all seven Infoceuticals.

Nearly a month later, Paula returned to Carter for a follow-up scan. She reported that she was smoking less and felt much better. Her peripheral circulation had improved, so her extremities felt warmer. The most marked improvement was in Paula's stamina and energy level, and she had been able to increase her daily activity level. She reported that her primary care physician was generally impressed with her improvement and asked what she was doing. (Paula soon put him in touch with Carter, who explained about NES.) Her current NES scan revealed that Polarity, Kidney Driver, Bone Driver, and Energetic Integrator 10 remained distorted, so she continued with those Infoceuticals. However, several other areas of her body-field showed distortions, and the scan revealed that she was ready to bioenergetically address her exposure to environmental chemicals, so Paula was given the appropriate Infoceuticals.

Between her next several visits to Carter, Paula continued to take the recommended Infoceuticals and continued to improve. Her energy level was up, and her platelet count was restored enough that her doctor advised her to prepare for the bypass surgery. Paula was feeling so much better that she requested another angiogram to see if the blockage in her heart artery was better, which might make the operation unnecessary, but that test was not repeated. Paula's doctor advised her to continue with NES as an adjunct treatment to his own prescribed allopathic treatment, and he had Paula come to his office to meet a colleague to tell him about her NES treatment and discuss the progress she had made.

On Paula's sixth visit with Carter, in late 2005, she reported that she had started exercising again, jogging for five minutes at a time throughout the day without any ill effects. She was walking up and down stairs with ease and had again increased her daily activity level without experiencing any chest pain. Paula's physician remained supportive of her NES treatment, and he asked for her scan results to be shared with him. Her blood platelets were close to normal level, and her blood pressure was the best it had been in twenty-six years.

Paula shifted into a maintenance program with NES, having a scan every couple of months to reveal and correct any severe body-field distortions as part of her continuing wellness program. Her doctor had agreed to do another angiogram to see if surgery was still necessary, but Paula, against both her doctor's and NES practitioner's advice, was resisting even doing that because she felt so much better. Her physician continued to monitor her heart.

In September 2006, Paula said, "I feel so much better. People have commented on how well I look now that I have had the bypass surgery, which I have not had! My doctor has found a great deal of difference in my health now and told me, 'Keep doing what you're doing.' That sounds good to me!"

14

DETAILS OF THE
ENERGETIC INTEGRATORS

PETER'S MATCHING TESTS have opened a window that allows you to see clearly the beauty and intricacy of your bioenergetic self. The Energetic Integrators reveal how your physical and energetic aspects are interconnected with and dependent on the field structures that make up your body-field. Although we can provide only a glimpse of the complexities of the Energetic Integrator system, even this overview should provide you with a wondrous sense of how energy and information work in concert to direct life processes.

ENERGETIC INTEGRATOR 1:
NEUROSENSORY/COLON MERIDIAN

When you think Energetic Integrator 1, think bioenergetically of correlations to your nervous system, cranial nerves, and the senses. This Integrator influences the bioenergetic information pathways of the prefrontal lobes of your brain and your nervous system in general. It connects with your skin and regulates the information processing coming to and from your sense receptors, including touch, pressure, heat and pain, taste, sight, and smell. It also covers your autonomic nervous system in general, which regulates the functions of your organs and their secretions and motility.

The precision with which Peter could make distinctions via his matching experiments allowed him to discover that although the cranial and spinal nerves are part of Energetic Integrator 1, the motor neurons to which they are attached are not. Motor neurons are part of Energetic Integrator 7. Also, although your sensory nerves are part of Energetic Integrator 1, the sense organs themselves (i.e., your eyes, nose, tongue, skin, and so on) are found in other Integrators. The nerves to the large bowel are part of Energetic Integrator 1, but the rectum, anus, and sigmoid colon are part of the information pathway of Integrator 6. The bronchial membranes are found in Integrator 1, but parts of the bronchial system are also part of Integrator 11. So, you can see that as with meridians in TCM, the Integrators connect many disparate systems, organs, nerves, and other anatomical and biochemical aspects of the body.

Energetic Integrator 1: Bioenergetic Connections at a Glance

Brain and Nervous System

- Frontal lobes (also Energetic Integrator 11)
- Sensory cortex, organs, and processes
- Autonomic nervous system
- Cranial nerves
- Spinal nerves: nerve plexuses, nerves to organs, and vasomotor nerves
- Motor neuron (also Energetic Integrator 10)

Other Bioenergetic Connections

- Large intestine: ascending colon, hepatic flexure, transverse colon, and descending colon mesentery (but rectum, anus, and sigmoid colon are in Energetic Integrator 6; also see Energetic Integrators 7 and 11)
- Skin: dermis layer (also Energetic Integrator 3)
- Bronchi: smooth muscles, mucosae (also Energetic Integrators 4, 5, and 11)
- Bone marrow in general

- Paranasal sinus
- Lymph vessels (also Energetic Integrator 5)

Minerals and Elements
- Boron
- Cobalt (also Energetic Integrator 6)
- Iodine (also Energetic Integrator 9)
- Molybdenum
- Sulfur

Although NES makes no claim for the diagnosis, treatment, prevention, or cure of physical disease, by inference from a bioenergetic perspective, distortions in Energetic Integrator 1 may be correlated to the following clinical conditions, among others: sensory cortex disturbances, ataxia and lack of coordination, convulsions, Ménière disease, sciatica, neuritis, and neuralgia.

In terms of emotions, Integrator 1 links via the colon meridian concept of TCM to organization, hopefulness, and consideration. It relates to the balance between letting go and grimly holding on. It also links to mental stagnation, especially as the tendency to avoid processing emotions.

ENERGETIC INTEGRATOR 2: HEART/LUNG MERIDIAN

Energetic Integrator 2 is linked primarily with the organs of your chest cavity, and secondarily its path runs through the entire upper midline of your body. This Integrator matches bioenergetically to heart tissue, especially the myocardium, and to the pulmonary valve, but not to pulmonary circulation. Energetic Integrator 2 deals with how energy flows between the left and right chambers of your heart. Because it links to the pacemaker aspects of heart cells, it has robust bioenergetic connections to the coronary artery, coronary sinus, and the arterioventricular (AV) and sinuatrial (SA) nodes of the heart.

There are cavities within cavities within cavities in the chest. The ribs, obviously, form the largest cavity, but there are also the chambers of the heart, the major arteries, the lungs, and the various smaller tubules within the lungs. We know that cavities attract, store, and amplify energy, so the chest is a primary area for Source energy. We know, too, that the heart is a major imprinter of information via the blood circulation to the entire body. So this area, and the related Energetic Integrators, including Integrator 2, have wide-reaching energetic and informational links in the body-field. However, Peter's research goes even deeper, indicating that the heart's chambers have direct bioenergetic links to cell organelles, a link that increases the heart's role as information imprinter even at the cellular and subcellular levels.

What's more, Peter has found that many parasites, or their energetic field signatures, gravitate to Energetic Integrator 2 and may spend part of their life cycles in the lungs or liver, so this Integrator may show up in a NES scan for that reason rather than because of any distortions in the lung or heart fields.

Energetic Integrator 2 also links to the germinal layers of the fetus: the ectoderm, endoderm, and mesoderm. So, it may be an important bioenergetic connection to embryological development. If the fetus's development is compromised through trauma or developmental disorders, the distortion may be most evident in Integrator 2.

Three female hormones also are contained bioenergetically in Energetic Integrator 2: estradiol, estrone, and pregnenolone. This fact offers tantalizing clues that disturbances in the levels of these hormones may bioenergetically affect heart function or, conversely, that the heart as imprinter of information may affect these hormones levels. This link may be especially important for the health of postmenopausal women, but much more research is needed before any conclusions can be reached.

Energetic Integrator 2: Bioenergetic Connections at a Glance
Heart and Cardiovascular System
- Right ventricle (also Energetic Integrators 3, 9, and 10)

- Pericardium
- Myocardium (also Energetic Integrator 8)
- Endocardium
- Pulmonary valve
- Coronary sinus
- Coronary arteries
- AV and SA nodes
- Circulation in chest area
- Hemoglobin (also Energetic Integrators 4 and 7)

Respiratory System

- Mediastinum (also Energetic Integrator 8)
- All lobes of the lungs
- Pulmonary tissue
- Trachea (but not bronchi or apex)

Germinal Layers of Fetus

- Ectoderm
- Endoderm
- Mesoderm

Hormones

- Estradiol (also Energetic Integrator 10)
- Estrone (also Energetic Integrator 8)
- Pregnenolone (also Energetic Integrator 10)

Minerals and Elements

- Osmium
- Rubidium (also Energetic Integrator 11)

Distortions in Integrator 2 could reveal themselves as bioenergetic correlations to problems such as angina, congestive heart failure, hormonal imbalances, congestive-obstructive pulmonary disease,

emphysema, bronchiectasis, parasitic infections, embryonic malforma-
tions, and developmental disorders such as autism.

Grief, in all its varied expressions, is the emotion most strongly correlated to Integrator 2. However, because the lungs are covered by this
bioenergetic pathway, Integrator 2 has a deep but subtle influence on
your entire emotional makeup. Ancient cultures the world over link
breathing patterns with emotions, noting that restricted and shallow
breathing tends to lead to restricted or suppressed emotions. So distortions in Energetic Integrator 2 may affect your emotions via its bioenergetic link to your lungs.

Of course, because the heart is found in this Energetic Integrator,
there is a powerful link to emotions. The heart as your "emotional
brain" yokes Energetic Integrator 2 to your sense of personal identity.
Consider, for example, the consequences on your health if you were
involved in many negative or stressful interpersonal relationships.
As a bioenergetic organ, your heart would be imprinting these stress
signals with every beat into the circulatory system, sending the messages throughout your body. For these reasons and others, the state of
Energetic Integrator 2 has especially wide-reaching consequences in
terms of balancing your physical and emotional health.

ENERGETIC INTEGRATOR 3:
MUCOSAE/SMALL INTESTINE MERIDIAN

Energetic Integrator 3 focuses on the back midline of the body, whereas Energetic Integrator 2 covered the front midline. Peter says that although
Energetic Integrator 3 is named for its link to the small intestine, it might
be more accurate to call it the Spine Energetic Integrator because so many
aspects of the spinal muscles are linked to it. Also, because Integrator 3
bioenergetically regulates calcium metabolism in general, it is strongly
linked to all of your bones, not just those of your spine. Hence, Integrator
3 is implicated bioenergetically in such conditions as osteoporosis. We
should note that Integrator 5 also is linked to the bones, but for different

reasons, which we will discuss when we describe that Integrator.

As with every Energetic Integrator, the bioenergetic influence of this one also reaches far and wide, influencing many different organs and physiological processes. For example, it links with endocrine function via the parathyroid gland and the metabolism of parathyroid hormone. Energetic Integrator 3 also has multiple connections to your digestive system, including the serous and muscular ileum, intestinal villi, and ileocecal as well as the ileocecal valve and appendix (both of which also have ties to Integrator 5). Because of these specific links, Integrator 3 is involved bioenergetically in your ability to absorb nutrients, especially various minerals and proteins. Finally, certain organ lining tissues show up in Integrator 3, including epithelial tissue and all of the mucosae of your nose, throat, bronchi, and stomach.

If you are familiar with TCM, you know that the small intestine meridian travels up to the neck and shoulder blades. Peter confirmed this pathway in Energetic Integrator 3 through his matching experiments. So, correcting this Integrator may affect the bioenergetic causes of complaints such as adhesive capsulitis, the medical name for what is commonly called frozen shoulder, a condition of inflamed connective tissue in the shoulder that causes severe pain and greatly reduced motion.

Energetic Integrator 3: Bioenergetic Connections at a Glance
Skeletal System
- Bone metabolism, especially calcium metabolism
- Vertebrae: atlas, cervical, dorsal, lumbar, and sacrum (also in Energetic Integrator 5)

Heart and Cardiovascular System
- Left ventricle (also Energetic Integrators 2, 9, and 10)

Endocrine System
- Parathyroid gland
- Parathyroid hormone

Lining Tissues

- Skin: epithelium (also Energetic Integrator 1)
- All mucosae of nose, throat, bronchi, and gut

Sensory System

- Ear canal (external auditory meatus)

Digestive System

- Ileum: serous and muscular coats
- Intestinal villi
- Ileocecal villi (also Energetic Integrator 5)
- Ileocecal valve
- Appendix (also Energetic Integrator 5)

Other Bioenergetic Connections

- Muscle fascia (also Energetic Integrator 12)
- Penis: glans (also Energetic Integrators 5 and 11)

Minerals and Elements

- Calcium (also Energetic Integrator 4)
- Carbon
- Hydrogen (also Energetic Integrators 4 and 6)
- Strontium
- Vanadium

Conditions in which Energetic Integrator 3 may be bioenergetically implicated include calcium metabolism and bone matrix issues in general, osteomyelitis or osteitis, osteoporosis (also affected by Energetic Integrator 5 distortions), and osteoarthritis. Other conditions that may be linked to an Energetic Integrator 3 distortion include irritable bowel syndrome, colitis, and Crohn disease, although because of the mucosa issues related to these conditions, Cell Driver distortions also are likely to play a role. The stomach and digestive issues associated with conditions such as CFS may be linked through Integrator 3, as are dietary problems such as food allergies and protein sensitivity and microbial issues related to candida or intestinal bacteria in general. Abdominal hernias, arteriosclerosis, and lithiasis (stones, as in kidney stones) may be associated bioenergetically with Integrator 3 distortions, although lithiasis would also likely correlate to Integrator 5.

The bioenergetic emotional components of Energetic Integrator 3 distortions are mostly involved with mental agility and concentration, or the lack of them. Short-term memory problems—as in difficulty holding a thought—and learning disabilities, especially in children, appear to have correlations to Integrator 3.

ENERGETIC INTEGRATOR 4: NEUROTRANSMITTERS/HEART MERIDIAN

Bioenergetically, the best way to think of Energetic Integrator 4 is as linking the heart of the thoracic cavity with the heart of the cranial cavity—the midbrain. The midbrain regulates your autonomic nervous system, which is responsible for maintaining many physiological processes, such as maintaining your blood pressure, temperature, pH balance, and blood sugar, and for coordinating certain motor and sensory skills. Energetic Integrator 4 also links to the temporal lobe, so it has connections to consciousness and emotional experience. The speech area and the primary auditory centers of the cortex also are found in Integrator 4, particularly as it relates to their levels of acuity.

In the thoracic cavity, Energetic Integrator 4 bioenergetically connects to specific parts of your heart. Whereas Energetic Integrator 2 is involved in gas exchange processes in the body, Integrator 4 is vital to the oxygenation of tissues, so it links the heart and the lung functions in this cavity. Although the physical tissue of your heart is found in Integrator 2, the bundle of His is found here in Integrator 4. Interestingly, Integrator 4 is linked to the nucleus of all nerve cells, which tightens the sensory ties between the heart and brain at a bioenergetic level.

In addition to its bioenergetic links to organs in the thoracic and cranial cavities, Energetic Integrator 4 also has links to organs of the lower abdominal cavity, specifically in the sacral, or pelvic, area of your body. Integrator 4 has bioenergetic ties in females to the ovaries (aspects of which are distributed among several Integrators), cervix, and uterus, so it is important to the proper bioenergetic regulation of menstrual cycles. Your bladder also finds a bioenergetic home in Integrator 4. Finally, this Energetic Integrator is energetically matched to many types of environmental chemicals and pharmaceuticals, so sensitivities can show up as a distortion here.

Energetic Integrator 4: Bioenergetic Connections at a Glance

Brain and Nervous System

- All neurotransmitters, including dopamine, serotonin, and L-dopa
- Midbrain (also Energetic Integrator 10)
- Substantia nigra
- Cerebral ventricles: all four
- Cerebrospinal fluid (also Energetic Integrator 6)
- Speech center of cortex
- Auditory areas of cortex
- Nerve cell nuclei (but not axon or dendrites; motor neurons are in Energetic Integrators 1 and 10)

Respiratory System

- Bronchi, bronchioles (also Energetic Integrators 1, 5, and 11)
- Alveoli
- Vagal bronchoconstrictor
- Sphenoid sinus

Reproductive and Genito-urinary Systems

- Uterus: myometrium, cervix (but not vagina)
- Ovaries: left, right, inner, and outer parts, corpus luteum (but not fallopian tubes); (also Energetic Integrators 8 and 10)

- Nerves to bladder: both sympathetic and parasympathetic (also Energetic Integrator 5)
- Muscle sphincters (also Energetic Integrator 12)

Cardiovascular System
- Blood plasma
- Hemoglobin (also Energetic Integrators 2 and 7)

Other Bioenergetic Connections
- Sphincter muscles (also Energetic Integrator 12)

Minerals and Elements
- Calcium (also Energetic Integrator 3)
- Fluorine
- Hydrogen (also Energetic Integrators 3 and 6)
- Iron (also Energetic Integrator 11)
- Magnesium
- Manganese
- Oxygen
- Potassium (also Energetic Integrator 10)

Common conditions bioenergetically associated with a distorted Energetic Integrator 4 include aphasia, stuttering, some types of hearing loss, and learning difficulties in general. Other problems correlated to distortions in this Integrator include chorea, delirium tremens, vertigo, Parkinson disease, and paralysis due to central nervous system conditions (but Energetic Integrator 7 also likely plays a role). In terms of problems correlated to toxins or microbes, there is a strong bioenergetic link in this Integrator to the *E. coli* bacterium and the *Aspergillus niger* fungus.

Energetic Integrator 4 is associated with the ability to manage emotional states (or being able to relate to others who are managing these states) such as depression (especially postpartum depression), grief, and brokenheartedness. Psychosomatically, health-related anxiety is linked to Integrator 4, especially in the form of self-sabotage through the unconscious belief that one gains attention or other benefits by being sick. Character rigidity also is linked to this Energetic Integrator. This could take any number of forms, such as inflexible attitudes and not achieving personal goals because of the fear of taking the necessary leaps of faith.

ENERGETIC INTEGRATOR 5: LYMPHATICS/BLADDER MERIDIAN

Energetic Integrators 1 through 4 all dealt with frequency ranges (in hertz) in the sound, or phonon, range. Energetic Integrator 5 is the first one whose frequency range reaches into the visible light range of the electromagnetic spectrum and for a ways beyond (see the NES Energetic Integrator Frequency and Phase Chart on page 268). Those Energetic Integrators whose frequency ranges span this portion of the electromagnetic spectrum are particularly sensitive to geopathic stress. In fact, geopathic stress may be the *single* most important cause of one of these Integrators becoming distorted.

Energetic Integrator 5 is one of the more complex Integrators because of its many bioenergetic links to parts of the brain and the immune system. Its areas of influence include the cerebellar cortex, pons, and medulla oblongata. Actually, every Energetic Integrator links to the medulla, but the connection is especially robust in Integrators 5 and 6. Bioenergetically, there is some evidence that shock and trauma can strongly affect the medulla, so for these types of psycho-physical issues, correcting Integrators 5 and 6 may be especially recommended.

Energetic Integrator 5 links to your immune system through the lymphatic and endocrine networks. It influences the broad scope of your immunity responses through bioenergetic connections to your lymph nodes, T-cells and B-cells, and cortisol. Lymphatic connections yoke it to the small organs of your body, such as your tonsils, bladder, kidneys, appendix, prostate or cervix, and gallbladder. It even connects to your teeth, which may explain why the condition of your gums correlates to aspects of your health, such as heart health, as many dentists have noted. It also communicates with the cochlea of the ear, so it has bioenergetic relevance for chronic hearing conditions or problems with the inner ear.

Energetic Integrator 5 may be called the Neural-Hormonal Integrator. Endocrine connections abound because of this Integrator's bioenergetic connections to so many nerves that go to glands and organs. It communicates with your thyroid gland (although evidence suggests it is more tightly yoked to the cartilage capsule than the gland itself). It bioenergetically influences fluid balance and inflammatory processes in your body through the adrenal hormones. Energetic Integrator 5 is the place of the male hormones (although these are linked to Integrator 11 as well) and of the prostate and penis.

We saw that Energetic Integrator 3 dealt with the bones of your spinal column, and we see the spine again in Energetic Integrator 5, only this time the focus is on the spinal nerves. Integrator 5 is sometimes called the Chiropractic Integrator because it communicates bioenergetically with your vertebra and discs via your spinal nerves. Balance is controlled, bioenergetically speaking, via this Integrator through its connection to the cerebellum and cochlear nerve.

Energetic Integrator 5: Bioenergetic Connections at a Glance

Brain and Nervous System

- Gray matter of the brain (also Energetic Integrator 7)
- White matter of the spine: cervical, dorsal, lumbar, and sacral nerves; spinal cord
- Cerebellum
- Medulla oblongata (also Energetic Integrator 6)
- Pons
- Cochlear nerve

Immune System

- Lymph vessels and fluids (also Energetic Integrator 1)
- Lymph nodes
- Lymphatic tissue of the pharynx
- Tonsils
- T-lymphocytes (also in Energetic Integrator 7)
- B-lymphocytes

Hepatic System

- Gallbladder (also Energetic Integrator 7)

Skeletal System

- Vertebral motor unit and vertebrae: atlas, cervical, dorsal, lumbar, and sacral (also Energetic Integrator 3); coccyx
- Spinal discs (also Energetic Integrators 6 and 12)

Respiratory System

- Bronchi: smooth muscles, mucosae (also Energetic Integrators 1, 4, and 11)

Genito-urinary System

- Bladder: mucosae, muscular coats, sphincter, and autonomic nerves (also Energetic Integrator 4)
- Urethra
- Penis and nerves to penis (also Energetic Integrators 3 and 11)
- Corpora cavernosa
- Prostate: tissue, veins, nerves, isthmus, and muscles

Digestive System

- Ileocecal valve (also Energetic Integrator 3)
- Appendix (also Energetic Integrator 3)

Endocrine System

- Anterior pituitary (also Energetic Integrator 9)
- Thyroid capsule (also Energetic Integrator 9)
- 5-Hydroxytryptophan
- Adrenocorticotropic hormone (ACTH)
- Cortisol
- Noradrenaline
- Diiodotyrosine
- Aldosterone

Other Bioenergetic Connections

- Frontal sinuses
- Teeth

Minerals and Elements

- Tantalum

Clinical conditions in which Energetic Integrator 5 distortions may be bioenergetically implicated run the gamut from appendicitis and tonsillitis to subluxations, neuralgia, prostate and impotency problems, inflammatory conditions of all kinds, thyroid problems, and balance disorders. Menstrual difficulties also can fall under the purview of Integrator 5, although distortions in Integrators 4 and 10 also may play a role.

In the emotional palette of this Energetic Integrator, you will find timidity and hypersensitivity and the propensity to be easily startled. If Energetic Integrator 5 is badly distorted, you also may suffer in general from lack of trust and be unable to feel grief and/or to express it.

ENERGETIC INTEGRATOR 6: KIDNEY/KIDNEY MERIDIAN

Energetic Integrator 6 holds a special place among the Energetic Integrators. In NES, we used to call this a "zero-tolerance" item, meaning that if Energetic Integrator 6 was distorted, it took precedence over other distorted Integrators in a correction program. Although we no longer identify it as zero tolerance because we know now that all the Integrators are equally important, we still consider Energetic Integrator 6 as having a bit of a special status. Generally, if many Energetic Integrators are distorted and there is no reason showing from the scan results to wait to correct Integrator 6, it will take precedence among the other Energetic Integrators. Why? Because of its numerous important brain connections, its bioenergetic link to the nucleus of every cell in your body, and its role in processing emotions.

The information pathway of Energetic Integrator 6 goes through the white matter of the brain and down the white matter of the spine. It bioenergetically connects to the thalamus, pineal gland, medulla oblongata, and the arachnoid membrane (lining of the skull). It relates to the skull as a cavity and its role in the attraction and storage of Source energy, which, of course, has immense ramifications for brain function. Energetic Integrator 6 also has strong connections to the emotional self, so it is important in maintaining physical-emotional harmony.

Energetic Integrator 6 generally adheres to the connections noted in TCM for the kidney meridian. Of course, it is bioenergetically connected to the kidneys themselves and all of the microtubules in the kidneys. However, it has many other functions, such as bioenergetically influencing the regulation of your body's pH balance, which is dependent on Energetic Integrator 6's connection to hydrogen. It also has a strong endocrine association, especially to your pineal gland, which controls your sleep-wake cycle, and to dehydroepiandrosterone (DHEA), which is a precursor to female hormones such as estrogens and progesterone, relating this Integrator bioenergetically to parts of the menstrual cycle. Trace minerals have an important link to Energetic Integrator 6, so this Integrator is involved bioenergetically in enzyme and hormone production and function. The thymus is also correlated to Integrator 6, making this Integrator important to your overall immune function. Interestingly, Energetic Integrator 6 links to the lower bowel, urethra, anus, and rectum, but not the bladder or other parts of the urinary system. Finally, Energetic Integrator 6 is connected bioenergetically to certain microbes and pathogens, including human papilloma virus and some forms of candida.

Energetic Integrator 6: Bioenergetic Connections at a Glance

Hepatic System

- Kidneys and fibrous capsules
- Glomerulus
- Renal calyx
- Renal tubules
- Ureter
- Blood plasma salts

Brain and Nervous System

- White matter
- Thalamus
- Hindbrain
- Cranial cavity
- Medulla oblongata (also Energetic Integrator 5)
- Cerebrospinal fluid (also Energetic Integrator 4)

Digestive System

- Sigmoid colon
- Rectum
- Anus

Endocrine System

- Pineal gland
- Androstenedione
- DHEA
- Thymus and serum thymic factor

Skeletal System
- Bones in general (also Energetic Integrator 10)
- Spinal discs (also Energetic Integrators 5 and 12)

Minerals and Elements
- Cobalt (also Energetic Integrator 1)
- Copper
- Germanium
- Hydrogen (also Energetic Integrators 3 and 4)
- Lithium
- Phosphorus
- Zinc (also Energetic Integrator 11)

Distortions in Energetic Integrator 6 might correlate bioenergetically to such problems as disrupted sleep patterns and insomnia, kidney disorders of all types, edema and problems with sodium-potassium balance (also Energetic Integrator 5), hypertension, arteriosclerosis (also Energetic Integrator 1), seasonal affective disorder, constipation, psychosis, bipolar disorder, and poor long-term immunity.

The emotions bioenergetically linked to Integrator 6 are those related to drive and performance and to personal characteristics such as charisma. Empathy also is found here.

ENERGETIC INTEGRATOR 7: BLOOD FIELD /GALLBLADDER MERIDIAN

Whereas Energetic Integrators 5 and 6 relate bioenergetically to the brain and/or spine's white matter, Energetic Integrator 7 connects to the gray matter. It especially is tightly linked to the motor cortex of the brain, so it is correlated clinically to all types of motor problems, from twitches and numbness to gait problems.

In TCM, the gallbladder meridian passes through the hip, in particular the great trochanter, and down the body to the toes. However,

Peter's matching experiments could not confirm this route. So whereas TCM would correlate gallbladder meridian blocks with conditions such as arthritis, NES cannot. For bioenergetic connections to arthritic inflammation, we look to the Cell Driver, not to Integrator 7.

When you think of Energetic Integrator 7, think hemoglobin (in addition to motor cortex and digestive system). There are two important cardiovascular correlations here: blood pressure regulation and hematopoietic stem cell activity as related to white and red blood cell production. This Integrator does not link bioenergetically to actual cells but instead is concerned with the virtual aspect of blood formation, the bioenergetic influences on immune function and disease resistance. This Integrator also is implicated bioenergetically in the formation of excess fibrin, which can clog arteries in the brain and contribute to increased susceptibility to stroke. For this reason, it may be correlated to problems that stem from aging. Blood pressure can be bioenergetically affected by this Integrator, although blood pressure regulation is enormously complex at both the physiological and bioenergetic levels, so there are no doubt many Integrators that correlate to pressure regulation problems. (In NES, Stomach Driver may play an important bioenergetic role in blood pressure because it is connected to the bone marrow, where heavy metals can accumulate and affect cell production and function.)

Energetic Integrator 7: Bioenergetic Connections at a Glance

Digestive System
- Stomach: peritoneal cavity in general and muscular coat of stomach
- Duodenum and jejunum
- Colon: muscular coat (also Energetic Integrators 1 and 11)
- Bile ducts
- Gallbladder and arteries (also Energetic Integrator 5)
- Peritoneum
- Epigastrum

Brain and Nervous System
- Motor cortex
- Gray matter of brain and spinal cord (also Energetic Integrator 5)
- Sympathetic control of blood pressure

Hematopoietic System
- Hemoglobin (also Energetic Integrators 2 and 4)
- Blastic cells
- Natural killer cells
- T-cells (also Energetic Integrator 5)

Other Bioenergetic Connections
- Ligaments (also Energetic Integrator 9)
- Cellular cartilage (also Energetic Integrator 12)

Minerals and Elements
- Antimony
- Nickel (also Energetic Integrator 10)

Field disturbances in Energetic Integrator 7 may correlate to stomach or duodenal ulcers, although ulcers also would likely involve Energetic Terrain 7 because they have a microbial connection. Diverticulitis also correlates to field disturbances in both Energetic Integrator 7 and an Energetic Terrain. Gallbladder conditions in general, including cholecystitis, find bioenergetic links to Integrator 7, as do such diverse conditions as headaches and glaucoma. Hypertension correlates to Integrator 7 but would also likely involve distortions in other Integrators, such as 2 and 6. Genetic causes of hypertension would bioenergetically involve Integrators 3, 4, 6, and 9. There appears to be a bioenergetic correlation between Energetic Integrator 7 and Parkinson disease, but such a connection would also likely involve Energetic Integrator 1. Integrator 7, however, also correlates to other types of motor neuron diseases. In terms of correlations to toxins, Integrator 7 is particularly susceptible to distortions from organochlorides and organophosphates.

Decisiveness, honesty, loyalty, and willpower are the emotions bioenergetically influenced by Energetic Integrator 7. A distortion in this Integrator also correlates to tendencies to vacillate or be indecisive as well as to not manage situations well in which these emotions and behaviors play a role.

ENERGETIC INTEGRATOR 8: MICROBES/LIVER MERIDIAN

The eyes and hormones most closely correlate to distortions in Energetic Integrator 8, although this Integrator also plays a major bioenergetic role in how your body handles microbes, especially pleomorphic organisms, which are microorganisms that can change shape and size. In frontier microbiology, pleomorphic organisms are believed to be the most elementary forms of precelluar life and may play a major role in the development of many diseases, including cancer. For this reason, Energetic Integrator 8 links to all of the Energetic Terrains. This Integrator also regulates fields that bioenergetically help the body deal with endogenous body waste and exogenous environmental toxins. In relation to the Terrains and the bioenergetic network for toxin and microbial response in the body, Energetic Integrator 8 correlates strongly to susceptible organs, such as your eyes, sinuses, liver, and myocardium. Note, however, that the field of the actual tissue of the myocardium is in Energetic Integrator 9 and that bioenergetic cardiovascular function also is associated with Integrator 2. Integrator 8 also plays a major role in bioenergetically addressing problems caused by overexposure to electromagnetic fields—what we call e-smog—both natural and man-made.

The optical system correlates to the Energetic Integrator 8 network, including the eyes themselves and the visual areas of the brain. In Integrator 8, we find a bioenergetic link to many hormones and to the hypothalamus, which also is linked to Energetic Integrator

10. Correcting distortions in Integrator 8 may have a wide-reaching bioenergetic effect on endocrine function. NES discourages any attempt to try to bioenergetically target individual hormones because the hormonal network of the physical body is just too complex. Instead, we can have a better effect by addressing the wider bioenergetic Driver and Integrator systems, which regulate the fields of the hormone-producing organs and glands themselves. When these organs and glands are fully powered, via the Drivers, and information flow is unrestricted through the Integrators, then problems can be addressed holistically rather than by using a reductionist approach.

Energetic Integrator 8 also has a profound influence on the myriad error fields that can arise around DNA and the genetic material in each cell. These are the sustained, inheritable genetic error fields that cause what homeopaths call "miasms." We won't go into particulars here because the theory of miasms is too complex to discuss with any rigor in limited space, but in classical homeopathy miasms are considered to be at the root of all disease, especially chronic diseases. In NES, we don't identify or name these error fields as homeopaths do, nor do we try to treat them individually. As we have said before, by correcting the distorted structure of the information regulation pathway—the structure in space that we call an Energetic Integrator—everything within that information pathway is corrected.

Energetic Integrator 8: Bioenergetic Connections at a Glance

Brain and Nervous System
- Hypothalamus (also Energetic Integrator 10)
- Supraoptic nucleus

Visual System
- Iris
- Retina
- Center of the optic nerve
- Visual cortex

Hepatic System

- General function and nerves to lobes in liver (liver cells are in Liver Driver)

Cardiovascular and Respiratory System

- Myocardium (also Energetic Integrator 2)
- Diaphragm
- Mediastinum of lungs (also Energetic Integrator 2)
- Maxillary sinus

Female Reproductive System

- Ovaries: corpus luteum (also Energetic Integrators 4 and 10)

Endocrine System

- Calcitonin
- Adrenaline
- Prolactin
- Estrogen
- Estrone (also Energetic Integrator 2)

Minerals and Elements

- Chromium

Disease states that correlate to distortions in Energetic Integrator 8 include optic nerve and general eye diseases. Macular degeneration is associated bioenergetically with this Integrator in conjunction with Cell Driver. Here we also may find bioenergetic links to conditions such as pneumonia, scarlet fever, postviral heart symptoms, myocarditis, renal colic, vertex headaches, arthritis of the hands, osteoporosis (along with Energetic Integrator 3), amoebic dysentery, candida infection, myco-plasma, and microbial problems in general. Hormonal imbalances, especially those related to the hypothalamus, correlate to Integrator 8. Finally, geopathic stress, especially that related to certain types of subterranean watercourses, can have a strong impact on the function of this Integrator.

In terms of emotions, Energetic Integrator 8 correlates to calmness and tolerance as well as the ability to deal with situations in which those qualities are lacking. Feelings of elation are tied to Energetic Integrator 8, as is verbal dexterity, particularly in terms of verbosity.

ENERGETIC INTEGRATOR 9: THYROID/TRIPLE BURNER MERIDIAN

Energetic Integrator 9 is especially noteworthy in the Integrator system because, like Energetic Integrator 4, it bioenergetically affects all of the major cavities—the cranial, thoracic, and abdominal—as well as the myriad smaller cavities distributed throughout the body, such as the capsules around each organ and the spaces around the joints. Through its relation to zero-point energy usage, this Integrator may affect the body's ability to regulate temperature.

Energetic Integrator 9 is associated conceptually with the triple burner meridian of TCM, a meridian that among other things helps the body maintain its thermal equilibrium. In the NES system, energy is produced by a fetus as it develops, as brain waves begin to course through the nervous system, but also through phonons, pressure waves, and electrical frequencies produced by the heart as it beats, the lungs and other bioenergetic mechanisms. It is only after birth that food metabolism and molecular biology (i.e., through adenosine triphosphate [ATP] and adenosine diphosphate [ADP] processes) become important in terms of cell energy production. So Energetic Integrator 9, through its ties to the major and minor cavities of the body, plays an important holistic role in the larger scope of body metabolism. Because fatigue is usually the first sign of illness, Integrator 9 tends to show up frequently on NES scans. It may be an indication that the body is unable bioenergetically to produce the energy it needs to mount an adequate healing response.

As with all the Integrators, however, Energetic Integrator 9 also is linked to specific organs, glands, and physiological processes. Through the endocrine system, Energetic Integrator 9 bioenergetically affects the entire thyroid gland, adrenal medulla, and serotonin production in the pituitary gland. It has widely distributed correlations to specific parts of the brain, heart, and the mucosae of the body, as reviewed in the following lists.

Energetic Integrator 9: Bioenergetic Connections at a Glance

Endocrine System
- Thyroid gland (also Energetic Integrator 5)
- Pituitary gland: posterior and medial (also Energetic Integrator 5)
- Adrenal medulla (also Energetic Integrator 10)

Brain and Nervous System
- Lateral ventricles
- Trigeminal nerve

Other Bioenergetic Connections
- Heart: mitral valve and right atrium (also Energetic Integrators 2, 3, and 10)
- Vagina (also Energetic Integrator 10)
- All mucosae
- Ligaments (also Energetic Integrator 7)
- Links cranial, thoracic, and abdominal cavities

Minerals and Elements
- Calcium-sodium relationship
- Iodine (also Energetic Integrator 1)
- Ionic chlorine
- Selenium

Physical complaints that correlate bioenergetically to an Energetic Integrator 9 distortion include thyroid conditions, autoimmune conditions including arthritis, delayed mental development, postpartum depression, CFS, fibromyalgia, environmental allergies and chemical sensitivities, temperature imbalances of all kinds, and diabetes insipidus.

The emotional correlations to a distorted Energetic Integrator 9 include courage and confidence (as in over- or underconfidence) and difficulty managing situations in which these responses might come into play. Other problems include difficulty verbalizing and a general tendency toward being withdrawn, timid, and silent. However, distortions in Integrator 9 also could display themselves as erratic mood swings, especially as expressed in hyperemotional behavior and a tendency toward fight-or-flight responses.

ENERGETIC INTEGRATOR 10: CIRCULATION/PERICARDIUM MERIDIAN

Energetic Integrator 10 bioenergetically correlates to cell respiration processes (as does Energetic Integrator 2) and a host of organs and their neuroendocrine functions. It has a significant bioenergetic influence on major portions of the circulatory system, and it is linked to digestion and respiration in general. It can be challenging to sort out distortions linked to Energetic Integrator 10, not only because its reach bioenergetically in the body-field, and hence the body, is so wide, but also because it pairs up with other Drivers and Integrators that also correlate to the same organs connected to this Integrator. For example, because of its influence on cell respiration, Energetic Integrator 10 pairs with Cell Driver and Muscle Driver. This Integrator also has a strong correlation to the hypothalamus, so it has a significant bioenergetic influence on that organ and its functions. It affects the midbrain, which also has a strong link to Energetic Integrator 4. It bioenergetically controls aspects of the vagina and ovaries, but they are also linked to Integrators 9 and 4, respectively. The tail of the pancreas is found in Energetic Integrator 10, but other aspects of the pancreas are in Energetic Integrator 12.

Energetic Integrator 10 is particularly susceptible to distortions correlated to physical or emotional shock and trauma, surgeries, chemotherapy, and exposure to chemicals including asbestos, dioxins, and PCPs.

Energetic Integrator 10: Bioenergetic Connections at a Glance

Neuroendocrine System

- Hypothalamus (also Energetic Integrator 8)
- Midbrain (also Energetic Integrator 4)
- Motor neurons (also Energetic Integrator 1)
- Adrenal cortex: corticosterone, 11-deoxycorticosterone, and melanocyte-releasing hormone
- Adrenal medulla
- Ovaries: 2-hydroxy estradiol and 16-hydroxy estrone
- Estradiol (also Energetic Integrator 2)
- Pregnenolone (also Energetic Integrator 2)
- Growth hormone

Cardiovascular System

- Venous and arterial circulation
- Heart: left atrium (also Energetic Integrators 2, 3, and 9)

Digestive System

- Pylorus
- Mucous coat of stomach (also Energetic Integrator 11)

Respiratory System

- Larynx
- Pharynx

Female Reproductive System

- Vagina (also Energetic Integrator 9)

- Ovaries (also Energetic Integrators 4 and 8)
- Clitoris

Other Bioenergetic Connections
- Lens of the eyes (but most of the eye is Energetic Integrator 8)
- Tail of the pancreas
- Bones (also Energetic Integrator 6)

Minerals and Elements
- Nickel (also Energetic Integrator 7)
- Potassium (also Energetic Integrator 4)
- Silicon
- Sodium

Energetic Integrator 10 field distortions correlate to such physical issues as arteriosclerosis, varicose veins (also influenced by Energetic Integrator 6 and Bone Driver), circulatory stasis, and inflammation and arthritis (these last two conditions are also linked to Muscle Driver and Cell Driver). Menstrual irregularities are found here and also in Energetic Integrator 4, as are menopausal problems and hormonal imbalances, which also are tied to Energetic Integrator 5, and conditions relating to the vagina, such as vaginismus. Adrenal insufficiency, CFS, and fibromyalgia are correlated to Energetic Integrator 10 distortions, as are laryngitis, pharyngitis, and other throat-pharyngeal conditions. Parkinson disease and other diseases of the central nervous system appear to correlate bioenergetically to Energetic Integrator 10 distortions, as do gout, calcium or uric acid stones and deposits, some types of diabetes, acid reflux, and ulcers.

The emotions that correlate bioenergetically to Energetic Integrator 10 distortions include thoughtfulness and either runaway thought patterns or problems with thinking coherently. Obsessiveness also is found here but is more generally correlated with distortions of Integrator 11. Premenstrual or menopause-related emotional swings, especially those that tend to be depressive, are linked to Integrator 10 distortions. However, the fluid ability to enter meditative states and to maintain calmness in general are influenced by this Integrator (along with Integrator 11).

ENERGETIC INTEGRATOR 11: BONE MARROW/STOMACH MERIDIAN

Although Energetic Integrator 11 broadly follows the pathway of the stomach meridian in TCM, Peter's matching tests have uncovered a host of specific bioenergetic correlations to areas of the body and physiology that are not accounted for in that system. In terms of the stomach and digestive system, Integrator 11 links only with the muscular lining of the esophagus, stomach, duodenum, and large bowel. Other aspects of these organs are found in other Integrators. For instance the stomach's muscular lining also is found in Energetic Integrator 7, as is the peritoneal cavity in general. Whereas TCM traces the pathway of the stomach meridian down the body to the dorsum of the foot and the middle toe, Peter's matching tests were not able to find any bioenergetic connections between Integrator 11 and those areas of the feet. Although Integrator 11 does follow the traditional meridian pathway through your sinuses to below the orbit of your eyes, Peter has found that there is no single bioenergetic correction possible for sinuses because different sinuses are correlated to different Integrators, with only the maxillary sinuses found in Integrator 11. This Integrator also links bioenergetically to a diverse web of other systems, organs, and related processes, including the throat in general, the lower jaw, the bronchi and the top of the lungs, and the male genitals.

Energetic Integrator 11 has an important bioenergetic correlation to bone marrow function and has an especially strong link to red marrow. It also has a robust correlation to the higher-processing areas of your brain, in particular your frontal lobes. As a consequence of its many connections to the digestive system, lungs, bone marrow, and brain, this Integrator is extremely vulnerable to bioenergetic distortions correlated to the accumulation of toxins, especially heavy metals. The marrow and sinuses are also prime areas for the formation of Energetic Terrains, which, you will remember, are environments amenable to hosting microbes, both real and virtual. The Energetic Integrator 11 pathway also crosses the breast area and moves through the genital area, although its plays a larger bioenergetic role in terms of the male reproductive system than the female system. Energetically, it is linked to the head of the penis, vas deferens, epididymis, scrotum, and other male organs, glands, and vessels. It also bioenergetically governs testosterone.

Energetic Integrator 11: Bioenergetic Connections at a Glance

Digestive System

- Abdominal cavity in general
- Stomach: mucous (also Energetic Integrator 10) and muscular coats
- Fundus: gastric acid production
- Pyloric glands: pepsin
- Duodenum: mucosae and muscles
- Colon: muscular coat (also Energetic Integrators 1 and 7)
- Esophagus

Ears, Nose, Throat, and Respiratory System

- Lungs: bronchi, branchioles, smooth muscles, and mucosae (also Energetic Integrators 1, 4, and 5)
- Maxillary sinuses
- Diaphragm
- Epiglottis

Male Reproductive System

- Head of penis (also Energetic Integrators 3 and 5)
- Testicles and lymph vessels to testicles
- Vas deferens

- Seminal vesicles and epididymis
- Spermatic cord
- Scrotum
- Testosterone and dihydrotestosterone

Brain and Nervous System
- Frontal lobes of brain (also Energetic Integrator 1)
- Sympathetic and parasympathetic nerves

Hematopoietic System
- Red bone marrow
- Yellow bone marrow

Other Bioenergetic Connections
- Groin
- Muscles to front of legs
- Teeth and gums of lower jaw

Minerals and Elements
- Iron (also Energetic Integrator 4)
- Rubidium (also Energetic Integrator 2)
- Silver (also Energetic Integrator 12)
- Tin
- Zinc (also Energetic Integrator 6)

Clinical conditions that correlate bioenergetically to distortions in Energetic Integrator 11 include maxillary sinusitis, myeloid leukemia, anemia, gastrointestinal disorders of all types, impotency, and other male genital/sexual function disorders (also relate to Integrator 5). Because this pathway includes the breast area, it may have a bioenergetic correlation to breast cancer. As the result of its bioenergetic connection to the brain (frontal lobes), this Integrator may link to schizophrenia and certain mental degenerative diseases, although conditions such as Alzheimer disease probably will include distortions in Stomach Driver as well. The bioenergetic effects of heavy metal poisoning and contamination also are expressed through this Integrator because of its robust links to the brain, blood marrow, and stomach, all places where heavy metals tend to accumulate when your body cannot process and expel them.

The emotional correlations to Energetic Integrator 11 relate to higher mental functions, particularly to the expression of memories and spatial awareness difficulties. Obsessive-compulsive disorders correlate bioenergetically to Energetic Integrator 11 distortions, as does the capacity—or the incapacity, as the case may be—to express benevolence and to maintain a calm attitude.

ENERGETIC INTEGRATOR 12: SHOCK/SPLEEN MERIDIAN

Energetic Integrator 12, coming as it does at the end, or adaptation point, of the big body-wave, bioenergetically correlates to serious and often chronic disease states and to what we in NES call field collapse, which is the result of extremely low energy flow or stagnant energy. When energy does not flow, neither can information. Shocks and trauma, both physical and emotional, can drastically affect Energetic Integrator 12, slowing the energy flow through all the Integrators so that the wave does not cycle properly from Integrator 12 back to Integrator 1 again. However, prolonged stress and exhaustion may have the same effect. When you say you are feeling "burned out," you may be speaking less metaphorically than you think! Geopathic stress also may slow the energy flow and scramble the information in this Integrator. When Integrator 12 is in a state of what amounts to energetic chaos, the body will eventually become compromised. However, this process can take a long time to make itself felt at the physical level.

In terms of specifics links to the body, Energetic Integrator 12 controls aspects of the pancreas, spleen, lymphatic system, nervous system, and several key female reproductive organs, as noted in the list below. In the case of pregnant women, it correlates to the fetus as well. Also, Energetic Integrator 12 connects to the neurilema, which is a sheath, sometimes called the sheath of Schwann, that covers the axons of nerve fibers.

Energetic Integrator 12: Bioenergetic Connections at a Glance

Pancreatic System and Spleen
- Head and tail of pancreas
- Pancreatic duct
- Islets of Langerhans
- Alveoli and centroacinar cells
- Spleen

Brain and Nervous System
- Corpus callosum
- Fourth cerebral ventricle

Immune System
- Lymphatic fluid

Female Reproductive System
- Uterus (also in Energetic Integrator 4)
- Cervix, including its lymph, veins, and arteries (also see Energetic Integrator 4)
- Fetus

Other Bioenergetic Connections
- Muscle sphincters (also Energetic Integrator 4)
- Cellular cartilage (also Energetic Integrator 7)
- Muscle fascia (also Energetic Integrator 3)
- Spinal discs (also Energetic Integrators 5 and 6)

Minerals and Elements
- Cesium

- Gold
- Nitrogen
- Silver (also Energetic Integrator 11)
- All twelve Schüssler tissue salts in homeopathy[1]

Physical problems that correlate to a bioenergetic distortion in Integrator 12 include benign and malignant neoplasms, pancreatic diseases, and diabetes (which are all likely to involve Integrator 11 also) as well as lymphatic congestion. In addition, immune deficiencies (also likely to involve distortions in the Immunity and Thymus Drivers), stroke (also correlated to Integrator 10), seizures and convulsions, and digestive ailments are linked to distortions in this Integrator. Learning difficulties also may be affected bioenergetically by an Integrator 12 distortion, especially in relation to right-left brain coordination (Energetic Integrator 4 would also play a role).

Energetic Integrator 12 is affected easily by radiation of all types, including microwaves, and by shocks and trauma. Because exhaustion in general is associated with a distorted Energetic Integrator 12, this Integrator links to conditions characterized by extreme fatigue, such as CFS. Energetic Integrator 12, along with Integrator 8, also communicates with all of the Energetic Terrains, so in a NES protocol these two Integrators are rarely used at the same time.

The predominant emotional correlation to Energetic Integrator 12 is the ability to experience pleasure. People with severe Integrator 12 distortions may lose their feelings of well-being and so lack joie de vivre. Other emotional overtones of chronic distortions in Integrator 12 correlate to mental and emotional exhaustion and an overarching but ambiguous sense of hopelessness. Long-term memory is also bioenergetically linked to this Integrator.

NES Case Overview: Jake

Three-year-old Jake came to Lynette Frieden, a naturopathic physician and chiropractor, in early 2006. Jake is severely disabled with Pelizaeus-Merzbacher disease, which is a rare hereditary disease of the nervous system that is progressive and degenerative. His motor skills and intellectual capacity are severely limited. Like most children with this disease, Jake is confined to a wheelchair, with his head stabilized because of lack of neck muscle tone. His vocal cords are partially paralyzed, and although he can make sounds, he is nonverbal. His hands are curled and clutched. His eyes lack focus. He must be fed through a gastrointestinal tube. Jake has had many surgeries, and he undergoes weekly physical, occupational, and speech therapy sessions. The only medications he is on are Xanax (an antianxiety medication) and an antihistamine for reflux and to somewhat dry up the mucus that he constantly struggles to clear. Beyond these therapies and medications, at present there is not much more that medical science can do for him.

Frieden provided chiropractic care to Jake but also counseled Jake's parents about nutritional options, for instance, suggesting they replace the brand-name liquid meal they were giving Jake with options containing less sugar, which might help the condition of Jake's teeth and generally improve his health. She also used a technique called Total Body Modification to help with a candida infection, improve his sinus problems, balance his body fluids, and address other general health concerns. When she scanned Jake with NES, Frieden noted body-field distortions including Skin Driver, Energetic Integrators 1 (Neurosensory/Colon Meridian) and 3 (Mucosae/Small Intestine Meridian), and several Energetic Terrains. Because of Jake's fragile condition, Frieden started him slowly on the NES Infoceuticals, suggesting he be given only the minimum number of drops of Skin Driver, taken every three days.

At his second visit many weeks later, Jake had not shown much improvement. His second NES scan showed that Energetic Integrator 3 was still a problem, and that Source, Polarity, Cell Driver, and Nerve Driver showed as distorted, as well as one Energetic Terrain. It was clear from the scan—with two Drivers and Source out of balance—that Jake's body-field was in drastic need of "repowering." So Jake went off of the Skin Driver Infoceutical and was started on the Source, Polarity, and Cell Driver Infoceuticals as well as Energetic Integrator 3 Infoceutical.

Jake continued using NES, and by the third visit, his bronchial problems were improving. By his fifth visit, in late summer, changes were evident. Jake was becoming more responsive and was even smiling. So much change was evident that even his physical and occupational therapists commented on the improvements.

As this book is being written, Jake's parents plan to continue using NES for him, noting that it and the adjunct therapies, particularly the new nutritional program, are making a difference in his functionality and quality of life. His mother said, "We have noticed a remarkable change in Jake since beginning his NES program. . . . Among the changes we have noticed are improvements in Jake's appearance: his skin coloring looks great, and his eyes are brighter. Jake tends to keep his hands fisted, and his hands often are sweaty and smelly, but now he is opening them more, and his hands are dry and clean and don't smell. He is making good strides with his physical, occupational, and speech therapy, with almost every appointment ending with therapists excitedly telling us about the good session with Jake that day. His prior normal behavior during therapy was to become easily agitated and frustrated. Now, at therapy and in general, he is calmer and seems more emotionally stable."

15

THE ENERGETIC
TERRAINS

IT'S NOT A NEW IDEA THAT there are such things as energetic environments within the body that can host pathogens. For instance, homeopathy has offered a theory that there are energetic terrains as well as chemical ones in the body, but homeopathic theory links these energetic terrains only to vaguely defined groups of toxins and microbes. The NES theory of Energetic Terrains goes much farther, linking specific microbes or families of microorganisms with specific tissues and providing an explanation of energetic pathology to explain how disease may develop in the body.

In the NES model of the body-field, an Energetic Terrain is the result of an energetic disturbance that causes body tissues to become suitable environments for microbes. However, NES is able to identify a chain of bioenergetic and physical events that leads to the conditions that cause Energetic Terrains. First, the body-field must be weakened—lose energy and strength—which can happen for any number of reasons, including genetic damage, geopathic stress, overexposure to electromagnetic and other types of fields, overuse of certain kinds of pharmaceuticals, emotional stress, and so on. When the body-field is compromised, breakdowns can occur in cell functioning, which affects the state of the surrounding tissue or the entire organ. This damage changes the energetic environment of the body generally or of specific tissues making them more suitable for hosting microbes. In the same way that conventional microbiologists recognize that certain classes of microbes gravitate to particular areas of the body—some kinds will infect your eyes but not your liver, or your muscles but not your lymph nodes—NES has found that certain types of microbes gravitate toward particular Energetic Terrains.

So far, NES Energetic Terrain theory is not so different from the conventional theory of microbial interaction. However, in the NES model, microbes do not have to be spread physically to be contagious. That is, the conventional theory of infectious disease says that microbes have to be spread by some physical mechanism—shaking hands with someone who has a cold, eating infected food, or drinking unclean water. The transmission of the infection is always via a physical route. In contrast, in the NES bioenergetic model, microbes have their own energy and information fields, and these fields can be transmitted and can affect the body-field and, thus, the body. Biologist Rupert Sheldrake has hypothesized that every life form has a morphogenetic field that shapes it and drives its evolution. In a similar vein, NES proposes that every family of virus—or other type of microbe—creates a field, and that field, as the bioenergetic template for that life form, transmits information that may be as real as the physical microbe. The organism's field—its information template—may be all that is necessary for the spread of viruses and other infectious microbes or for the appearance of symptoms associated with the real microbe. However, to be *susceptible* to that field, your body-field has to be compromised in some way. There has to be an environment—an Energetic Terrain—in which that information has meaning and, consequently, can affect the physical body.

THE NES THEORY OF ENERGETIC TERRAINS

According to conventional microbiology, organisms such as bacteria and viruses reproduce inside the body using our cells as mediums for thriving, and in some cases they even hijack our DNA to reproduce. What if this is not the whole picture? We know that at the quantum level, everything is mediated by energy and information exchanges. Why should microorganisms, the very earliest forms of life in most cases, be any different? The NES model says that they are not. It outlines a possible energetic transmission for disease that may be as real in its effects on the body as are the effects of physical bacteria, viruses, or mold spores. We are suggesting that the body and its many immune systems may not be able to distinguish between a real disease-causing microbe and the energetic/informational field of one.

All chemical reactions—even those that happen inside a cell when it is infected with a disease-causing microorganism—are dependent on the way molecules form hydrogen bonds, on how those bonds form and how they break. Peter has discovered from his decades of matching experiments that hydrogen bonding directly connects to body-field structure and functioning, so the effects microorganisms have on our cell functioning link directly to the state of our body-field as well. Some microorganisms upset the normal functioning of our body-field to the point that we feel ill. Their effect, then, is both physical and energetic.

Peter described how the structures in space he discovered through his matching experiments related to Energetic Terrains. "It became quite clear to me that, energetically speaking, the body could arrange its own field—the big body-field—naturally into what could be a protective system, and one of those systems was a protection against microorganisms. In other words, there is the immune system of the physical body where we've got cells hunting things down and killing them, but then there is the purely energetic aspect of the immune system, which also has protective aspects, but also can hide things from the physical immune system. It's a truly revolutionary concept, and it boggled my mind for quite some time, but it looks as if there is an energetic distortion in the body-field that can host the *information* related to disease from microorganisms, and in NES we call these environments Energetic Terrains."

Peter's contention is that although drugs, such as antibiotics, can kill the physical pathogens, in this case bacteria, they may not affect the energetic imprint—the field distortions—left by the bacteria or other microorganisms. So, disease can remain present or can appear as if out of nowhere, long after the physical microbes have been cleared from the body. This NES theory provides one possible explanation for why some people appear to have all the symptoms of a microbial-related disease—such as hepatitis A or even human immunodeficiency virus (HIV)—but lab tests cannot detect the actual disease-causing agent.

ENERGETIC TERRAIN INFOCEUTICALS AND ENERGETIC TERRAINS IN THE NES SCAN

The Energetic Terrain Infoceuticals are designed to address the energetic imprints of specific families of microbes. Each Energetic Terrain Infoceutical both corrects one of the bioenergetic subfields of the larger body-field that are identified as the sixteen individual Energetic Terrains and energetically tags the microorganisms that each Terrain may be shielding, making those microbes recognizable to the body's immune system. In general, however, you can think of the Energetic Terrain Infoceuticals as providing the body-field with information about what the body should look like in its normal state and directing the body back from its distorted state to its proper, natural state of function. As with all the NES Infoceuticals, because order or sequence is important, the Energetic Terrain Infoceuticals are taken from the lowest number to the highest. (The first Terrain Infoceutical is actually numbered zero because it was discovered after many of the others but needed to come first in the sequence, and it was too late into the development of NES to renumber all the other Terrain Infoceuticals that were already in use by NES practitioners.)

Although Energetic Terrains sometimes can show up on a first scan with the NES system, they are not addressed until other aspects of the body-field have been corrected. In general, Energetic Terrains are more complicated to correct than are the Big Field, Drivers, or Integrators because they may hide in the body. That is, they may not be immediately detectable. Just as real microbes can hide in the body undetected by the immune system for long periods of time, Energetic Terrains can be masked in the body. These energetic environments hide the field signature of the microbe from the physical immune system—and even may disguise it from the body-field. Here's how that may happen. Because Energetic Terrains are set up as the result of tissue damage, it is very likely that the damage will show up as a distorted Energetic Driver and/or Energetic Integrator, although Drivers seem to be more affected by Terrains than Integrators. You may try correcting that Driver or Integrator using the appropriate Infoceutical, but the field pattern set up by the microbes will persist, so the Driver or Integrator will keep showing up as distorted. When a Driver or Integrator resists correction over time, that is a clue that a Terrain is hiding in the wings as the real culprit of the distortion.

We have said over and over that one of the unique aspects of the NES system of health care is that sequence is important to getting to the root bioenergetic cause of problems and should always be followed; however, with Terrains sometimes the sequence must be varied slightly. There are two scenarios that become important in this respect: Terrains may not begin to show up as distorted until Driver and Integrator distortions are corrected, so Terrains usually are not addressed at all until about the fourth visit to a practitioner. But if a persistent pattern emerges where the same Drivers and Integrators resist correction, a Terrain has to be considered as the underlying problem and so may have to be addressed a bit earlier. NES practitioners are trained to consider these and other possible scenarios when interpreting NES scans.

Energetic Terrains have a tendency to shield each other from detection. There are sixteen Energetic Terrains, designated by number. Terrains 0, 1, 2, and 3 have a tendency to mask the presence of the higher-numbered Terrains. So, when you clear a lower-numbered Terrain, suddenly other, high-numbered ones may appear in a later

NES scan. They were there all along, but they were masked by the lower-numbered Energetic Terrains.

Energetic Terrains help explain why people may not recover their strength and overall wellness even long after the disease-causing microorganism is gone. For instance, it is not uncommon for people, especially the elderly, who already may have compromised immune systems and body-fields, to suffer weakness, fatigue, and many other symptoms long after they have recovered from an illness. The story of Randolph, presented early in part 3, is a case in point. His pneumonia was cleared and he was released from the hospital, but he never regained his strength. For all intents and purposes, he was still ill long after his doctors declared his pneumonia cured. Taking the Polarity Infoceutical was all that was needed to regenerate the integrity of his body-field, which in turn restored his body to proper functioning. In this case, we may never know if a Terrain was the cause. As we have said so many times throughout this book, with NES you don't have to worry about physical diagnosis, all you have to do is pay attention to what your body-field is telling you it needs. In all likelihood, however, Randolph probably retained the informational template—the Energetic Terrain—for the pneumonia microbe in his body, and by aligning his field (which is what the Polarity Infoceutical does) his body was able to clear it.

Peter explained, "The model we have been taught in school is that a pathogen invades and there is a battle between antigens and the pathogen, and lymph cells and the pathogen, and the macrophages and the pathogen—or whatever. These processes are real, and we can see them under the microscope. We don't have any problem with microbiology in that respect, but there is another aspect to healing, which is energetic. From past and present research, we are suggesting that the body can create ETs—these energetic environments—after exposure to triggering events, such as prolonged exposure to geopathic stress or electromagnetic fields or some other factor, and so host a microorganism, but—and this is a pretty big statement—it can do this even when there has been no invasion by an actual microorganism at all! In a sense we are getting phantom diseases, but, of course, what we call phantom is just another way of saying bioenergetic—nonphysical. It's information—the field of the microorganism. This may explain the otherwise unexplained rapid appearance of disease in various parts of the world at nearly the same time. There are no real physical explanations—no good ones, anyway—for that kind of epidemiological variation, the nearly simultaneous appearance of the same disease in widely separated parts of the world. Perhaps the mechanisms are energy and information fields. We don't know for sure. It's perfectly okay to say, 'We don't know for sure,' but we can't ignore the hints, and we are unwise when we don't follow the pointers wherever they lead us.

"For instance," Peter continued, "consider chronic fatigue syndrome and many other of those so-called 'mystery' diseases. Perhaps we will never find a single or even a host of physical mechanisms for them. Perhaps the real causes are at the level of energy and information fields. That's what we are thinking; it's what the matching tests are telling us is possible. For instance, take multiple sclerosis, or really many of the degenerative nervous-system diseases. I have found that one of the Energetic Terrains may affect the outside of the axon in the Schwann cells of the nervous system. That's something not even considered in mainstream medicine—that there is an energetic connection to the physical symptoms. These types of complex diseases are very hard to assess, but maybe we can get a bit farther with them if we factor in the body-field, the Energetic Terrains, and such."

THE DYNAMICS OF ENERGETIC TERRAIN FORMATION

Peter's matching tests with the Energetic Terrains explored a variety of aspects of these energetic structures in space. One part of his research that is important to every aspect of bioenergetics and the body-field—including the Energetic Terrains—relates to microtubules. These tiny tube-shaped structures are found throughout the body as part of many major organs. Bioenergetically, it appears that they attract, store, amplify, and tune energy. In addition, there are myriad microtubules, called centrioles, inside our cells, and they may be like a collection of tiny tuning forks for energy. So when a cell or its DNA is affected by a microbe, it is not unrealistic to think that the energy being broadcast to the body-field from that cell changes. The signal will now include the distortion caused by the microbe, or by the energetic imprint of the microbe if the physical microbe is not there.

What's more, the arrangement of the microtubules matters to our bioenergetic health. If some tubules or even the cells themselves are arranged spatially at different angles from others, then energy and information is affected. Imagine you have an array of transmitters all sending out signals that build up into a coherent picture, like a picture on a TV screen. Shift the spatial arrangement or angle of some of the transmitters, and the part of the picture that they encode will become distorted.

Peter discovered that the centrosome of the cell, and the centrioles within it, can become misaligned from exposure to distorted magnetic fields. According to conventional cell biology, the centrosome and centrioles are only active during cell division, a process called mitosis, whereby one cell divides to become two separate but fully functioning cells. During mitosis, pairs of centrioles separate and migrate toward opposite poles of the cell. Other microtubules in the cell form what is known as the mitotic spindle, and then these spindles, together with the centrioles, form a larger structure called the mitotic apparatus. The mitotic apparatus plays a central role in chromosome division. During this process, the centrioles move so that they are aligned at 90 degrees to each other but the mictotic apparatus forms a circle, or tubule, made of even tinier tubules. These tubules can act as spatial resonators, tuned to different frequencies and forming a mechanism for projection.

Peter's matching experiments revealed that the centrosome, when subject to a QED field, may be affected by magnetic forces from the Earth, sun (especially solar flares), and moon. Under these magnetic influences, centrioles appear to communicate with DNA through exchanges of light (photons). Through this exchange, they can project "informational images" of microbes, creating what amounts to energetic and informational structures in space. When a collection of similar cells all project the same information structure, they create what we in NES call an Energetic Terrain. Because similar cell types cluster to form distinct organs, the Energetic Terrains tend to be localized environments in specific body tissues and organs. Energetic Terrains, from a bioenergetic perspective, are what amount to the manifestations of the body's own DNA interacting with external fields.

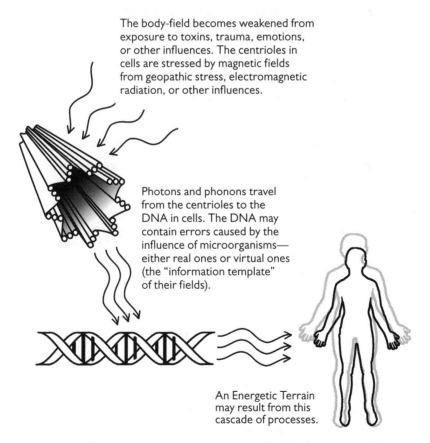

The body-field becomes weakened from exposure to toxins, trauma, emotions, or other influences. The centrioles in cells are stressed by magnetic fields from geopathic stress, electromagnetic radiation, or other influences.

Photons and phonons travel from the centrioles to the DNA in cells. The DNA may contain errors caused by the influence of microorganisms— either real ones or virtual ones (the "information template" of their fields).

An Energetic Terrain may result from this cascade of processes.

Figure 15.1. The primary bioenergetic process for the formation of Energetic Terrains.

Peter's matching experiments also yielded another startling insight: Energetic Terrains may encode different phase shifts, thereby affecting the way the body-field is transmitting its information. The Terrains are numbered from 0 through 15, and Peter found that Energetic Terrain 0 carried what he calls an "error" of 2 degrees from its optimal phase range. As Peter moved up the Energetic Terrains, the deviation increased, until it was 60 degrees at Energetic Terrain 15. So because of phase shift errors, the individual Terrains can have huge impacts on the functioning of the body-field, and hence on the body as well. A phase shift error from an Energetic Terrain can have an especially drastic impact on the Energetic Drivers, which are the fields that are linked to the physical organs and organ systems. Peter explained, "The Drivers power the organs; they are a source of energy for them to function properly, so you can imagine that an Energetic Terrain can cause a lot of trouble. The Terrains stop the organ Energetic Drivers from doing their job. That's why we get so tired when we first get sick. All disease starts with a loss of energy."

It should be clear by now that if a Terrain shows up on your NES scan, it does not mean you have the associated viruses, bacteria, molds, or whatever pathogen is associated with that particular Energetic Terrain in your system. It means that your body-field has set up an environment that is amenable to the microorganism should you be exposed to it or that if your immune systems (physical and energetic) are weakened, then you could display symptoms that are associated with diseases caused by those microorganisms and/or their own fields.

Geopathic stress appears to be a major cause of Energetic Terrain formation. It also accounts for the appearance of a whole string of Terrains showing up on a scan, what we at NES call "ET soup." The Infoceuticals can correct the Terrains, but the problem is likely to recur if you don't also take precautions against your exposure to geopathic stress. Because geopathic stress is not a disease-causing mechanism accepted by conventional science, it is not something the general public is educated about, so it can seem strange and even outlandish to address it as part of a natural health care program. However, NES and other natural health modalities, such as homeopathy and acupuncture, acknowledge the effects of geopathic stress on health.

The Energetic Terrains, especially the theory behind them, can get quite complex, but we trust that the information provided so far gives you at least a preliminary understanding of them and their role in bioenergetic health. Let's quickly outline several key points we've already covered about Energetic Terrains and add a few words more to elaborate on and clarify each point. Then we will go on to highlight the specifics of each of the sixteen Energetic Terrains.

Energetic Terrains Overview

• Energetic Terrains are energetic disturbances associated with specific body tissues that are highly disruptive to the body-field. They are caused by many factors but primarily by geopathic stress, DNA and genetic damage, and electromagnetic smog.

• Parasites, bacteria, molds, viruses, and other microorganisms can create patterns of energy and information, forming what might aptly be called "pictures" or "templates" of themselves. The Energetic Terrains are environments in the body-field that are amenable to both real and virtual microbes.

• These virtual microbe patterns can affect the physical body, often expressing themselves as diseases that defy diagnosis by conventional pathology tests. They are bioenergetic disease patterns and thus will respond only to bioenergetic corrections.

• Errors in the body-field, including Energetic Terrains, tend to accumulate slowly, usually over months and years, and even sometimes decades. The formation of Energetic Terrains generally takes place more slowly than does formation of distortions in Energetic Drivers and Energetic Integrators, and they can persist for decades before causing noticeable problems in the physical body. However, as with other bioenergetic errors, they can appear suddenly as the result of a significant shock or trauma.

- The NES Energetic Terrain Infoceuticals help correct body-field distortions caused by virtual microbes. However, geopathic stress factors also must be addressed. Energetic Terrain corrections can take time to clear, often up to three months, and sometimes longer.

- Energetic Terrains can be masked in the body, especially if the body is out of alignment with Earth's magnetic fields. Thus, the Big Field in the NES scan should be corrected first or else Terrains can be masked. However, Energetic Terrains also may not show up on a scan until Drivers and Integrators are corrected. Driver correction is closely tied to Energetic Terrains, for when a deviated Driver (and sometimes an Integrator) fails to correct itself over time, that is a clue that a Terrain is lurking as an influencing factor in the background. Energetic Terrains also can mask other Terrains, so by correcting one Terrain, especially a lower-numbered one, you may find that a whole host of other Terrains suddenly reveal themselves in subsequent scans.

THE ENERGETIC TERRAINS AT A GLANCE

Now we will provide brief descriptions of the sixteen Energetic Terrains and their bioenergetic correlations to the physical body and to actual microbes. You will note that Terrains 1, 2, and 3 are almost identical in their links to the physical body and correlations to micro-organisms, especially retroviruses, but they are separated into distinct Terrains because of their particular energetic signatures and their degree of phase shift error. Additionally, each Terrain is connected to the energetic imprint of a huge number of organisms, although in the following information we for the most part list only the general microbial types or families. It is worthwhile to note that although each Terrain is correlated bioenergetically with particular types of tissues or aspects of the physical body, a Terrain may encroach on surrounding tissue and cells. Also, because every Terrain has the potential to adversely affect organs or organ systems, they can have a damaging impact on the Energetic Drivers for those organs. We urge you to remember that the presence of an Energetic Terrain in a scan does *not* mean that your body is hosting the actual microbe. It means only that there are field disturbances in tissues that can be amenable to either real or virtual microbes. Likewise, vaccines are included in the descriptions because there is some evidence from Peter's matching experiments that the ingredients of particular vaccines may contribute to energetic disturbances that govern Energetic Terrain formation. It does not mean that having a vaccine will result in the formation of an Energetic Terrain or contraction of a physical disease. Vaccines can save lives, and the decision to have vaccinations is up to each individual as a matter of personal choice in consultation with a health care professional.

Energetic Terrain 0

This Energetic Terrain is generally bioenergetically correlated to tissues of the central nervous system and myocardium. It can occur specifically in the sphincter muscles, midbrain tegmentun, auditory nerve, vestibular nerve, thalamus, optic thalamus, medulla oblongata, inner testes, and renal tubules. Energetic Terrain 0 is linked bioenergetically to specific viruses and multiple vaccines, particularly live-virus vaccines such as the polio and measles-mumps-rubella vaccines.

Energetic Terrain 1

This Energetic Terrain correlates bioenergetically to blood and bone marrow, and it is generally associated with people who have chronically weak immune function. It is bioenergetically associated with viral particles and the entire retrovirus family, with an especially strong bioenergetic correlation to lentivirus. Generally, this Terrain masks slow-onset viruses, which take a long time to grow and may persist for decades in the body.

Energetic Terrain 2

Energetic Terrain 2 bioenergetically may affect the bone marrow, and it is bioenergetically associated with viral particles and the entire retrovirus family.

Energetic Terrain 3

This Energetic Terrain is the third one that bioenergetically affects the bone marrow specifically, and it is associated with viral particles and the entire retrovirus family. Energetic Terrain 3 can be thought of as a distinct Terrain that forms from the combination of Terrains 1 and 2 when both exist simultaneously in the body. When Terrains 1, 2, and 3 all show on a scan, it is the body-field's way of bioenergetically indicating a deep problem that should be addressed as soon as possible in the NES protocol sequence.

Energetic Terrain 4

Host tissues that bioenergetically correlate to this Terrain include the brain and the central and peripheral nervous systems. It is linked with the energetic imprint of viruses and prions, which are aberrant proteins that fold bizarrely and turn into disease-causing agents. Prions are most familiar to the public as the cause of bovine spongiform encephalopathy, or mad cow disease.

Energetic Terrain 5

Energetic Terrain 5 is associated bioenergetically with the skin and lungs and links to the energetic template of a broad spectrum of viruses, including the many strains of human papilloma virus and the Bunyavirus family, particularly herpes-related and wart-related viruses.

Energetic Terrain 6

The nose, throat, lungs, and bronchi are all host sites bioenergetically for Energetic Terrain 6. The real or virtual microbes correlated to this

Terrain include those in the wide variety of families of viruses that cause the common cold and flu, so most people will at one time or another show this Terrain in their NES scan. Correcting this Terrain can bring on flulike episodes, lasting on average from a few hours to about three days, as the virtual imprint of these ubiquitous viruses tend to persist in the body-field. This Terrain also is bioenergetically linked to more virulent viral families that cause such illnesses as severe acute respiratory syndrome (SARS).

Energetic Terrain 7
Energetic Terrain 7 has a wide bioenergetic reach, encompassing the encephalon of the brain, the central nervous system, pituitary gland, thyroid, pancreas, small intestine, and liver. The Flaviviridae viral family bioenergetically links to this Terrain, which means it may be implicated in CFS. It is a particularly difficult Terrain to correct, so it may take time, and your immune system may have to be bolstered by first using other NES Infoceuticals.

Energetic Terrain 8
This Energetic Terrain bioenergetically affects the coating of axons, the bladder, and most organs and tissues found in Energetic Integrator 5, including the appendix, ileocecal valve, parts of the endocrine system, tonsils, some of the lymphatic tissues, many vertebrae, cerebellum, medulla oblongata, gray matter of the brain and spine, spinal nerves, and parts of the male genitalia.

Energetic Terrain 9
The stomach and duodenum bioenergetically host this Energetic Terrain, which is correlated to bacteria such as *Heliobacter pylori*, *Escherichia coli* (*E. coli*), and *Salmonella*. It also may be associated bioenergetically with gastric reflux and acid stomach in general.

Energetic Terrain 10

This Energetic Terrain corresponds bioenergetically to the liver, chest, and gastrointestinal tract. It is correlated to the Picornaviridae virus family, which includes those that cause hepatitis A. It also bioenergetically links to some rhinoviruses, coxsakie viruses, and adenoviruses.

Energetic Terrain 11

The liver and large bowel are both bioenergetically affected by Energetic Terrain 11. It is correlated to the Hepadnaviridae virus family, which includes those that cause hepatitis B.

Energetic Terrain 12

This Energetic Terrain bioenergetically hosts the Flaviviridae virus family, including those that cause hepatitis C, and like Energetic Terrain 11 correlates to the liver and large bowel. It is implicated bioenergetically in CFS and related types of illnesses.

Energetic Terrain 13

Energetic Terrain 13 is linked bioenergetically to a wide array of cells, tissues, organs, and other aspects of the body, including the blood, large bowel, chest cavity, skin, lungs, nasal cavity, pancreas, bones, and various kinds of neurons. It bioenergetically correlates to microbes including yeast, molds, fungi, and protozoa, including amoebas. Because this is a particularly robust Terrain in terms of its web of bioenergetic connections, dealing with more families of microorganisms than any other Terrain, the related Infoceutical can have a strong effect when you take it, so it always should be taken in minimum dosages to start.

Energetic Terrain 14

The skin and lungs tend to host this Energetic Terrain, so bioenergetically it is associated particularly strongly with low Source energy. It tends to show up most in people who work indoors for extended periods, especially in air-conditioned rooms, or those who are not exposed to enough natural sunlight and fresh air. In terms of microbes, it correlates bioenergetically to many bacteria strains, including *Staphylococcus, Streptococcus,* and *Legionella,* so it is implicated in ulcers of the ears, nose, skin, tonsils, and bladder, and in dental root canal infections, gastrointestinal catarrh, and other associated conditions.

Energetic Terrain 15

As the last Energetic Terrain in the sequence, this is a general Energetic Terrain, called a GET in NES. When it comes up on the NES scan it indicates a need for a specially designed Infoceutical rather than identifying a distortion correlated to a particular tissue or correlated to a specific family of microorganism. The Energetic Terrain 15 Infoceutical is used mostly as an adjunct Infoceutical when the other Terrain Infoceuticals do not seem to be having an effect.

Bioenergetically, this Infoceutical helps to correct Terrains as a whole and tends to have a generalized correcting effect on all Energetic Terrains that may be present in the body-field. It tends to stimulate the thymus and the secretion functions of the kidneys and bladder, so it is important to drink extra fluids when taking this Infoceutical. In addition, NES research has shown that all Terrains tend to distort the functioning of the nuclei of cells everywhere in the body, and Energetic Terrain 15 addresses this damage, bioenergetically assisting the nuclei to return to full functioning.

---◆---

When addressing Energetic Terrains in your body-field, it is wise to proceed slowly and with discretion, generally using no more than two Terrain Infoceuticals in a single protocol because clearing the bioenergetic imprint of microorganisms may correlate to the appearance of uncomfortable physical symptoms. Both NES and homeopathy support the concept that disease, especially a chronic problem, must go through at least a brief acute phase before it is cleared. Although it is not true in every case, it occurs often enough to become a signature of the healing process.

Remember, energy cannot be created or destroyed. It has to go somewhere. On its way out of your body-field or as it is rearranged within your body-field, energy and information can express themselves physically, most commonly in mild flulike episodes, fevers, or skin rashes that last from a few hours to a few days. As always with NES, or with any treatment, if you become uncomfortable, you should consult with your NES or other health care professional. Your NES practitioner may recommend that you discontinue the protocol for a few days or reduce the number of Infoceutical drops or the frequency with which you take them.

NES Case Overview: Cass

Cass is an author and the mother of two active children whose normal, hectic routine came crashing to a halt when she was felled by a contaminated dietary supplement. In the late 1980s, she had taken a supplement containing L-tryptophan, touted as a natural sleep aid. However, the Japanese manufacturer had cut corners in production, resulting in contaminated capsules, and also had inserted genetically modified bacteria to enhance its effectiveness. Before the product was banned, thirty-seven people died and more than fifteen hundred were incapacitated, many permanently, by crippling health breakdowns that included debilitating fibromyalgia-like muscle pain and intense fatigue. Doctors named this new, chronic disease eosinophilia myalgia syndrome (EMS), because sufferers have very high blood counts of eosinophilia, a type of white blood cell the body produces in response to toxins or parasitic infections. There are still no tests to diagnose this syndrome conclusively, and as of this writing, there is no cure.

Cass was one of the unfortunate victims of this product. Over the last nearly two decades, she has developed other serious health problems that her doctors believe are related to the EMS. She was put on medication for very high cholesterol, she developed thyroid problems and colitis, and her short-term memory became so severely compromised that her neurologist advised her that going back to school, which was something she had been planning to do, was going to be an enormous challenge. At one point, the counts for her liver enzymes skyrocketed, which could have been a symptom of the EMS or could have been related to a severe case of mononucleosis that had gone undiagnosed for a long time when she was a young adult. She also suffered from periodic bronchial infections.

Cass's sister-in-law, Randi Eaton, is a NES practitioner, and she persuaded Cass to give NES a try because conventional medicine was not helping and her quality of life had deteriorated so severely. Cass used NES regularly for seven months, and then intermittently after that. Her scans during that time showed a pattern of severe distortions in stomach-related and nervous system fields. She also showed a host of bioenergetic problems correlated to nutritional issues, including malabsorption. In addition, a pattern emerged of continually distorted Cell and Source Drivers. Over the seven-month period, Cass was given a number of different NES protocols, and she experienced healing reactions (which some call "detoxification effects") to many of the Infoceuticals. Eaton treated her as a "sensitive client," and she rarely took more than three drops of any Infoceutical.

The positive changes in Cass's health and her life occurred relatively quickly. Although her high cholesterol and thyroid problems remained, her short-term memory and mental clarity improved and her energy skyrocketed. Whereas for years she had experienced difficulty carrying out the tasks of a normal day, she now reported to Eaton:

"I just can't believe how much more energy I have! This morning I had devotions, ate breakfast, went to a workout, came home and showered and did my hair, went to the school to mentor an at-risk 10-year-old, met a friend for lunch and then went shopping with her on the spur of the moment, came home, rested for 30 minutes, met [my husband] for dinner, went to a one-hour rumba dance class, came home, rested, showered, and now I am e-mailing you. You have no idea how impossible that would have been anytime in the last sixteen years. I'm just afraid to believe it is true! There is no way to thank you for all you are doing for me."

Looking back, Cass said that the emotional shifts she experienced were among the most beneficial effects of her NES therapy. She said, "The energy shift was phenomenal, but the emotional shift was as important. I was able to make my health and personal needs a priority, free from feelings of guilt and selfishness, something I had never been able to do before. Whereas before I had wondered how I would get through the day, now I couldn't wait to start a new day. Everything seemed possible that before had seemed impossible."

16

THE ENERGETIC STARS

THE FINAL SUBSYSTEM of the body-field that Peter has identified so far are the Energetic Stars, which represent the field equivalent of metabolic pathways that govern energy and information usage in the body. The Stars are addressed only after all other energetic systems in the sequence of the body-field have been corrected initially. As with all of the other subsystems of the body-field, the Energetic Stars are arranged in a sequence—in this case from Stars 1 through 15—and they roughly follow a "survival" hierarchy in the body, with the lowest number representing the most important energetic and informational mechanism for the body's proper functioning. In addition, the Stars can be thought of as unblockers, so they are used to restart or reinvigorate energy and information flows that have resisted correction by the other classes of Infoceuticals or when the body-field needs to reestablish energetic and informational processes at the deepest, most fundamental levels.

You can think of the Energetic Stars as the bioenergetic counterparts to metabolic pathways. They represent flows of information and energy that regulate broad systems in the body, but those influences also converge to affect specific aspects of the body's bioenergetic functioning, such as immunity or enzyme production processes. The Stars underlie the chemical metabolic processes, providing the energetic and informational template to drive those systems. NES research shows that they synthesize two high-level energy systems—zero-point energy (Source energy) and electromagnetic energy influences on the body—but they don't stop there. Through his matching tests, Peter has been able to reveal a complex web of connections in each Star, so the Stars affect or are affected by just about everything that goes on in the body.

The Energetic Star Infoceuticals are made from precise combinations of Driver and Integrator Infoceuticals. When Infoceuticals are combined, as they are in the Star Infoceuticals, they are not merely an additive mixture of the ingredients but instead form whole new complexes. To use an analogy, when you mix blue and yellow dyes, you don't get a swirling mass of blue and yellow streaks. You get green dye. The Star Infoceuticals work in a similar way, creating something new from a mixture of ingredients. For this reason, and others, NES clients are cautioned by their practitioners never to mix different Infoceuticals in the same glass of water but always to take them separately.

ENERGETIC STAR 1:
LYMPHATIC IMMUNITY AND GENERAL RADIATION

Without a strong immune system, you cannot survive. Your immune system is your alert and warning system as well as your defense against anything from the environment that threatens your health or survival. Even your emotions affect the strength of your immune system because depression, negativity, worry, and stress dampen it. Energetic Star 1, therefore, takes priority in the Star series.

There are many components to a versatile, well-functioning immune system, and the Energetic Star 1 Infoceutical addresses most of them on an energetic level, helping to catalyze the immune system to full function and power. However, it is robustly linked specifically to the lymphatic immune system. This Infoceutical also is designed to address the bioenergetic consequences of overexposure to electromagnetic radiation, or e-smog, from both man-made sources such as computers, mobile phones, and radio waves—and natural ones, such as solar radiation. It also has a bioenergetic impact on the nervous system, specifically addressing issues correlated to many of the bacteria, fungi, parasites, viruses, and viral particles—both real and virtual—that may disrupt the nervous system and affect other tissues. Therefore, this Energetic Star has a robust connection to Energetic Terrains. It specifically correlates energetically to those viruses or viral particles that are implicated in slow-moving, chronic diseases such as CFS and perhaps even HIV. The field associated with this Star also appears energetically correlated to a range of diverse physical and emotional conditions that include manic depression, bipolar disorder, hypersensitivity to light and sound, glaucoma, hernia, and migraines.

ENERGETIC STAR 2: MEMORY IMPRINTER

According to conventional biology, you wouldn't think of memory as either a metabolic pathway or a survival mechanism for the body, but in bioenergetics memory means patterns of information, and the body depends on this systemic, bodywide memory to perform at all levels of functioning. Memory is not only a function of your brain/mind but also of every aspect of your body, of those processes taking place at the cellular and even the DNA levels as well as those at the larger systems level, such as in your nervous system or immune system.

For example, if you experience an emotional or physical shock or trauma, that experience and its related emotions may be bioenergetically stored in your muscles, forming a memory that can affect your biology. If many years later you have a deep-tissue massage, you may experience the spontaneous release of that long dormant memory and the accompanying emotions. As another example, when you are exposed to a virus, your immune system makes antibodies against it, protecting you from that virus should you be exposed to it again, even decades later. The various antibodies in your system form what amounts to a storehouse of information—a reservoir of memories—of past infections and responses.

It is not too far-reaching to say that health and illness are processes that reveal memory at work. Our bodies remember how to carry out millions, even trillions, of processes every minute of every day, usually without a glitch, but when a glitch does occur, we begin to experience the loss of homeostasis or the advent of the symptoms of illness. You could say that illness occurs when the body forgets. You will recall that Energetic Terrains tend to hide microorganisms and even other Terrains in the body. You might say Terrains are expert at making the body forget. Shingles is a good example. It is a painful skin condition caused by the virus that initially gives you chicken pox. After you recover from chicken pox, the virus remains hidden away in your nerves, dormant (another word for forgotten!) until something triggers your body's response to it. That "remembering" manifests as painful skin lesions when the virus becomes active again. So, even though you overcome your initial illness, the physical or bioenergetic imprint of that breakdown can linger for decades and manifest later in wholly different ways. When we say that certain illnesses have triggers—whether they are environmental, biological, or emotional—we are really saying that the body stores patterns. It remembers both the trigger and the response to the trigger. So, Energetic Star 2 represents both personal memory (what amounts to your personal identity) and this kind of functional bioenergetic and body-oriented memory system. The Energetic Star 2 Infoceutical is designed to help correct distortions in your overall body-field memory network.

Specifically, Energetic Star 2 has a strong bioenergetic correlation to triglycerides and other lipids or fats. Peter's testing shows that emotions and experiences are imprinted via the heart onto certain types of fats, which then circulate in the blood, reaching every part of the body. Energetic Star 2 Infoceutical is a mixture of Infoceuticals, mostly Drivers, that link to all the major memory systems of the body, including those for Emotional Stress Release, Nervous System Driver, Imprinter Driver, Triglycerides (an Infoceutical that was once used by itself but is no longer offered as a stand-alone Infoceutical), and others.

The Energetic Star 2 Infoceutical in general is designed to energize and reestablish processes of energetic recording of data for later recall by the body. Because learning is dependent on memory, it is no surprise that Peter found bioenergetic correlations between Energetic Star 2 and conditions such as mental lethargy, slow language skills development, and learning difficulties in general, both for children and adults. However, it also affects at a bioenergetic level our ability to express ourselves, to be clear in our identity, and to be the unique individuals that we are.

ENERGETIC STAR 3: NERVE FUNCTION

Bioenergetically, this Star links robustly to the central nervous system, to neurotransmitters of all kinds, and to specific aspects of the nerves such as axons, neurons, and dendrites. Because many types of toxins, but especially environmental toxins, may adversely affect nerve function, this Star has a strong bioenergetic correlation to heavy metals, such as lead, cadmium, and mercury. Heavy metals can have drastically deleterious effects on nerve function, so they may be implicated, at least on a bioenergetic level, in such nervous system conditions as Parkinson disease, neuritis, and narcolepsy, although there does not appear to be a bioenergetic correlation between this Star and multiple sclerosis. It also bioenergetically affects ear function, so it may be related to auditory acuity.

Although Energetic Star 3 Infoceutical generally may help address bioenergetic distortions in neural-cell-generation processes, particularly the excretion of heavy metals, it also plays a protective energetic role in how the nerve field deals with molds, fungi, protozoa, and yeast. Energetic Star 3 also connects bioenergetically to triglycerides, bioenergetically correlating to the detoxification of these fats and aiding their metabolism in the body. Because nerve endings assist in the body's production of enzymes and hormones, this Star also may be involved to some degree in hormone regulation, although a lot more research needs to be done. The hormonal system is vastly complex, so it is not well understood by either conventional or bioenergetic researchers.

ENERGETIC STAR 4: TRIPLE CAVITY

Although the physical body and its biochemistry are powered directly by the breakdown of hydrogen bonds in sugars, the body-field relies on Source energy (also called zero-point energy), which is collected in your body's cavities. The concept of the Triple Cavity, or Triple Burner, comes from TCM, and NES concurs with this ancient healing tradition that the three major body cavities (the cranial, thoracic, and abdominal) play a critical role in how the body stores and uses energy. Energetic Star 4 is concerned with the network of energy and information dependent on the dynamics of this triple-cavity system.

NES research shows that the Triple Burner system has a particularly strong link to the hormonal system, but in NES we don't try to influence the hormonal system directly because it is simply too complex. However, Peter's research shows that Source energy has a bioenergetic influence on enzyme and hormone molecules, and the Energetic Star 3 and 4 Infoceuticals are designed to have indirect bioenergetic effects on our hormonal system, providing energy to the most basic mechanisms that contribute to proper hormone production and regulation. Specifically, the Energetic Star 4 Infoceutical is designed to influence the dynamics of the three cavities and their integration and to reestablish their integrity as repositories of Source energy and dynamos for the body's use of this energy. By increasing the efficiency of how Source energy is stored and used, the Energetic Star 4 Infoceutical may bioenergetically address issues of fatigue and energy depletion. It also correlates bioenergetically with detoxification of the organs within the three cavities and the restoration of proper function, especially to the pituitary, thalamus, thymus, heart, suprarenal glands, digestive glands, and gonads. The thyroid and parathyroid, which lie at the border of the cranial and thoracic cavities, also benefit from the restoration of the proper functioning of these two cavities.

As you might imagine, mental function is deeply connected to how efficiently your body stores and uses Source energy. Therefore, the

Energetic Star 4 Infoceutical correlates bioenergetically with increasing mental agility and clarity of thought as well as aiding with better sleep. It also appears to correlate bioenergetically with the lifting of depression. If you remember back to the Energetic Integrator information, mental and emotional function, and even consciousness itself, may be dependent on the unobstructed movement of energy and information along the Integrator structures. Bioenergetically, depression may be viewed as stuck energy and/or information, and the Energetic Star 4 Infoceutical appears to aid in getting them moving again. This Star also bioenergetically correlates to conditions ranging from obesity (not linked to overeating), vessel-specific blood pressure problems, and sluggish mental processing.

Interestingly, we can do a lot ourselves to aid our body's absorption and use of Source energy. It's as easy as breathing deeply. Most of us tend to be shallow breathers, not often fully expanding our lungs and diaphragm as we breathe. If you practice yoga or the martial arts, you know how important proper breathing is to overall physical strength and agility. It may be just as important to your health at a bioenergetic level. On the negative side, one interesting hint from NES research is that spending a lot of time in air-conditioning may deplete your Source energy.

ENERGETIC STAR 5: AUTOIMMUNE

Contrary to its name, this Star is not correlated only to autoimmune disorders, for it also has a bioenergetic antiallergy effect, especially when used with Thymus Driver in the same protocol. Energetic Star 5, as a bioenergetic pathway, generally correlates to the cell-destroying mechanisms of your immune system, mechanisms that when they go awry—mistakenly attacking healthy cells—can have wide-ranging negative effects on the body, particularly in your joints.

NES matching tests show that this Star is correlated bioenergetically to allergic conditions of all types, including lupus (which is normally thought of as only an autoimmune disease), urticaria (hives), colitis, soft-tissue rheumatism, and asthma, among other things. However, the Energetic Star 5 Infoceutical does not appear to have a clear bioenergetic link to arthritis. Although arthritis may have an autoimmune component to it, NES research shows that is far from the whole bioenergetic story. We have hints that an important contributory factor may be a malfunction in how the body uses calcium and regulates carbohydrates. Simply put, cells are not using energy correctly, particularly in the joint capsules. Inflammation results, and over time cartilage and tissue begin to break down. Hence, the Cell Driver Infoceutical and to some extent also the Source Driver Infoceutical are primary correctors for the bioenergetic links to arthritic conditions, although the Energetic Star 6 Infoceutical, described in the following section, may prove beneficial as well.

Additional NES research suggests that many childhood disorders may have bioenergetic ties to inflammatory responses provoked by viral infections or even live inoculations. There are several Driver Infoceuticals that bioenergetically correlate to these types of problems more directly, provided the NES scan shows them as distorted, so the Energy Star 5 Infoceutical, in almost all cases, is better used as a fallback if relief is not achieved using other Infoceuticals.

ENERGETIC STAR 6: CIRCULATION/LIPIDS

Energetic Star 6 correlates to specific arteries that are prone to narrowing from fat deposits or the buildup of calcium plaque. These include many of the major coronary arteries (especially the left pulmonary artery), neural and cerebral arteries, and the penile artery. NES research suggests that not all arteries are the same bioenergetically, and this Star links to those that develop in the early stages of embryological development. It is interesting to note that NES matching tests reveal that Energetic Star 6 does not link to cholesterol in terms of the "good" and "bad" fats in the bloodstream. Further research needs to be conducted, but in this regard NES's understanding of bioenergetic physiology is at odds with the widely accepted conventional view that cholesterol levels play a major contributory role in narrowing of the arteries.

Bioenergetically, Energetic Star 6 correlates to blood flow, and the related Infoceutical may help in this regard. In addition, this Star, as a communication pathway, links to the tissue of ligaments, tendons, and cartilage, so it might be implicated bioenergetically in arthritis and other diseases of these tissues. It also correlates to a host of anti-inflammatory hormones. For these reasons (increased blood flow and anti-inflammation) Energetic Star 6 might correlate to the alleviation of the pain associated with arthritis, but it is not considered a bioenergetic corrector in its own right for this condition.

ENERGETIC STAR 7: MUSCLES/ENZYMES

Energetic Star 7 correlates primarily to striated muscles, fascia, and triglycerides. The bulk of body tissue is in the musculoskeletal system, which is a major repository for environmental toxins. We have already mentioned that muscles, from a bioenergetic perspective, can store memories such as physical or emotional shocks and traumas. So this Star serves bioenergetically as a major unblocker on many levels for the entire musculoskeletal system, especially concerning muscle metabolism and excretion capabilities.

Metabolic errors also can affect muscles, and NES matching tests show that some hormones and neurotransmitters—including but not limited to gamma-aminobutyric acid (GABA), serotonin, dopamine, norepinephrine, and melatonin—have strong bioenergetic connections to muscles. Triglycerides have a bioenergetic link through the heart's ability to imprint information via the lipids into the blood. Our research also has indicated that Energetic Star 7 correlates to enzyme production and use, which bioenergetically may play a role in Alzheimer disease and conditions related to premature aging.

This Star bioenergetically links to particular types of physical symptoms and conditions such as myasthenia gravis, muscular dystrophy, and other muscle-wasting diseases as well as muscular fibrosis. Many of the Infoceuticals that are combined to make the Energetic Star 7 Infoceutical have influences on the central nervous system and so this Infoceutical may help bioenergetically address problems with sleep or depression, lessen pain sensitivity, and increase feelings of relaxation and calm.

ENERGETIC STAR 8: CHILL

This Star's name says it all—not in relation to temperature but to emotions. Energetic Star 8 deals with what Peter likes to call "emotional tangles." Emotions form a powerful communication network that reaches throughout your physical body, imprinting either helpful or harmful information and energies into your body. Just as a positive attitude and a sense of hopefulness can aid your recovery from illness, a pessimistic attitude can hinder it. However, the connections go much deeper than that, for all of your emotions, both conscious and unconscious, have an effect on your body.

Energetic Star 8 bioenergetically connects with the ways that your emotions block information and energy flow in your body. The related Infoceutical is designed to aid, on a bioenergetic level, the way in which your cerebral cortex processes thoughts and emotions, and it bioenergetically assists in clearing blockages of energy and information that result from a sensory or mental overload. It has a particularly noticeable effect on aiding sleep because one of the most common causes of insomnia is excessive thought—the endless review of past problems, the ceaseless parade of concerns, and the projecting forward to the future.

The NES Infoceuticals are not chemical in nature, so the Energetic Star 8 Infoceutical's relaxing effect occurs at the bioenergetic level only. This Infoceutical also is not used to relieve physical stress. Its focus is almost entirely on your emotional state, helping to settle out-of-control emotions. Interestingly, this Infoceutical appears to have the ancillary bioenergetic effect of helping with learning difficulties. Because of its calming effect, it is best taken in the evening, and many people have reported having meaningful dreams or clear insights while using it. These reports make sense in light of NES research that suggest this Infoceutical can bioenergetically stimulate the recovery of conscious awareness of emotional problems and concerns, bringing them into the light of knowing if you are ready, so it may stimulate self-knowledge and awareness. Overall, it has been called the "feel-good" Infoceutical. Need we say more!

ENERGETIC STAR 9: SHOCK—AUDIO PROCESSING

This Star correlates with clearing bioenergetic blocks primarily caused by shock and trauma, which get imprinted into your body via the energetic memory systems that affect your cells, muscles, and nerves. Such shock can upset low-frequency waves, which power the Energetic Drivers. When the Drivers are distorted, overall function decreases as your ability to store and use Source energy lessens. Bioenergetics, at least in the way NES is able to explore it using the matching tests, reveals that shocks that are perceived primarily through auditory perceptual routes have specific ramifications for the body, so Peter was able to develop the Energetic Star 9 Infoceutical to help address these auditory shock issues. However, this Infoceutical does not address functional or structural auditory difficulties.

Sometimes the only aspect of a shock or trauma that you may register is the sound associated with it. For example, soldiers suffering from post-traumatic stress syndrome may dive for cover at the sound of a backfiring truck even decades after they have left the war zone. Bioenergetically and emotionally, they still fear for their life, and a specific type of sound is a trigger for that fear response. The same type of reaction can be seen in adults who were subject to protracted and severe verbal abuse as children. The sound of a raised voice from an authority figure can set them on edge. All that many of us can remember from a bad car accident is the crashing sound. Each of these examples explains what we mean by auditory shock.

The Energetic Star 9 Infoceutical is designed to address bioenergetic distortions at the level of the temporal lobe, which is the primary area of the brain that processes sound, and specific sound and speech recognition centers of the brain, such as Broca's area.

ENERGETIC STAR 10: STRESS—VIDEO PROCESSING

This Star deals with shock and trauma generally associated with sight and the visual processing of information. Just as you might retain only the sounds associated with an extremely stressful event, such as a car accident, you also might focus on its visual aspects—the shock of the car veering into your path or your body being flung forward toward the windshield or dashboard. The Energetic Star 10 Infoceutical is designed to deal with shock-induced bioenergetic problems that may result from visual trauma and with the often unconscious emotions that accompany the event. It does not deal with anatomical visual problems, but with the bioenergetic function of shock as related to the visual cortex, thalamus, and motor neurons (but not the motor cortex). It also correlates with the optical interpretation center of the cortex. Both auditory and visual shock can, if severe enough, badly disrupt the big body-wave, eventually leading to field collapse in the most extreme cases.

ENERGETIC STAR 11: MALE ENERGY

Despite its name, this Star is not about male sexual potency in the functional sense. Instead, it addresses the emotional issues that surround being male and all the cultural, emotional, and psychological baggage you may carry because of it. It is directed toward maleness not only in terms of gender but also as a foundation for identity. The Energetic

Star 11 Infoceutical's effect is positive in nature, bioenergetically reinforcing what Peter calls "male charisma." It works bioenergetically at a mostly emotional level, helping to clear blocks to such feelings as confidence, willpower, social warmth, and well-being.

This Infoceutical does not directly affect the physical aspects of the endocrine glands but instead helps strengthen the communication link between these glands and Source Driver. It also may bioenergetically stimulate circulation to the endocrine glands, but hormones are only part of the bioenergetic story of gender and identity.

ENERGETIC STAR 12: FEMALE ENERGY

This Star is the female counterpart to Energetic Star 11, Male Energy. Everything we have said about Energetic Star 11 Infoceutical's bioenergetic effects applies to this Infoceutical as well, only in terms of the female gender and social identity. However, Peter admits that the female field is more difficult to influence bioenergetically because it is made more complicated by the menstrual cycle and the complex hormonal cascade of events, at both the physical and bioenergetic levels, that females experience every month. The Energetic Star 12 Infoceutical can have a regulating effect, at the bioenergetic level, on irregular or dysfunctional menstrual cycles but is not intended as a correction for those kinds of problems. Its bioenergetic correlation is not so much to the endocrine system as it is to increasing blood supply, and its focus is less about function than it is about facilitating the integration of mind and body.

Use of either the Male or Female Energetic Star Infoceuticals may stimulate physical and bioenergetic detoxification because the endocrine glands can store toxins and when these glands begin to work more effectively they can more easily excrete those toxins. Peter's matching experiments indicate that tin and lead both are particularly deleterious to sexual function.

ENERGETIC STAR 13: C–O–H

Carbon, oxygen, and hydrogen are staple elements related to aspects of your body's chemical physiology, so they are the focus of Energetic Star 13. Their respective roles in carbohydrate and sugar metabolism, which regulate your body's energy use, are among their most important functions to the relative state of your health. They also affect the way the body uses fats, so Energetic Star 13 correlates bioenergetically with the production of energy generally and is intimately tied to the citric acid cycle (Krebs cycle), which plays a role in many diseases. Peter's matching tests reveal that this Star correlates to many crucial elements and compounds related to the body's energy-production process. For example, it talks to lipotropin, a hormone that promotes the body's use of fats; ATP, a nucleotide that is a major player in how cells get and use chemical energy; thyroxin, an essential mineral in thyroid hormones; and pyruvic acid, a compound important in the metabolism of carbohydrates, proteins, and fats.

Energetic Star 13 also affects the body's ability, on a bioenergetic level, to excrete toxins, which aids cellular metabolism. For this reason, it correlates to the liver and pancreas, which play dominant roles not only in the elimination of toxins but also in sugar and fat metabolism. Additionally, it connects via the body-field to lactic acid production in muscles and calcium metabolism, especially in relation to the creation of stones, such as kidney stones.

Interestingly, NES matching tests have revealed that osteoarthritis may be a consequence of impaired carbohydrate metabolism at the bioenergetic level. Practitioners of allopathic medicine admit that the causes of arthritis are unknown and speculate that it may have a hereditary genetic factor or be the result of an injury or disease processes that eventually cause the cartilage in joints to deteriorate. They identify aging as a major factor because the joints wear over time, especially in people who are obese. However, NES has gleaned clues from our own testing procedures that arthritis may occur as a bioenergetic consequence of compromised carbohydrate metabolism. Although NES recognizes that the body-field is a complex, interconnected web of energy and information and that chronic diseases such as arthritis are bound to involve multiple processes, our research provides a clue that is worth exploring on many fronts because arthritis is so ubiquitous a problem among the general population.

Because of its bioenergetic effect on sugar metabolism, the Energetic Star 13 Infoceutical should be used cautiously by anyone with blood sugar instability or known pancreas or liver disease. As we have explained previously, even though we are dealing only with the energy and information of the body-field, NES practitioners rarely if ever seek to stimulate a diseased organ directly. The NES protocol calls for following the sequence of the body-field according to the scan results but allows deviations in the case of stressed organs (as identified by an allopathic or other diagnosis), which should not be further stimulated even at a bioenergetic level. The advantage of the bioenergetic approach to health is that your NES practitioner can support related organs, which through their interconnections with the stressed organ can help restore proper function to that organ. When used appropriately, the Energetic Star 13 Infoceutical can influence proper cell metabolism throughout the body, and many types of problems can be alleviated naturally as a consequence.

ENERGETIC STAR 14: CELL METABOLISM

Although this Star is called Cell Metabolism, its primary bioenergetic effect is on general cell detoxification. From a bioenergetic perspective, and from an allopathic one as well, most disease results from cell function gone wrong. Almost every pharmaceutical is directed at the cell. Because cell function is so complex, it is difficult, if not impossible, to target only one aspect of cells, which is why many drugs have a plethora of side effects. The Energetic Star 14 Infoceutical is designed to help cells excrete or resist the effects of environmental toxins bioenergetically so that they work more effectively and efficiently. This Star, then, is energetically connected to a wide range of detrimental effects from a variety of environmental toxins, including but not limited to those commonly found in dyes, car exhaust, fungicides, some pesticides, and the like. Specific compounds it bioenergetically correlates to include PCPs and PCBs (polychlorinated biphenyls), vinyl acetates and chlorides, dioxins, methyl mercury and methyl tin, and nitrates. It also may address field damage caused by chronic exposure to artificially created electromagnetic fields (e-smog). Any detoxification process is going to be long term because as creatures of technologically advanced societies we have extreme difficulty controlling our exposure to environmental toxins and electromagnetic pollution.

ENERGETIC STAR 15: HEAVY METALS

As with Energetic Star 14, this Star correlates bioenergetically to detoxification. Heavy metals present a special problem for most of us because we live in highly industrialized areas, where the toxin load is high. The Energetic Star 15 Infoceutical provides body-field correction for cellular metabolism, and your entire physiology in general, from the bioenergetic effects of heavy metals, especially the residue of lead, mercury, and cadmium salts in your circulatory system, nervous system, and body organs. As with any detoxification involving environmental toxins, the process can take many months and will likely have to be periodically addressed over the long term because it is next to impossible to limit your exposure.

NES Case Overview: Mark

Lynette Frieden, a naturopathic physician and chiropractor, began seeing Mark when he was seven years old, and he has been under her care for a year. Although he has never been medically diagnosed with autism or attention deficit disorder, Mark displays most of the symptoms. His mother tells his story in her own words.

"Mark was born twenty-three days before his due date. He had a variety of odd health problems, such as weight loss, vomiting (from just a little to projectile), and nonstop crying. He had an upper GI [imaging scan of the upper part of the digestive tract] at six weeks of age. They saw no deformity and said he had reflux. Mark was started on three medications for reflux, taken four times a day. He often took antibiotics for the ear and sinus infections he always seemed to have. We were told not to put him on his back, that he was never to lie flat at all. He could not swing or be bumped up and down on your knee. Basically you could hold him at a 45-degree angle and look at him. He never had the opportunity to develop upper body muscles or equilibrium and balance. . . . He never crawled. He scooted for a couple of months, then walked at about thirteen months.

"When Mark was two he had his tonsils and adenoids removed. This seemed to help his reflux a little. Mark did not talk until he was three. At this time, it was still mostly grunts and pointing, with some sign language he had learned.

"Mark seemed to be sick all the time, so he was not up to date on immunizations. At one point when he was not running a fever, we went to have them administered. A short time after this I began to see changes. He no longer wanted to be touched or held. He startled easily, did not like loud noises, would sit for long periods of time in a room by himself. If we could get him outside, then we could not get him back in. He would fixate on one toy or TV show, and you could not get him away from it.

"Around the time Mark was four years old, we enrolled him in prekindergarten. Mark did not go to school a complete year because he was always sick, and his behavior and social skills got worse. We began home schooling . . . and began looking for ways to treat his health and behavior. We took him off all reflux medicines but continued to use antibiotics and sinus medicines.

"I had been to Dr. Frieden in the past when I needed a chiropractor, and I went back to see her again for some problems I was having. My dad was on NES, and so I discussed Mark's health and NES with Dr. Frieden, and we made him an appointment. Dr. Frieden used Total Body Modification and helped us deal with nutritional issues, with what turned out to be a gluten intolerance. We immediately started Mark on a gluten-free diet. He also had a NES scan and started on the Infoceuticals.

"There has been incredible improvement in his health and behavior. Since Mark has been on NES over the past year, he has begun to read at sixth- or seventh-grade level, and he is on track with all his other subjects and is taking riding lessons and guitar lessons. He still has some issues with dyslexia and auditory processing, but he is a completely different child. He is outgoing and makes friends everywhere he goes. We don't have to use antibiotics anymore, and Mark is finally gaining weight. We believe this is all due to NES and Total Body Modification."

CONCLUSION

A New Direction
in Healing

IN THIS BOOK we have provided an overview of an emerging paradigm in biology and medicine—one that explores and seeks to engage the quantum processes in the body. Bioenergetics as envisioned and practiced by NES is truly an integrative approach to wellness, seeking as it does to validate the reality that we are more than matter, we are beings of energy and information as well. We are in integral interconnection with the vast web of relationships that underlie the natural world. Our bodies are subject to influences far beyond our biochemistry, and our ability to heal from illness, whether emotional or physical, is dependent on more than alleviating symptoms. Root causes of illness exist at the subcellular level, where quantum waves—and forces, fields, energy, and information—provide the instruction manual for our physiological functioning. At this level, we find that we are not separate from our environment, that our thoughts and beliefs affect our health, and that we are cocreators of the conditions of our lives.

This new paradigm is still considered very much frontier science. There are dozens more studies we could have cited to demonstrate the richness of inquiry that is taking place around the world and the evidence that supports our model of the quantum body-field, but space limitations precluded us from doing so. Our focus by necessity has been reduced to the intersection of physics and physiology, but even this area of exploration is beyond the means of one person, or one company, except in the most rudimentary of ways. We hope we have motivated readers to enlarge the scope of their understanding of what it means to be healthy and how they can better contribute to their own state of health. Quantum medicine is at its best as preventive medicine—used for correcting the body-field before the physical body becomes compromised. If NES clinical results are any indication, the bioenergetic approach to health care works. While no health care system is perfect, the fact is that thousands of people have found their health and well-being immeasurably improved by using the NES Infoceuticals. Many have found relief from chronic conditions that allopathic medicine could not treat.

We hope, too, that we have whetted the appetite of frontier researchers to join us in exploring these intriguing new directions in biology and health care. The field is rich almost beyond imagining. We at Nutri-Energetics Systems—a young company of people dedicated to changing the paradigm in health care—think big. Our vision for the possibilities of quantum health care is more than ambitious, it is daring. We don't fear the dismissal, or even the ridicule, of academics or shy away from the potential obstacles thrown up by the related politics or bureaucracy. Our focus is on helping people just like you find the most direct path to health and well-being in the most natural and supportive way.

Quantum health is natural health to its core. It is not that we dismiss conventional health care. We don't. Surgery has its place. In acute and emergency situations, allopathic medicine works. The modern world is immeasurably improved by conventional improvements in medicine, especially in public health areas, but conventional biology and medicine are not the whole story, by any stretch of the imagination. Just as the birth of microbiology revolutionized medicine at the turn of the twentieth century, physics is revolutionizing medicine at the start of the twenty-first century. And NES is on the forefront of that revolution.

Nearly every week Peter uncovers some new, and often startling, information about the body-field through his matching experiments. We will continue to explore, test, and probe for answers and puzzle things out to add to our knowledge of how the body-field is the master control system of the physical body. Outcome studies and other kinds of clinical research about the NES clinical system and Infoceuticals are beginning in earnest. Conversations and visits with such diverse researchers and visionaries as Milo Wolff, Fritz-Albert Popp, and Lynne McTaggart are opening new doors and stimulating new ideas. Peter can barely keep up with his own rush of ideas, but he has always welcomed collaboration and conversation with others. These kinds of encounters will continue and no doubt will stimulate the ongoing refinement of the NES system.

While Peter toils away, furthering the theory, Harry continues as the company visionary, turning theory into practice. On the drawing board are several ambitious plans for other kinds of biotechnologies and tools that can help you improve your health and well-being, and no doubt by the time this book is in your hands several of these technologies will have moved from concept to reality. Future plans include creating a way to infuse nutrients and vitamins with encoded body-field information, so that your body not only gets what it needs physically but also uses it more efficiently and directly. It makes no sense to take a B complex vitamin or calcium supplements if your body cannot process those vitamins or compounds properly. Combining the nutrient with the functional quantum information to improve how your body uses that nutrient may enhance the efficacy of vitamins and supplements.

Plans also include a home device for imprinting your environment with supportive and restorative information. Imagine being able to add Source energy to your workspace, bedroom, or den, or better yet, to a hospital room or nursery. Imagine being able to infuse your bath water with the restorative information of Source energy or the Chill or Emotional Stress Release Infoceuticals. NES research, and research by others, such as William Tiller, show that space can be imprinted with information and that information in the environment can persist over time and affect those who enter the space. We have said that you are not separate from your world, that your body, at its deepest, most fundamental quantum core, is in constant interaction with the external environment. Soon it may be possible to make your environment a truly healing environment.

These and other wonders are coming from NES, but most important is our focus on changing the way you—and the public at large—think about health and wellness. It is only a matter of time until health is not something you forget about until you lose it, and then turn over to someone else to fix, but is something that you exert conscious influence over and foster to a vibrant fullness as a matter of everyday living. The new health care paradigm is one defined by the integrative, holistic, conscious approach to health. NES is at the forefront of ushering in this new century of quantum biology. We invite you—from this very minute forward—to join us and to begin your own journey toward the fullness of bioenergetic health.

RESOURCES

Remember, NES as a company and its distributors do not offer health care advice or recommendations. If you have a specific health concern, please consult a licensed health care professional.

www.nutrienergetics.com

This site provides comprehensive information for both NES practitioners and the public about the NES–Professional System, NES theory, the Infoceuticals, and how to locate a certified NES practitioner in your area.

www.energetic-medicine.net

This site offers information about a range of energetic biotechnologies, modalities, and products related to bioenergetics, biophysics, and complementary health care.

www.thelivingmatrix.tv

This site offers information about a forthcoming documentary, whose working title is *The Living Matrix,* that will lead you on a journey of exploration into complementary health care, discussing many traditions and modalities, from traditional Chinese medicine to NES. You will learn about the mysteries still facing biologists and theories about how the body has a healing intelligence of its own, such as demonstrated in cases of spontaneous remission from disease. Plus, scientists and visionaries on the leading edge of alternative health care will discuss how twenty-first-century medicine must address more than biochemistry, but also the bioenergetic and quantum aspects of health.

GLOSSARY

big body-field: *See* body-field.

big body-wave: The systems-level quantum waveform for the entire body-field, in contrast with the countless signal waves from all the smaller, subsystem waves from the individual organs or different types of cells, and from the individual Energetic Drivers and Energetic Integrators and other body-field subsystems.

Big Field: The energy field that comprises the natural Earth and cosmic energies that affect your body-field. It consists of the energy grids/fields of Earth (vertical, equatorial, and magnetic polar axes).

bioenergetics: As used by NES, the study of the energy and information that informs the physical body at the subcellular level, including the possible quantum aspects of physiology as correlated to the body-field.

biophoton: A unit of ultraweak light emitted by cells in humans and other living organisms.

body-field: The network of energies and information that form a self-organizing, coherent, intelligent whole as a correlate to the physical body. As described by NES, the body-field is a complex system of structures in space, a vast web of relations and space resonances that ultimately determines the state of the physical body. It encompasses not only the physical aspects of the self but emotions, beliefs, memories, and other qualities of the self. The body and its body-field are interdependent, each arising from the other and interacting with each other. The body-field regulates the body's physiology at a possibly quantum level, providing the subcellular instructions the body needs to work properly. Distortions in the body-field, if left uncorrected, correlate to the symptoms of illness. It is not to be confused with the aura, chakras, or other metaphysical descriptions of an "energy body."

carrier: That which contains or helps transfer information. For instance, the carriers in Infoceuticals are plant-derived microminerals, which are imprinted with QED information that can be used by the body-field to correct distortions.

cavities: The more or less hollow structures of the body, as in its organs and glands, as well as the structural hollow spaces created by bones or fascia—such as the cranial, thoracic, and abdominal cavities. In NES theory, cavities attract, store, and amplify Source energy. (*Also see* microtubules.)

decoherence: The theory that quantum processes cannot be detected at the macroscopic level because the quantum-mechanical state of the macroscopic system cannot be untangled from its environment and so no separate measurement of that system's qualities can be taken.

emergence: The manner in which novel, coherent, and self-organizing patterns arise in dynamic, complex systems from simpler interactions.

Energetic Drivers: Fields that arise from organs and organ systems according to fetal development. The powerhouses of the body-field. There are sixteen individual Driver fields, which together power the full body-field. If a Driver field weakens, then the organ system itself becomes compromised.

Energetic Integrators: Information structures in the body-field that, like meridians in the body, regulate specific physiological processes. There are twelve Integrators, and together they coordinate the information that drives millions of chemical processes, ensuring that the correct information gets to a specific place in the body at the precise time it is needed.

Energetic Stars: Mini-information networks in the body-field, in which multiple information channels converge to address a single issue (forming a hypothetical starlike shape). There are sixteen Energetic Stars, each of which represents specific metabolic pathways or multiple influences in the body-field that converge on one major function or mechanism.

Energetic Terrains: Bioenergetic field errors that create environments in body tissues that are amenable to hosting the energetic imprint of viruses, bacteria, and other microbes. There are sixteen Energetic Terrains, each of which correlates not to the actual physical pathogen or microorganism but to the energetic imprint of a particular pathogen or family of microorganisms. In the causative chain, the field error comes first, not the microbe.

entanglement: A curious quantum property of certain types of particles that yokes them together. When entangled, the particles act not as separate entities but rather as a correlated system—even when the individual particles are separated by vast distances.

e-smog: Electromagnetic radiation or pollution, both natural and man-made. Overexposure to e-smog correlates to body-field distortions that may affect the immune system and other aspects of the physical body.

field effect: The concept that fields of information permeate the universe in a vast, interconnected web of relations, linking people (and all entities and even objects) in ways that researchers have only begun to explore.

frequency: The number of cycles, occurrences, or other predefined units as measured against an independent variable—in waveforms, the number of repetitions of that waveform during a predetermined unit of time. In the electromagnetic spectrum, each type of energy (e.g., radio waves, visible light, gamma rays) falls within a distinct frequency range.

geopathic stress: The negative effects, both physical and emotional, on the human body of particular types of vibrations and fields that emanate from Earth's interior and flow across its surface. Energies from many kinds of natural formations and environments—such as caves, mineral deposits of particular types, and some subterranean watercourses—are considered detrimental by some traditions, such as the feng shui tradition.

hologram: An image created on a photo plate such that when coherent light (such as laser light) is shined on the photo plate, the two-dimensional image appears as three dimensional. More generally, something is said to be holographic when it is three-dimensional and every part of it contains information about the whole of it.

homeostasis: The body's ability to maintain physiological equilibrium, a process that is dependent on the body's own self-healing intelligence. Illness can be considered to be a loss of homeostasis.

human body-field: *See* body-field.

Infoceutical: In NES, a mixture of purified water and plant-derived microminerals that are encoded with information that directly influences the body-field to correct distortions in how it processes and regulates the information that is vital to the physical body.

magnetic confetti: The tiny bits of magnetic-like energy left over from the forming and breaking of bonds, especially hydrogen bonds, and other biochemical processes. In NES theory, magnetic confetti is considered necessary for making and sustaining a human body-field.

masking: A phenomenon that occurs when the body is not ready or able to deal with a specific distortion and so does not reveal that distortion in the body-field scan, even though the client and practitioner might expect to see evidence of that problem based on allopathic diagnostic standards. As the sequence of correcting the body-field is followed, distortions that were masked are revealed. Energetic Terrains especially are involved in masking.

matching: The process by which two items or processes link within the vast network of relations that make up the body-field. This process may be dependent on the change of the resistance or permittivity of space. If two items match, they can "talk" to each other, or share information, within the dynamic body-field.

microtubules: Hollow structures within cells, organs, and other structures of the physical body that in NES theory are thought to create their own fields and to attract, store, and amplify energy. (*Also see* cavities.)

NES–Professional System: The biotechnology created by Harry Massey and Peter Fraser and used by NES practitioners to detect distortions in the body-field to determine both their severity and their priority for correction.

Nutri-Energetics Systems (NES): The system of health care developed by Peter Fraser and Harry Massey, which integrates physics and biology to reveal a revolutionary understanding of how the body works. According to the NES model, everything in the physical body has an energetic and informational counterpart in the body-field. The loss of homeostasis in the physical body starts at the level of the body-field, and thus detecting and correcting those body-field distortions correlates to improvement in the way the body works and, by extension, to improved health.

phase-conjugate-adaptive-resonance theory: A theory of consciousness and perception, two of whose main proponents are Edgar Mitchell and Peter Marcer, that says that resonant wave interactions account for all acts of conscious perception of three-dimensional, macroscopic (everyday) reality. They propose that a nonlocal quantum hologram underlies all of reality, and there must be an incoming wave from the object that carries quantum-level information about the object and also an outgoing wave from the person perceiving the object, which is like a wave of attention. The outgoing attention wave of the viewer meets the incoming wave carrying the information about the object, and if the two resonate (essentially match vibrations), then perception takes place. According to NES theory, something similar may be going on at the level of the human body-field and the body (and its physiology and interaction with the environment). The associated physics theory would be Milo Wolff's space resonance theory.

phase shift: In NES theory, the wave's change in a periodic signal in relation to a reference signal. In terms of two or more matter waves, phase can be thought of as how the waves line up or match in relation to each other. The two waves can be said to be in phase with respect to their amplitudes (the size of their peaks and troughs is the same), but displaced (shifted out of phase) in relation to time (where one wave is moving ahead of the other).

phase transition: A process by which a system changes its energy state, usually according to certain well-defined parameters. For example, below a certain temperature (energy level) liquid water undergoes a phase transition to become ice, whereas above a certain temperature, it boils and undergoes a phase transition from liquid to vapor.

phonon: A quantum of acoustic or vibrational energy, rather like a particle of sound, that occurs in a rigid crystal lattice of a solid and can be used to calculate the thermal and vibrational aspects of the solid. In terms of energy, it also refers to the absorption of light by its conversion to vibrational energy. As a photon is to light, a phonon is to sound.

photon: A quantum of electromagnetic energy. The name of the quantum particle associated with light, although light has both particle and wave characteristics.

photo-repair: The mechanisms by which cells repair the damage done to them by ultraviolet rays from the sun and other sources.

Polarity: In NES, a slightly negatively charged electrostatic field that permeates the physical body. It is formed in part from the overall biological and energetic activity of the body and plays a vital role in the formation and functioning of the human body-field.

quantum electrodynamics (QED): The area of physics devoted to the study of the interaction of matter (quantum particles) and light. It generally concerns itself with the wave (or field) aspects of nature. At the level of the quantum realm, QED demonstrates that everything is connected. The world is a vast web of relationships, with everything affecting everything else.

Source energy: In NES theory, the natural or cosmic energy, perhaps even zero-point energy, that your body uses to power itself, similar to constitutional or life force energy. Without adequate Source energy, it is difficult to stay well or to restore wellness.

space resonance theory: An interpretation of quantum physics proposed by astrophysicist Milo Wolff, in opposition to the Standard Model, that says that waves, not particles, make up the fundamental, underlying nature of the cosmos. The heart of the theory is that the universe is awash with In waves and Out waves, which, when they meet, interact and change the resonance of quantum space. The different possible characteristics of those resonances account for the different types of particles the Standard Model has cataloged, with only the electron, neutron, and proton being fundamental particles and all the rest of the more than four hundred particles of the Standard Model's particle zoo being different kinds of space resonances. In other words, all but three of the particles of the Standard Model are simply appearances caused by these space resonances. Wolff's theory can explain away most of the paradoxes that now plague quantum mechanics, and it can be derived from core principles and equations already accepted as part of the Standard Model of quantum physics.

Standard Model: The most widely accepted interpretation of high-energy particle physics. It integrates classical theory, relativity and special relativity theory, and others with quantum mechanics to describe and explain nature and natural laws. It does not yet integrate gravity into its model and has a number of other flaws that have caused theorists to propose alternative theories. But so far it is the most widely tested theory in the history of modern science and it has been able to make predictions that have been borne out to exquisite degrees of accuracy through experiment and testing.

succussion: In homeopathy, a method of making homeopathic remedies through a process of shaking and dilution. Minute particles of matter, chosen for their healing attributes, are suspended in water, and then the mixture is put through a series of dilutions and succussions until only the imprint of the energetic signature of the substance, rather than the physical substance itself, is left in the solution.

superposition of states: The state in which quantum entities take on all possible allowable characteristics until measured or otherwise constrained. It is a formal way of saying, for example, that a subatomic entity is both a wave and a particle until something, such as a measurement taken during an experiment, collapses its wavefunction and makes it appear as either a wave or a particle.

transactional interpretation of quantum theory: A theory by physicist John Cramer, who proposes that quantum mechanical wavefunctions have not only a mathematical reality, as is proposed by the Copenhagen interpretation, but a physical reality as well. His theory explains the complex state vector of quantum mechanics and mechanisms that leads to the collapse of the wavefunction, turning quantum events into observable macroscopic reality. His theory is primarily a wave-based picture of quantum, based on "advanced" and "retarded" waves, in contrast to the particle-dominant theory of the Standard Model.

wave-particle duality: In quantum mechanics, the view that subatomic entities have both wave and particle natures simultaneously—they are in a superposition of states—and that how that quantum entity appears when it is measured depends only on the type of experiment carried out.

NOTES

CHAPTER 1. THE UNIVERSE OF THE BODY

1. The MS story is cited in Larry Dossey, *Reinventing Medicine: Beyond Mind-Body to a New Era of Healing* (San Francisco: HarperSanFrancisco, 1999), 141–43.

2. The example about the student with reduced brain matter is cited in many websites about British neurologist John Lorber's work with hydrocephalus patients and in Bruce H. Lipton, *The Biology of Belief: Unleashing the Power of Consciousness, Matter and Miracles* (Santa Rosa, Calif.: Mountain of Love/Elite Books, 2005), 161–62.

3. The case of the girl with lupus is from Amit Goswami, *The Quantum Doctor: A Physicist's Guide to Health and Healing* (Charlottesville, Va.: Hampton Roads, 2004), 184–85.

4. Mark Buchanan, "Beyond Reality: Watching Information at Play in the Quantum World Is Throwing Physicists into a Flat Spin," *New Scientist,* March 14, 1998, 26.

5. Jacob D. Bekenstein, "Information in the Holographic Universe," Special issue, "The Frontiers of Physics," *Scientific American* 15, no. 3 (2005): 75.

6. For Zeilinger's comments about information, see Buchanan, "Beyond Reality."

7. For a more detailed review of the characteristics of systems and nonsystems concepts, see Gary E. R. Schwartz and Linda G. S. Russek, *The Living Energy Universe: A Fundamental Discovery That Transforms Science and Medicine* (Charlottesville, Va.: Hampton Roads, 1999), 219. Their theory proposes that memory is inherent in many natural systems, and indeed in the universe at large.

8. For a primer on the science of sync, see Steven Strogatz, *Sync: The Emerging Science of Spontaneous Order* (New York: Penguin, 2003).

9. Bill Bryson, *A Short History of Nearly Everything* (New York: Broadway Books, 2004), 371. Of course, the actual number of cells in the body cannot be determined precisely, and the methods used to extrapolate a total count vary, which results in differing estimates. The range of 50 trillion to 100 trillion represents the consensus among biologists.

10. The calculation for one trillion seconds in ordinary clock time is (60sec/min) × (60 min/hr) × (24 hr/day) × (365.25 day/yr) = 3.16×10^7 sec; therefore, $(10^{12} \text{ sec})/(3.16 \times 10^7 \text{ sec/yr}) = 31{,}546$ years.

11. The miscellaneous facts about the body are from Bryson, *Short History of Nearly Everything*; Eric P. Widmaier's *The Stuff of Life: Profiles of the Molecules That Make Us Tick* (New York: Henry Holt & Company, 2002); Franklin M. Harold's *The Way of the Cell: Molecules, Organisms and the Order of Life* (Oxford: Oxford University Press, 2001).

12. The example of how many cells fit into a one-inch space came from coauthor Joan Parisi Wilcox's correspondence with scientist Steve Mack, via the MadSci network question-and-answer website, www.madsci.org. When it comes to creating word-based illustrations about cell size, information differs wildly. For example, Christopher King, editor of *Science Watch,* wrote in the Encarta Online Encyclopedia http://encarta.msn.com, "Cell (Biology)," that ten thousand average-size human cells can fit on the head of a pin. However, in a 1997 PBS-TV interview, science writer Boyce Rensberger said that two hundred cells, arranged side by side, will fit into the dot on this letter *i.* Public Broadcasting Service, "The Realm of the Living Cell," www.pbs.org/newshour/gergen/april97/rensberger_4-25/html.

13. Bryson, *Short History of Nearly Everything,* 377.

14. Harold, *Way of the Cell,* 35.

15. P. W. Atkins, *Molecules* (New York: W. H. Freeman and Company, 1987), 3.

16. Ibid., 2.

17. Deepak Chopra, *Quantum Healing: Exploring the Frontiers of Mind/Body Medicine* (New York: Bantam Books, 1990), 85.

18. Kevin Davies, *Cracking the Genome*: *Inside the Race to Unlock Human DNA* (New York: The Free Press, 2001), 14–15.

19. For information about how linguistic theory has been applied to the study of junk DNA, see F. Flam, "Hints of a Language in Junk DNA," *Science* 271 (5245) (January 5, 1996): 14–15.

20. The statistics about colon cancer are from David Ewing Duncan, "Gene Test Report Card" in the news section "Frontiers of Science: Genomics," *Discover* 26, no. 10 (October 2005): 63.

21. National Institutes of Health, National Genome Project, http://science .education.nih.gov/supplements/nih1/genetic/guide/genetic_variation2.htm.

22. Davies, *Cracking the Genome,* 222. The cancer and twins study was originally reported in the *New England Journal of Medicine.*

23. Kenneth W. Ford, *The Quantum World: Quantum Physics for Everyone* (Harvard University Press, 2004), 1.

24. The general consensus is that a typical atom is about 10^{-8} centimeters, but we should mention that scientists have not measured atoms or fundamental quantum particles with any precision. The problem with the atom is that there are different kinds of atoms, so size might vary slightly, but more importantly no atom has a precisely defined outer boundary. The problem in terms of quantum entities such as the fundamental particles (e.g., the electron) is that they cannot *ever* be measured directly—all of their characteristics and properties have to be inferred from indirect measurements taken through various kinds of tests and experiments.

    Most quantities in science, especially physics, are written in standard scientific notation, which uses the metric system. A centimeter is equivalent to about 0.39 inches, or just over one-third of an inch. A meter is about 3.28 feet. The superscript number indicates the power of ten (the number of zeros) when the number is written out. For example, the quantity 1,000 is written as 10^{3}; the quantity one billion (1,000,000,000) is written as 10^{9}. For very small quantities, those less than 1, the superscript becomes a negative number and indicates the places after the decimal point rather than the number of zeros (the number 10^{-8} would be written as 0.00000001).

25. Ford, *Quantum World,* 1.

26. Davies, *Cracking the Genome,* 34.

27. Ian Stewart, *Nature's Numbers: Discovering Order and Pattern in the Universe* (London: Phoenix, 1995), 168.

28. Robert B. Laughlin, *A Different Universe: Reinventing Physics from the Bottom Down* (New York: Basic Books, 2005), 200. For examples of emergent and self-organizing behavior in the natural world, see Stuart Kaufman, *At Home in the Universe: The Search for the Laws of Self-Organization and Complexity* (New York: Oxford University Press, 1995).

29. James Oschman, *Energy Medicine in Therapeutics and Human Performance* (Edinburgh, Scotland: Butterworth Heinemann, 2003), 204.

30. The discussion about the quantum nature of biological water and all accompanying quotations come from Robert Matthews, "The Quantum Elixir," *New Scientist,* April 8, 2006, 32–37.

31. For more information about water and memory, see the work of the late Dr. Jacques Benveniste and the less rigorous but no less intriguing work of Masaru Emoto. Benveniste has published dozens of scientific journal papers about his work, but for the layperson an accessible summary of his work can be found in Lynne McTaggart's *The Field: The Quest for the Secret Force of the Universe* (New York: HarperCollins, 2002), 60–73 ff. The book that launched Emoto's work is *Hidden Messages in Water,* written by Emoto and translated into English by David A. Thayne (Hillsboro, Oreg.: Beyond Words Publishing, 2004). He has since written several other books about his work.

32. Gilbert N. Ling, *Life at the Cell and Below-Cell Level* (New York: Pacific Press, 2001), 274.

33. Bryson, *Short History of Nearly Everything,* 158.

34. John Gribbin, *Schrödinger's Kittens and the Search for Reality* (Boston: Little, Brown and Company, 1995), 194.

35. Maggie Mahar, *Money-Driver Medicine: The Real Reason Health Care Costs So Much* (New York: HarperCollins, 2006), 243.

36. Ling, *Life at the Cell and Below-Cell Level,* 110.

CHAPTER 2. THE MICROWORLD AND THE MACROWORLD

1. Harold, *Way of the Cell,* 7.

2. Dossey, *Reinventing Medicine,* 16–26.

3. Mehmet Oz, *Healing from the Heart: A Leading Surgeon Combines Eastern and Western Traditions to Create the Medicine of the Future* (New York: Plume, 1998).

4. Michael Wayne, *Quantum-Integral Medicine: Towards a New Science of Healing and Human Potential* (Saratoga Springs, N.Y.: iThink Books, 2005).

5. Goswami, *Quantum Doctor.*

6. In his book *Quantum Healing* Chopra set the stage for ideas that Dossey and other visionary and frontier medical professionals would later espouse in terms of what Dossey calls Era III medicine. The bold ideas offered here

were instrumental in introducing the concept of nonlocality in terms of healing and of the quantum aspects of health to the general public.

7. For reader-friendly accounts of the history of quantum physics, we recommend Robert Gilmore, *Alice in Quantumland: An Allegory of Quantum Physics* (New York: Springer-Verlag, 1995) or Ford, *Quantum World.* For an explanation of quantum theory and its application to a host of scientific disciplines, from technology to cosmology, see Tony Hey and Patrick Walters, *The New Quantum Universe* (Cambridge: Cambridge University Press, 2003).

8. A new particle accelerator, called the Large Hadron Collider, which is located in Geneva, Switzerland, and is run by CERN, the European Organization for Nuclear Research, began operation in late 2007. It, and other accelerators not yet built but in the planning stages, may be able to achieve the energies that could verify certain aspects of string theory.

9. We should point out that in terms of energy, some particles, such as electrons orbiting around the nucleus of an atom, can occupy only certain discrete levels of energy, or certain quanta of energy. The orbit of an electron around a nucleus is called a "shell," and the electron can be in only certain shells, although it can move from one shell to another as it either emits or absorbs a photon. However, quantum weirdness rules here as well because the electron moves from one allowable energy level (shell) to another without ever having traversed the energy states or space in between! It simply is in one state, then it is in another state, blinking out of existence at one point/energy level and then appearing again at another. This is not so strange if you consider the electron as a field, not a particle, as some current quantum physics models do. The allowable energy state, the shell, is as a kind of density within the field that indicates the region the electron is currently occupying.

10. Gordon Kane, "The Dawn of Physics Beyond the Standard Model," Special issue, "The Frontiers of Physics," *Scientific American* 15, no. 1 (2005): 4–11.

11. Ibid., 10.

12. Ibid.

13. Until recently, scientists believed that information (as in a meaningful message) could never be exchanged between entangled systems because there would have to be a signal transmitting that information and it would have to travel faster than the speed of light, which is a violation of accepted natural law. In the standard entanglement experiments, particles are correlated

through their *inherent* characteristics, such as spin, so that when one particle's spin is changed, the other, entangled particle has to change accordingly. Inherent correlative factors such as spin have no real physical expression and so require no information transfer to affect them. With two entangled particles, if one has spin up, the other must have spin down. They must be opposite, under all circumstances, as a matter of their inherent relationship as a pair. So changing one changes the other, and no message is needed to precipitate the change. (Who said scientists are not philosophers!) However, recent experiments have shown that information may in fact be imparted through entanglement. See, for instance, the work of Charles Bennett, whose experiments are mentioned in Amir Aczel, *Entanglement: The Greatest Mystery in Physics* (New York: Four Walls Eight Windows, 2001). Also see the newswire story by Will Knight and Nicola Jones, "Long-Distance Quantum Teleportation Draws Closer, *New Scientist,* February 12, 2003; and Michael Brooks, *New Scientist,* "The Weirdest Link," March 27, 2004, 32. A search of the Internet (for instance, via www.Googlescholar.com) also turns up other articles relating recent experiments in teleporting information via entanglement. In addition, one cannot dismiss the evidence from parapsychology research, which shows entangled states, and the transfer of information, between two people or a person and an object. See, for example, Dean Radin, *Entangled Minds: Extrasensory Experiences in a Quantum Reality* (New York: Paraview, 2006).

14. The buckyball is the shortened name for the buckminsterfullerene molecule ($C_{60}F_{48}$), which was discovered in 1985 by researchers at Rice University. They named the biomolecule after Richard Buckminster Fuller, the architect who invented the geodesic dome, because the molecule has a similar geodesic shape.

15. Marcus Arndt, Klaus Hornberger, and Anton Zeilinger, "Probing the Limits of the Quantum World," online at PhysicsWeb, http://physics web.org/articles/world/18/3/5. Originally published in *Physics World* 18 (March 2005): 35.

16. Shahriar S. Afshar, "Sharp Complementary Wave and Particle Behaviours in the Same *Welcher Wag* Experiment," *Proceedings of SPIE* 5866 (July 2005): 229–44. Available online, www.irims.org/quant-ph/030503. For an overview of Afshar's experiment and its implications in nontechnical language, see Marcus Chown, "Quantum Rebel," *New Scientist,* July 24, 2004, 30. All quotations attributed to Afshar are from this arti-

cle, available online at www.NewScientist.com/channel/fundamentals /quantum-world/mg18324575.300.

17. David Gross, "Physics' Greatest Endeavour Is Grinding to a Halt," *New Scientist,* December 10, 2005, 5. Available online, www.NewScientist .com/channel/fundamentals/quantum-world/msg18825293.200.

CHAPTER 3. THE INTELLIGENCE OF THE BODY

1. Koichiro Matsuno and Raymond C. Paton, "Is There a Biology of Quantum Information?" *BioSystems* 55 (February 2000): 39–46.

2. Holograms were first created in the late 1940s by Hungarian physicist Dennis Gaber. He received the Nobel Prize in physics in 1971 for this work. For holography's implications in consciousness studies, see Peter Marcer, Edgar Mitchell, and Walter Schempp, "Self-reference, the Dimensionality and Scale of Quantum Mechanical Effects, Critical Phenomena, and Qualia," *International Journal of Computing Anticipatory Systems* 13 (2002): 340–59. Karl Pribram was a pioneer in applying the principles of holography to consciousness, and his work has now been extended by many others. Michael Talbot's book, *The Holographic Universe* (New York: Harper Perennial, 1992), was among the first books for nonscientists about the cosmos as a giant hologram. For a more recent scientific discussion, see Bekenstein, "Information in the Holographic Universe," 74–81.

3. Recent matter-wave experiments indicate that there is no clear-cut or fixed boundary between the classical and quantum worlds, as reported in Arndt, Hornberger, and Zeilinger, "Probing the Limits of the Quantum World."

4. Buchanan, "Beyond Reality," 26.

5. Radin's work and reports on the research of others is catalogued in his book *Entangled Minds.* The brain-imaging experiment is described on pages 137–41.

6. Ibid., 225.

7. Lipton, *Biology of Belief,* 73.

8. Popp's research is recounted for the nonscientist in McTaggart, *The Field,* 39–55. For the technical science of biophotonics and other aspects of biophysics, we recommend Mae-Wan Ho, Fritz-Albert Popp, and Ulrich Warnke, eds., *Bioelectrodynamics and Biocommunication* (Singapore: World Scientific, 1994); and Fritz-Albert Popp and Lev Beloussov, eds., *Integrative Biophysics: Biophotonics* (Drodrecht, The Netherlands: Kluwer Academic Publishers, 2003).

9. McTaggart, *Field,* 50–51.

10. C. Choi, W. M. Woo, M. B. Lee, et al., "Biophoton Emission from the Hands," *Journal of the Korean Physical Society* 41.2 (August 2002): 275–78.

11. In a review of Ling's *Life at the Cell and Below-Cell Level*, Dr. Mae-Wan Ho wrote, "According to Ling, cell membranes do exist, but they are not the barriers to diffusion into and out of the cell, which, for far too long, has been regarded as little more than a 'bag of enzymes' in free solution that would instantly disintegrate were the membrane to disappear. Rather, the cell membrane is more like the skin of an apple which itself constitutes a phase similar to the bulk phase it encloses: the major constituents of membranes are also proteins that behave in a similar way as proteins in the cytoplasm. They too, preferentially bind K^+ over Na^+ in the resting state. Membrane potentials are local surface potentials, while action potentials simply reflect the changes of state that involves a release of bound water and the temporary exchange of Na^+ for K^+ bound to the carboxylic acid groups in the protein side chains. . . . The picture of what Ling has referred to as the 'resting' living state with ATP and lots of associated water is very much like the liquid crystalline state that I and my colleagues have discovered in cells and organisms . . . , which is another reason why I believe Ling may be largely correct. The living state—as opposed to the state of death in which ATP is exhausted, and *rigor mortis* sets in—is maximally hydrated by polarized layers of bound water, and hence flexible and full of energy." Institute of Science in Society, www.i-sis.org.uk/SMFCB/php.

    For more about the Ling theory, see his book *Life at the Cell and Below-Cell Level* and visit his website, www.gilbertling.org, where he has posted numerous papers. Also see Eric Armstrong, "How Cells Really Work: The Ling Hypothesis," www.treelight.com/health/nutrition/Cells.html.

12. Lipton, *Biology of Belief*, 65–66.

13. Ibid. For more about Lipton's views about epigenetics and the role proteins play in regulating genes, see pages 67–69.

14. W. R. Adey, "A Growing Scientific Consensus on the Cell and Molecular Biology Mediating Interactions with Environmental Electromagnetic Fields," in *Biological Effects of Magnetic and Electromagnetic Fields,* ed. S. Ueno, 45–62 (New York: Plenum Press, 1996).

15. Oschman, *Energy Medicine in Therapeutics,* 61–62. We would like to acknowledge this Oschman book as a major source for the information in chapter 3.

16. The most well-known theory about the quantum aspect of consciousness (via microtubules and a process called quantum tunneling) is called

orchestrated object reduction (Orch-OR), developed by Roger Penrose and Stuart Hameroff. Strong refutation of this theory has come from Swedish cosmologist Max Tegmark, but Hameroff claims Tegmark's comments are based on a number of incorrect assumptions about his and Penrose's theory. Although the debate rages, this work has stimulated others to begin serious inquiries into the quantum nature of consciousness.

17. Becker's work on the perineural system is recounted in James Oschman, *Energy Medicine: The Scientific Basis* (Edinburgh, Scotland: Butterworth Heinemann, 2000); and Oschman, *Energy Medicine in Therapeutics*. Becker's books *The Body Electric* and *Cross Currents* have been popular bestsellers and brought the electromagnetic properties of the body—and the dangers of electromagnetic overexposure to health—to the attention of the public at large. See Robert O. Becker, *The Body Electric: Electromagnetism and the Foundation of Life* (New York: William Morrow, 1985); and Robert O. Becker, *Cross Currents: The Perils of Electropollution, The Promise of Electromedicine* (1989; repr., New York: Tarcher/Penguin, 1990).

18. For information about the neuronlike behavior of immune system cells, see Daniel M. Davis, "Intrigue at the Immune Synapse," *Scientific American* 294, no. 2 (February 2006): 48–55. All quotations in this section are from this article.

19. For an overview of Albert Szent-Györgyi's work, see Oschman's books *Energy Medicine in Therapeutics* and *Energy Medicine.*

20. The Pienta and Coffey research is mentioned in Oschman, *Energy Medicine in Therapeutics,* 102. The original paper is K. J. Pienta and D. S. Coffey, "Cellular Harmonic Information Transfer Through a Tissue Tensegrity-Matrix System," *Medical Hypotheses* 34 (1991): 88–95.

21. For three of Fröhlich's major papers, see Herbert Fröhlich, "Long-Range Coherence and Energy Storage in Biological Systems," *International Journal of Quantum Chemistry* 2 (1968): 641–49; Herbert Fröhlich, "The Extraordinary Diaelectrical Properties of Biological Molecules and the Action of Enzymes," *Proceedings of the National Academy of Sciences of the USA* 72 (1975): 4211–15; and Herbert Fröhlich, "Coherent Electrical Vibrations in Biological Systems and the Cancer Problem," *IEEE Transactions on Microwave Theory and Techniques, MIT* 26 (1978): 613–17.

22. See note 1 in chapter 12 for more references about the heart as a sensory organ.

CHAPTER 5. GLIMPSES INTO THE VIRTUAL BODY

1. Homeopathy is a complex subject, and there are various disciplines or schools. Fundamentally, it is a healing therapy based on the law of similars, a premise that "like treats like." Part of its theory is based on how the immune system springs into action when it identifies a foreign substance and makes antibodies against the substance, making homeopathy similar in theory to vaccines. With vaccines, for example, you would give the immune system a "taste" of yellow fever, so if it were ever infected with the yellow fever virus, it would already have the antibodies to recognize the threat and mount a vigorous defense. The homeopath takes a detailed history to identify the circumstances that may be contributing to the person's lack of immune response, then gives a homeopathic remedy that will stimulate the immune system. Although this is a vastly oversimplified explanation of homeopathy, it provides a basis for understanding its method.

   Homeopathic remedies are dilutions of tiny bits of plants, minerals, or other natural substances. A substance is put in a liquid, usually a mixture of water and alcohol, and then succussed. Then the mixture is diluted further and succussed again. The procedure continues until the mixture has been diluted many, many times. Sometimes it has been diluted so that there are no molecules of the original substance in the remedy. Only its energetic imprint remains.

   A homeopathic imprinting machine is able to make a homeopathic remedy electronically, without the need to go through the succussion process.

2. Electrodermal measurement systems, of which there are several types, are based largely on the work of German physician Helmut Schimmel. They all work in a similar manner, basically by sensing the changes in galvanic skin response or electromagnetic state at the acupuncture points of the body. Schimmel's machine itself is based on earlier work by physician Reinholdt Voll, who was trained in medicine, homeopathy, acupuncture, and electronics and was instrumental in developing EAV machines (short for "ElectronicAcupuncture according to Voll"). Their shared premise as they developed these technologies was that the body's electromagnetic signature changes when disease is present. By detecting specific electromagnetic shifts in organs, tissues, and so on (usually via the skin), the machines can pick up related health problems. Practitioners who use EAV or electrodermal equipment even claim to be able to screen for potential problems because

the electromagnetic signature can be detected *before* the body has expressed the problem as a disease. However, a common problem with these technologies is that the operator can have a major influence on the test results and must be extremely competent at knowing how to screen out noise from the signals to get an accurate reading. In addition, to achieve the best results, practitioners must have expertise in TCM and acupuncture.

3. Although Peter used blood, saliva, and sometimes hair samples in this early work to test people who could not be present in his lab, today NES does not endorse distance-testing using such samples. There are several reasons, but the primary one is that the NES scan will not be as accurate as if the person were there in the practitioner's office being scanned. That said, if distance-testing must be used for some reason, it is always best to first have at least one scan with the client in person.

4. For a paper on Peter Fraser's work, see Julian Kenyon, "A Method of Cancer Diagnosis Using Samples of Saliva Based on Quantum Biology." Available online, www.doveclinic.com (under the Research & Resources section and Papers subsection).

5. See note 1 for an understanding of how homeopathic remedies are made from tissue samples and other kinds of matter.

6. We have provided only the most rudimentary information about acupuncture and the meridian system of TCM in this book. It is quite a complex subject, and its detailed discussion is beyond the scope of this book. There are other, more modern interpretations of acupuncture that designate hundreds of additional acupuncture points in the meridian system.

7. For a discussion of the latest advances in understanding the connective tissue matrix of the body in relation to the electromagnetic and quantum energies of the body and to health, see Oschman, *Energy Medicine in Therapeutics,* especially pages 76–79.

8. For a short time, Peter was part of a research group formed by Reid that was exploring a way to diagnose cancer using bioenergetics. His main contribution was his theory of the body-field, although at that time it was not fully formulated. They achieved some promising results in diagnosing cancer using their biotechnology, but the data is proprietary to the organization that initiated the blind study and has never been released publicly. The group eventually disbanded, and no commercial products resulted from their efforts.

9. Other research corroborates the findings that space itself has a memory and can be imprinted with information. See, for example, the work of Stanford professor and materials scientist William Tiller, who has conducted experiments that show that space can be imprinted with information as a consequence of running energy exchange experiments in the same place over a period of time. Even when the machines are removed, the space around where they were contains residual signals that can imprint a liquid. Although the books are highly technical and difficult for the nonscientist, if you are interested in learning more, see William Tiller, *Science and Human Transformation: Subtle Energies, Intentionality and Consciousness* (Walnut Creek, Calif.: Pavior, 1997); and William Tiller, *Conscious Acts of Creation: The Emergence of a New Physics* (Walnut Creek, Calif.: Pavior, 2001).

10. For intriguing information about the orientation of epithelial cells, see Guenter Albrecht-Buehler, "Can Cells See Each Other?" Available online, www.basic.northwestern.edu/g-buehler/cellint0.htm.

11. Cavities are important in physics because they tend to amplify energy. They have theoretical implications for optics, cryptography, lasers, and quantum computing, to name only a few areas of study. There is even a discipline called cavity quantum electrodynamics. For a technical take on the subject, see Sergio Dutra, *Cavity Quantum Electrodynamics: The Strange Story of Light in a Box* (New York: Wiley-InterScience, 2004).

CHAPTER 6. CALIFORNIA COLLABORATION

1. Ervin Laszlo, *Science and the Akashic Field* (Rochester, Vt.: Inner Traditions, 2004), 106.

2. Ibid., 107.

3. For a basic paper on his model of holographic consciousness, see Edgar Mitchell, "Nature's Mind: The Quantum Hologram." Available online, http://www.edmitchellapollo14.com/naturearticle.htm. For a related article, and a more scientifically rigorous account, about phase-conjugate-adaptive-resonance, see Peter Marcer, "A Quantum Mechanical Model of Evolution and Consciousness." Available online, www.secamlocal .ex.ac.uk/~mwatkins/zeta.marcer.htm.

4. The healing response is neither understood by nor generally accepted by allopathic medical professionals. However, it is widely recognized by complementary health care providers that a healing response is a primary indicator of the body's ability to fight disease. Such responses are most

commonly seen in people who have suffered from chronic disease in which their body has been compromised for a long time.

Ayurvedic medicine, which is the ancient Hindu system of healing; TCM, which includes acupuncture, massage, herbs, breathing, and exercise in its system of healing; and more recent schools of healing such as Hahnemanian homeopathy, all have insights into healing dynamics or healing processes. In some cases, these systems are based on thousands of years of careful observation. The healing reaction is one of these dynamics of the return toward health.

Peter was well-versed in many of these traditions of healing, and when his clients who were using the early versions of the Infoceuticals began reporting healing reactions, such as flulike symptoms for several days, he was able to make connections to these ancient systems. For example, the Chinese sages had written treatises about intermittent fevers occurring as disease left the body. He knew, too, that homeopaths for more than two hundred years have reported on a process they called the "retracing" of the disease. There is a core teaching in homeopathy that says during the healing process a disease moves from the chronic to the acute state. The flulike episodes, and other healing reactions, indicate that movement.

Most complementary healing traditions include within their philosophy the tenet that the body will begin to detoxify itself as it begins the healing phase. Stalled physiological processes of the skin, liver, kidneys, bladder, and bowels begin to work again or to work more effectively. The healing reaction is evidence of the body's resumption of its own healing capabilities. Because the symptoms of this healing process can be acute, some people call this period a "healing crisis," but there usually is no crisis. The disease is resolving itself and the body is returning to normal.

It should be stressed, however, that a client might *not* experience a healing reaction. This does not mean that healing is not taking place. *It only means that the process is not externalizing itself as physical symptoms.* In fact, not having a healing reaction can present a challenge to patients who are trying complementary medicine for the first time. If they don't feel anything, they don't think the treatment is working. That simply is not the way it works, especially when you are dealing with the energies and information of the body-field. The healing process is as individual as patients are. The ultimate criterion of efficacy is how the patient is feeling overall—if his or her problem has resolved itself and he or she feels restored to well-being. However, it may take time to achieve results, especially if the problem has been chronic.

CHAPTER 8. NES AND THE FRONTIERS OF PHYSICS

1. Wolff's theory also is called the wave structure of matter theory, which is the name you will find commonly used on the Internet. However, Wolff refers to his theory as space resonance theory in his book, so that is the name we use.
2. Milo Wolff, *Exploring the Physics of the Unknown Universe* (Manhattan Beach, Calif.: Technotran Press, 1990), 147.
3. Ibid., 133.
4. The Feynman quotation and the Weinberg quotation about renormalization are both from James Gleick, *Genius: The Life and Science of Richard Feynman* (New York: Vintage, 1992), 348.
5. Quotation from a paper posted by Washington University professor John Cramer at the university's website, www.npl.washington.edu.ti. For the original publication of his theory, see J. G. Cramer, "An Overview of the Transactional Interpretation of Quantum Mechanics, *International Journal of Theoretical Physics* 27, no. 227 (1988).
6. For the list of point particle pros and cons, see Wolff, *Exploring the Physics of the Unknown Universe,* 133–34.
7. Strogatz, *Sync,* 3. This book provides an excellent overview of how coupled oscillators and sync are revolutionizing our understanding of natural and biological phenomena and even of human activities.
8. The quotation is from an article posted on the Wolff-related website www.spaceandmotion.com/Wolff-Wave-Structure-Matter.htm, which was created by Geoff Haselhurst.
9. The claim that the wave amplitude is a scalar quantity is from Wolff, *Exploring the Physics of the Unknown Universe,* 182. Purists in physics usually talk about scalar fields, not scalar waves. The notion of scalar waves as proposed by Wolff and some other frontier theorists, including those who apply them to health, such as Oschman, is controversial within the mainstream physics community. However, many physicists intentionally or unintentionally refer to scalar waves all the time themselves.

A wave-dominant view of the universe is not unique to Cramer or Wolff. William Clifford, back in the late 1800s, proposed that matter arises from undulations in space. Physicists John Wheeler and Richard Feynman, among the most respected scientists in the history of modern physics, while seeking the cause of radiation from an accelerated charge, devised calculations that assumed spherical waves radiating inward (advanced) or outward (retarded). However, they assumed these were electromagnetic waves. In hindsight, later scientists reviewing their work clarified that they had suppressed the vector characteristics of their electromagnetic waves, so what they were really calculating were scalar waves. Cramer's transactional interpretation is an outgrowth of Wheeler and Feynman's work in this area. There are an increasing number of scientists (physicists, cosmologists, systems theorists, and chaos and sync researchers) who are exploring the implications of a universe arising out of the interaction of spherical standing scalar waves.

10. Wolff, *Exploring the Physics of the Unknown Universe*, 188.
11. For the complete list of space resonance conditions, see Ibid., 190.
12. Ibid., 195.
13. Ibid., 192–94.
14. Ibid., 194.
15. Ibid., 190.
16. Ibid., 213.
17. Ibid., 23.
18. See the caption for figure 4 in Wolff's article "The Origin of Instantaneous Action in Natural Laws," online at www.quantummatter.com/articles/the_origin_of_instantaneous.html. Wolff also wrote in this article, in Section J, under the heading "Spin of the Electron": "Spin is a result of rotation of the inward (advanced) quantumwaves of an electron at the electron center in order to become the outward (retarded) waves. Rotation is required to maintain proper phase relations of the two wave amplitudes, similar to mirror reflection of e-m waves. The spherical rotation, which is a unique property of 3D space, can be described using SU(2) group theory algebra. In SU(2), the IN and OUT waves of the charged particle are the elements of a Dirac spin or wave function. Thus all charged particles satisfy the Dirac Equation. . . ."
19. For an overview of Mitchell's position, see Mitchell, "Nature's Mind."
20. For interesting but technical discussions about how space can be imprinted by energy and hold a memory of that energy for extended periods of time, see Tiller, *Science and Human Transformation,* and Tiller, *Conscious Acts of Creation.*

CHAPTER 9. OVERVIEW OF THE HUMAN BODY-FIELD

1. For the statistics on how nonlocal healing effects diminish with distance, see Radin, *Entangled Minds,* 191–93.

CHAPTER 10. INFORMATION FLOW
IN YOUR BODY AND BODY-FIELD

1. You can hear normal and abnormal heart and lung sounds at a website for medical students, http://www.med.ucla.edu/wilkes/intro.htm. Listening may make it easier for you to imagine how different sounds can encode different information in the body.

2. For an abstract of her research on the inner ear, see Adrian Cho, "Math Clears Up an Inner-Ear Mystery: Spiral Shape Pumps Up the Bass," *Science* 311, no. 5764 (February 24, 2006): 1087. Also available online, www .sciencemag.org/cgi/content/summary/311/5764/1087a.

3. Avtar S. Ahuja and William R. Hendee, "Effects of Red Cell Shape and Orientation on Propagation of Sound in Blood, *Medical Physics* 4, no. 6 (November 1977): 516–20. Available online, link.aip.org/link/ ?MPHYA6/4/516/1.

4. To review a controversial theory about the heart's role in the body, see Ralph Marinelli, Branko Fuerst, Hoyte van der Zee, et al., "The Heart Is Not a Pump: A Refutation of the Pressure Propulsion Premise of Heart Function," *Frontier Perspectives* 5, no. 1 (1995). Available online, Rudolph Steiner Archive, www.rsarchive.org (under the Archive link). For research about the heart as a sensory organ, see note 1 in chapter 12.

5. For more about how memory may be adversely affected by certain statins and cholesterol-lowering drugs, see Duane Graveline, *Lipitor: Thief of Memory* (West Conshohocken, Pa.: Infinity Publishing, 2004). Since the publication of his book, Graveline reports being contacted by hundreds of people who have experienced memory deficits while taking statins.

6. For information about heart rate variability, see the work of the HeartMath Foundation, http://www.heartmath.com. A search of the Internet reveals dozens of university studies about heartbeat variability and health status. For example, see Misia Landau, "Healthy Heart Keeps Polyrhythmic Beat," *Focus,* http://focus.hms.harvard.edu/2002/March8_2002/cardiology.html.

7. Candace Pert, *Everything You Need to Know to Feel Go(o)d* (Carlsbad, Calif.: Hay House, 2006), 109.

8. For Claire Sylvia's full story, see Claire Sylvia and William Novak, *A Change of Heart* (New York: Warner, 1997).

CHAPTER 11. BIG FIELD INFLUENCES

1. The US Navy conducts most of the research into the Schumann resonance because it uses extremely low-frequency bandwidths to communicate with submarines. Those signals can be disrupted by disturbances in the ionosphere.

2. For overviews of his work, see Neil Cherry, "Cherry on Safe Exposure Levels," http://pages.britishlibrary.net/orange/cherryonexplevel.htm; and Neil Cherry, "Schumann Resonances, A Plausible Biophysical Mechanism for Human Health Effect of Solar," *Natural Hazards* 26, no. 3 (July 2002): 279–331. For a brief discussion of the Schumann resonance and bioenergetics, see Oschman, *Energy Medicine,* 184–86.

3. The cancer-dowsing research is mentioned briefly in Oschman, *Energy Medicine,* 187. The German medical study, "Earth Currents: Causative Factor for Cancer and Other Diseases," is by G. F. von Pohl and was translated by I. Lang. See Oschman, *Energy Medicine,* 192.

4. Nicola Jones, "Feel the Force," *New Scientist,* April 4, 2002, 8. Available online at www.newscientist.com/article/mg17423370.500-feel-the-force.html.

5. Polarity in NES therapy is not related to the energy balancing therapy called Polarity Therapy, which was developed by naturopathic physician Randolph Stone.

CHAPTER 12. THE ENERGETIC DRIVERS

1. For more about the findings of the heart as sensory organ, a kind of second brain in the body, and a center of memory, learning, and emotion, see the work of the Institute of HeartMath, www.heartmath.org. See particularly two online papers, available through the HeartMath website under Research/Research Publications/Intuition Research, by Rollin McCraty, M. Atkinson, and R. T. Bradley, "Electrophysiological Evidence of Intuition: Part 1. The Surprising Role of the Heart," originally published in *Journal of Alternative and Complementary Medicine* 10, no. 1 (2004): 133–43; and "Electrophysiological Evidence of Intuition: Part 2. A System-Wide Process," originally published in *Journal of Alternative and Complementary Medicine* 10 no. 2 (2004): 325–36.

2. For more about how emotional and physical shock can cause disease, see the work of Dr. Ryke Geerd Hamer, who theorizes that emotional shock is the root cause of cancer and many acute and chronic illnesses. The English translation of Hamer's book on this topic is *Summary of the New Medicine,* Ryke Geerd Hamer, trans., updated edition (Fuengirola, Spain: Amici di Dirk, 2000). See also Hamer's website, www.newmedicine.ca. Also review the work of Dr. Ida Rolf, the creator of Rolfing, a deep-tissue massage technique that is known for releasing the imprint of emotional shocks held in the muscle and fascial system. The official website is www.rolf.org. A basic book to review the work of Ida Rolf is Ida Rolf's *Rolfing and Physical Reality* (Rochester, Vt.: Healing Arts Press, 1990) originally published as *Ida Rolf Talks About Rolfing and Physical Reality* (New York: Harper & Row, 1978).

CHAPTER 14. DETAILS OF THE ENERGETIC INTEGRATORS

1. Dr. Wilhelm Schüssler was a German homeopath who developed a theory that mineral deficiencies may lead to illness. He developed homeopathic remedies for twelve biochemical tissue salts to address deficiencies in the body.

BIBLIOGRAPHY

Aczel, Amir D. *Entanglement: The Greatest Mystery in Physics.* New York: Four Walls Eight Windows, 2001.

Adey, W. R. "A Growing Scientific Consensus on the Cell and Molecular Biology Mediating Interactions with Environmental Electromagnetic Fields." In *Biological Effects of Magnetic and Electromagnetic Fields,* edited by S. Uneo. New York: Plenum Press, 1996.

Afshar, Shariar S. "Sharp Complementary Wave and Particle Behaviours in the Same *Welcher Wag* Experiment." *Proceedings of SPIE* 5866 (July 2005): 229–44. Available online. www.irims.org/quant-ph/030503.

Ahuja, Avtar S., and William R. Hendee. "Effects of Red Cell Shape and Orientation on Propagation of Sound in Blood." *Medical Physics* 4, no. 6 (November 1977): 516–20. Abstract available at Medical Physics Online. link.aip.org/link/?MPHYA6/4/516/1.

Albrecht-Buehler, Guenter. "Can Cells See Each Other?" www.basic .northwestern.edu/g-buehler/cellint0.htm.

Armstrong, Eric. "How Cells Really Work: The Ling Hypothesis." www .treelight.com/health/nutrition/Cells.html.

Arndt, Markus, Klaus Hornberger, and Anton Zeilinger. "Probing the Limits of the Quantum World." Available online at PhysicsWeb. http://physics web.org/articles/world/18/3/5. Originally published in *Physics World* 18 (March 2005): 35.

Atkins, P. W. *Molecules.* New York: W. H. Freeman and Company, 1987.

Becker, Robert O. *The Body Electric: Electromagnetism and the Foundation of Life.* New York: William Morrow, 1985.

————. *Cross Currents: The Perils of Electropollution, The Promise of Electromedicine.* 1989. Reprint, New York: Tarcher/Penguin, 1990.

Bekenstein, Jacob D. "Information in the Holographic Universe." Special issue, "The Frontiers of Physics," *Scientific American* 15, no. 3 (2005): 74–81.

Brooks, Michael. "The Weirdest Link." *New Scientist,* March 27, 2004, 32.

Bryson, Bill. *A Short History of Nearly Everything.* New York: Broadway Books, 2004.

Buchanan, Mark. "Beyond Reality: Watching Information at Play in the Quantum World Is Throwing Physicists into a Flat Spin." *New Scientist,* March 14, 1998, 26.

Cherry, Neil. "Cherry on Safe Exposure Levels." The British Library. http://pages.britishlibrary.net/orange/cherryonexplevel.htm.

————. "Schumann Resonances, a Plausible Biophysical Mechanism for Human Health Effect of Solar." *Natural Hazards* 26, no. 3 (July 2002): 279–331.

Childe, Doc, Howard Martin, and Donna Beech. *The HeartMath Solution.* San Francisco: HarperSanFrancisco, 1999.

Cho, Adrian. "Math Clears Up an Inner-Ear Mystery: Spiral Shape Pumps Up the Bass." *Science* 311, no. 5764 (February, 24, 2006): 1087. Also available at the News of the Week section at *Science* magazine's website. www.sciencemag.org/cgi/content/summary/311/5764/1087a.

Choi, Ch., W. M. Woo, M. B. Lee, et al. "Biophoton Emission from the Hands." *Journal of the Korean Physical Society* 41, no. 2 (August 2002): 275–78.

Chopra, Deepak. *Quantum Healing: Exploring the Frontiers of Mind/Body Medicine.* New York: Bantam Books, 1990.

Chown, Marcus. "Quantum Rebel." *New Scientist,* July 24, 2004, 30.

Cramer, John G. "An Overview of the Transactional Interpretation of Quantum Mechanics." *Journal of Theoretical Physics* 27, no. 227 (1988).

Davies, Kevin. *Cracking the Genome: Inside the Race to Unlock Human DNA.* New York: The Free Press, 2001.

Davis, Daniel. M. "Intrigue at the Immune Synapse." *Scientific American* 294, no. 2 (February 2006): 48–55.

Dossey, Larry. *Reinventing Medicine: Beyond Mind-Body to a New Era of Healing.* San Francisco: HarperSanFrancisco, 1999.

Duncan, David Ewing. "Gene Test Report Card." *Discover* 26.10 (October 2005): 63.

Dutra, Sergio. *Cavity Quantum Electrodynamics: The Strange Story of Light in a Box.* New York: Wiley-InterScience, 2004.

Emoto, Masaru. *Hidden Messages in Water.* Translated by David A. Thayne. Hillsboro, Oreg.: Beyond Words Publishing, 2004.

Flam, F. "Hints of a Language in Junk DNA." *Science* 271, no. 5245 (January 5, 1996): 14–15.

Ford, Kenneth W. *The Quantum World: Quantum Physics for Everyone.* Cambridge, Mass.: Harvard University Press, 2004.

Fröhlich, Herbert. "Coherent Electrical Vibrations in Biological Systems and the Cancer Problem." *IEEE Transactions on Microwave Theory and Techniques, MIT* 26 (1978): 613–17.

———. "The Extraordinary Dielectrical Properties of Biological Molecules and the Action of Enzymes," *Proceedings of the National Academy of Sciences of the USA* 72 (1975): 4211–15.

———. "Long-Range Coherence and Energy Storage in Biological Systems." *International Journal of Quantum Chemistry* 2 (1968): 641–49.

Gerber, Richard. *Vibrational Medicine: The #1 Handbook for Subtle-Energy Therapies.* Rochester, Vt.: Bear & Company, 2001.

Gilmore, Robert. *Alice in Quantumland: An Allegory of Quantum Physics.* New York: Springer-Verlag, 1995.

Gleick, James. *Genius: The Life and Science of Richard Feynman.* New York: Vintage Books, 1992.

Goswami, Amit. *The Quantum Doctor: A Physicist's Guide to Health and Healing.* Charlottesville, Va.: Hampton Roads, 2004.

Graveline, Duane. *Lipitor: Thief of Memory.* West Conshohocken, Pa: Infinity Publishing, 2004.

Gribbin, John. *Schrödinger's Kittens and the Search for Reality.* Boston: Little, Brown and Company, 1995.

Gross, David. "Editorial: Physics' Greatest Endeavour Is Grinding to a Halt." *New Scientist,* December 10, 2005: 5.

Hamer, R. G. *Summary of the New Medicine.* Updated English translation, Fuengirola, Spain: Amici di Dirk, 2000.

Harold, Franklin M. *The Way of the Cell: Molecules, Organisms and the Order of Life.* Oxford: Oxford University Press, 2001.

Hey, Tony, and Patrick Walters. *The New Quantum Universe.* Cambridge: Cambridge University Press, 2003.

Ho, Mae-Wan. "Strong Medicine for Cell Biology: A Review of Gilbert Ling's *Life at the Cell and Below-Cell Level.*" www.i-sis.org.uk/SMFCB.php.

Ho, Mae-Wan, Fritz-Albert Popp, and Ulrich Warnke, eds. *Bioelectrodynamics and Biocommunication.* Singapore: World Scientific, 1994.

Jones, Nicola. "Feel the Force." *New Scientist,* April 4, 2002: 8.

Kane, Gordon. "The Dawn of Physics Beyond the Standard Model." Special issue, "The Frontiers of Physics," *Scientific American* 15, no. 1 (2005): 4–11.

Kaufman, Stuart. *At Home in the Universe: The Search for the Laws of Self-Organization and Complexity.* New York: Oxford University Press, 1995.

Kenyon, Julian. "A Method of Cancer Diagnosis Using Samples of Saliva Based on Quantum Biology." www.doveclinic.com (Research & Resources section, Papers subsection).

Knight, Will, and Nicola Jones. "Long-Distance Quantum Teleportation Draws Closer." *New Scientist.* Online News Service report, February 12, 2003. www.NewScientist.com. The research this news item was based on was originally published in Jian-Wei Pan, Sara Gasparoni, Markus Aspelmeye, et al. "Experimental Realization of Freely Propagating Teleported Quibits." *Nature* 421: 721–25.

Koichiro, Matsuno, and Raymond C. Paton. "Is There a Biology of Quantum Information?" *BioSystems* 55 (February 2000): 39–46.

Landau, Misia. "Healthy Heart Keeps Polyrhythmic Beat." http://focus.hms.harvard.edu/2002/March8_2002/cardiology.html.

Laszlo, Ervin. *Science and the Akashic Field: An Integrated Theory of Everything.* Rochester, Vt.: Inner Traditions, 2004.

Laughlin, Robert B. *A Different Universe: Reinventing Physics from the Bottom Down.* New York: Basic Books, 2005.

Ling, Gilbert N. *Life at the Cell and Below-Cell Level.* New York: Pacific Press, 2001.

Lipton, Bruce H. *The Biology of Belief: Unleashing the Power of Consciousness, Matter and Miracles.* Santa Rosa, Calif.: Mountain of Love/Elite Books, 2005.

Mahar, Maggie. *Money-Driver Medicine: The Real Reason Health Care Costs So Much.* New York: HarperCollins, 2006.

Marcer, Peter. "A Quantum Mechanical Model of Evolution and Consciousness." Abstract available online. http://secamlocal.ex.ac.uk/~mwatkins/zeta/marcer.htm#zeta.

Marcer, Peter, Edgar Mitchell, and Walter Schempp. "Self-reference, the Dimensionality and Scale of Quantum Mechanical Effects, Critical

Phenomena, and Qualia," *International Journal of Computing Anticipatory Systems* 13 (2002): 340–59.

Marinelli, Ralph, Branko Fuerst, Hoyte van der Zee, et al. "The Heart Is Not a Pump: A Refutation of the Pressure Propulsion Premise of Heart Function." *Frontier Perspectives* 5, no. 1 (1995). Available online. www.rsarchive.org.

Matthews, Robert. "The Quantum Elixir." *New Scientist,* April 8, 2006, 32–37.

McCraty, Rollin, M. Atkinson, and R. T. Bradley, "Electrophysiological Evidence of Intuition: Part 1. The Surprising Role of the Heart," *Journal of Alternative and Complementary Medicine* 10, no. 1 (2004): 133–43. Also available online at www.heartmath.org under Research/Research Publications/Intuition Research.

———. "Electrophysiological Evidence of Intuition: Part 2. A System-Wide Process," *Journal of Alternative and Complementary Medicine* 10, no. 2 (2004): 325–36. Also available online at www.heartmath.org under Research/ Research Publications/Intuition Research.

McTaggart, Lynne. *The Field: The Quest for the Secret Force of the Universe.* New York: HarperCollins, 2002.

Mitchell, Edgar. "Nature's Mind: The Quantum Hologram." www .edmitchellapollo14.com/naturearticle.htm.

National Institutes of Health. "Teacher's Guide: Understanding Human Genetic Variation." National Human Genome Research Institute. http://science.education.nih.gov/supplements/nih1/genetic/guide/genetic _variation1.htm.

Oschman, James L. *Energy Medicine: The Scientific Basis.* Edinburgh, Scotland: Butterworth Heinemann, 2000.

———. *Energy Medicine in Therapeutics and Human Performance.* Edinburgh, Scotland: Butterworth Heinemann, 2003.

Oz, Mehmet. *Healing from the Heart: A Leading Surgeon Combines Eastern and Western Traditions to Create the Medicine of the Future.* New York: Plume, 1998.

Pert, Candace B. *The Molecules of Emotion: The Science Behind Mind-Body Medicine.* New York: Simon & Schuster, 1999.

Pert, Candace B., and Nancy Marriott. *Everything You Need to Know to Feel Go(o)d.* Carlsbad, Calif.: Hay House, 2006.

Pienta, K. J., and D. S. Coffey. "Cellular Harmonic Information Transfer

Through a Tissue Tensegrity-Matrix System." *Medical Hypotheses* 34 (1991): 88–95.

Popp, Fritz-Albert, and Lev Beloussov, eds. *Integrative Biophysics: Biophotonics.* Drodrecht, The Netherlands: Kluwer Academic Publishers, 2003.

Radin, Dean. *Entangled Minds: Extrasensory Experiences in a Quantum Reality.* New York: Paraview, 2006.

Rolf, Ida. *Rolfing and Physical Reality.* Rochester, Vt.: Healing Arts Press, 1990.

Schwartz, Gary E. R., and Linda G. S. Russek. *The Living Energy Universe: A Fundamental Discovery That Transforms Science and Medicine.* Charlottesville, Va.: Hampton Roads, 1999.

Stewart, Ian. *Nature's Numbers: Discovering Order and Pattern in the Universe.* London: Phoenix, 1995.

Strogatz, Steven. *Sync: The Emerging Science of Spontaneous Order.* New York: Penguin, 2003.

Sylvia, Claire, and William Novak. *A Change of Heart: A Memoir.* New York: Warner Books, 1997.

Talbot, Michael. *The Holographic Universe.* Reprint, New York: Harper Perennial, 1992.

Tiller, William. *Conscious Acts of Creation: The Emergence of a New Physics.* Walnut Creek, Calif.: Pavior, 2001.

———. *Science and Human Transformation: Subtle Energies, Intentionality and Consciousness.* Walnut Creek, Calif.: Pavior, 1997.

Wayne, Michael. *Quantum-Integral Medicine: Towards a New Science of Healing and Human Potential.* Saratoga Springs, N.Y.: *i*Think Books, 2005.

Widmaier, Eric P. *The Stuff of Life*: *Profiles of the Molecules That Make Us Tick.* New York: Henry Holt & Company, 2002.

Wolff, Milo. *Exploring the Physics of the Unknown Universe: An Adventurer's Guide.* Manhattan Beach, Calif.: Technotran Press, 1990.

———. "The Origin of Instantaneous Action in Natural Laws," www.quantummatter.com/articles/the_origin_of_instantaneous.html.

INDEX